Infectious Diseases and Microbiology

snova
New York

Infectious Diseases and Microbiology

Psychological Consequences of the COVID-19 Pandemic on Children, Teenagers and Adults
Jean-Pascal Assailly, PhD
2022. ISBN: 978-1-68507-963-5 (Softcover)
2022. ISBN: 979-8-88697-072-2 (eBook)

COVID-19 Contracting: Opportunities, Actions and Reimbursements
Eric Neudorf
2022. ISBN: 978-1-68507-710-5 (Hardcover)
2022. ISBN: 978-1-68507-733-4 (eBook)

The Aviation Industry and COVID-19
Stefan Schneider
2022. ISBN: 978-1-68507-712-9 (Hardcover)
2022. ISBN: 978-1-68507-729-7 (eBook)

Diseases Transmitted by Ticks
Hacer İşler, Metin Özdemir, MD (Editors)
2021. ISBN: 978-1-68507-359-6 (Hardcover)
2021. ISBN: 978-1-68507-383-1 (eBook)

Impacts and Implications of COVID-19: An Analytical and Empirical Study
Anand Sharma, Prateek Agrawal,
Vishu Madaan, and Anuj Agarwal (Editors)
2021. ISBN: 978-1-53619-670-2 (Hardcover)
2021. ISBN: 978-1-68507-081-6 (eBook)

More information about this series can be found at
https://novapublishers.com/product-category/series/infectious-diseases-and-microbiology/

Jamie Isaacson
Editor

Racial Inequities Exposed by COVID-19

snova
New York

Library of Congress Cataloging-in-Publication Data

ISBN: 979-8-88697-153-8

Published by Nova Science Publishers, Inc. † New York

Contents

Preface

This book discusses how the COVID–19 pandemic is exacerbating racial inequalities in education, labor, and health and the steps needed to address these disparities.

Chapter 1

Inequities Exposed: How COVID–19 Widened Racial Inequities in Education, Health, and the Workforce*

Committee on Education and Labor

Monday, June 22, 2020
House of Representatives,
Committee on Education and Labor,
Washington, DC

The committee met, pursuant to call, at 12:02 p.m., via Webex, Hon. Robert C. "Bobby" Scott (Chairman of the committee) presiding.

Present: Representatives Scott, Davis, Grijalva, Courtney, Fudge, Wilson, Bonamici, Takano, Adams, Norcross, Jayapal, Morelle, Wild, Harder, McBath, Schrier, Underwood, Hayes, Shalala, Levin, Trone, Stevens, Trahan, Foxx, Thompson, Walberg, Byrne, Grothman, Stefanik, Allen, Smucker, Banks, Cline, Watkins, Meuser, Johnson, Keller, and Van Drew.

Staff Present: Tylease, Alli, Chief Clerk; Ilana, Brunner, General Counsel; Ijeoma, Egekeze, Professional Staff; Christian, Haines, General Counsel; Sheila, Havenner, Director of Information Technology; Carrie, Hughes, Director of Health and Human Services; Eli, Hovland, Staff Assistant; Andre, Lindsay, Staff Assistant; Jaria, Martin, Clerk/Special Assistant to the Staff

* This is an edited, reformatted and augmented version of Hearing before the Committee on Education and Labor, U.S. House of Representatives, One Hundred Sixteenth Congress, Second Session, Serial No. 116–59, dated June 22, 2020.

In: Racial Inequities Exposed by COVID-19
Editor: Jamie Isaacson
ISBN: 979-8-88697-153-8

Director; Richard, Miller, Director of Labor Policy; Katelyn, Mooney, Associate General Counsel; Max, Moore, Staff Assistant; Mariah, Mowbray, Staff Assistant; Jacque, Mosely, Director of Education Policy; Veronique, Pluviose, Staff Director; Lakeisha, Steele, Professional Staff; West, Rachel, Senior Economic Policy Advisor; Cyrus Artz, Minority Staff Director; Gabriel Bisson, Minority Staff Assistant; Courtney Butcher, Minority Director of Member Services and Coalitions; Rob Green, Minority Director of Workforce Policy; Jeanne Keuhl, Minority Legislative Assistant; John Martin, Minority Workforce Policy Counsel; Hannah Matesic, Minority Director of Operations; Carlton Norwood, Minority Press Secretary; Brad Thomas, Minority Senior Education Policy Advisor.

Chairman SCOTT. The Committee on Education and Labor will come to order.

And welcome to everyone. I note that a quorum is present. The committee is meeting today on a hearing to hear testimony on "Inequities Exposed: How COVID–19 Widened the Racial Inequities in Education, Health, and the Workforce."

This is an entirely remote hearing pursuant to House Resolution 965 and the regulations thereto. As a general rule, I will ask that microphones including those of Members and witnesses be kept muted to avoid unnecessary background noise. Members are responsible for un-muting themselves when they are recognized to speak or when they wish to seek recognition.

And somebody is not muted right now. Can you check to see if you are muted?

Further, Members are required to leave their cameras on the entire time they are in an official proceeding, even if they step away from the camera, in which case we should see an empty chair. As this is an entirely remote hearing, the committee's hearing room is officially closed.

Members who chose to sit with their individual devices in the hearing room must wear headphones to avoid feedback, echoes, and distortion resulting for more than one person on the platform, sitting in the same room.

We are also expected to adhere to the social distancing healthcare guidelines, including the use of masks, gloves, and wiping down the area before and after their presence in the hearing room. And I will also note that when you ask questions, if you are in the hearing room, if the witnesses also in the hearing room, it would help if you mute while the answer is taking place, because the answer is picked up by your mike and then that echoes back and there is usually distortion.

While the roll call is not necessary to establish a quorum in an official proceeding conducted remotely, whenever there is an official proceeding, with remote participation, the clerk will call the roll to help make clear who is present at the start of the proceeding.

And so I will ask the clerk to call the roll.

The CLERK. Chairman Scott.

Chairman SCOTT. Present.

The CLERK. Mrs. Davis.

Mrs. DAVIS. Present.

The CLERK. Mr. Grijalva.

Mr. GRIJALVA. Present.

The CLERK. Mr. Courtney.

Mr. COURTNEY. Present.

The CLERK. Ms. Fudge.

Ms. FUDGE. Present.

The CLERK. Mr. Sablan.

Ms. Wilson.

Ms. WILSON. Present.

The CLERK. Ms. Bonamici.

Ms. BONAMICI. Present.

The CLERK. Mr. Takano.

Ms. Adams.

Ms. ADAMS. Present.

The CLERK. Mr. DeSaulnier.

Mr. Norcross.

Mr. NORCROSS. Present.

The CLERK. Ms. Jayapal.

Mr. JAYAPAL. Present.

The CLERK. Mr. Morelle.

Mr. MORELLE. Present.

Mr. HAWKINS.

Ms. Wild.

Mr. Harder.

Mrs. McBath.

Mrs. MCBATH. Present.

The CLERK. Ms. Schrier.

Ms. SCHRIER. Present.

The CLERK. Ms. Underwood.

Ms. UNDERWOOD. Present.

The CLERK. Mrs. Hayes.

Ms. Shalala.

Mr. Levin.

Mr. LEVIN. Present.

The CLERK. Ms. Omar.

Mr. Trone.

Ms. Stevens.

Ms. STEVENS. Present. Thank you.

The CLERK. Mrs. Lee.

Mrs. Trahan.

Mrs. TRAHAN. Present.

The CLERK. Mr. Castro.

Ms. Foxx.

Ms. FOXX. Present.

The CLERK. Mr. Roe.

Mr. Thompson.

Mr. Walberg.

Mr. WALBERG. Present.

The CLERK. Mr. Guthrie.

Mr. Byrne.

Mr. BYRNE. Present.

The CLERK. Mr. Grothman.

Ms. Stefanik.

Mr. STEFANIK. Present.

The CLERK. Mr. Allen.

Mr. ALLEN. Present.

The CLERK. Mr. Smucker.

Mr. Banks.

Mr. Walker.

Mr. Comer.

Mr. Cline.

Mr. CLINE. Present.

The CLERK. Mr. Fulcher.

Mr. Watkins.

Mr. WATKINS. Present.

The CLERK. Mr. Wright.

Mr. Meuser.

Mr. MEUSER. Present.

The CLERK. Mr. Johnson.

Mr. JOHNSON. Present, ma'am.

The CLERK. Mr. Keller.

Mr. KELLER. Present.

The CLERK. Mr. Murphy.

Mr. Van Drew.

Mr. VAN DREW. Present.

The CLERK. Chairman Scott, this concludes the roll call.

Ms. WILD. Excuse me. Susan Wild, present.

Chairman SCOTT. Thank you.

Does anyone else want to note their presence?

Ms. UNDERWOOD. Lauren Underwood, present.

Mr. TRONE. David Trone, present.

Chairman SCOTT. David Trone.

Ms. Underwood.

Ms. FOXX. Mr. Chairman.

Chairman SCOTT. Hello?

Ms. FOXX. Mr. Chairman, it is Congresswoman Foxx.

I just want to note that Congressman Thompson was here and stepped out for just a moment and also that we have several members at Mrs. Barr's funeral today, both Kentucky people as well as other States. So there are several absent because of that funeral going on right now.

Chairman SCOTT. That is certainly understandable. Thank you very much.

Pursuant to Committee Rule 7(c), opening statements are limited to the Chair and Ranking Member. This allows us to hear from our witnesses sooner and provides all members with adequate time to ask questions.

I now recognize myself for the purpose of making an opening statement.

First, following up on the Ranking Member's comment, I want to express my deepest condolences to our colleagues who are mourning the loss of loved ones. Our thoughts and prayers are with Representative Omar for the loss of her father, Representative Bonamici for the loss of her mother, Representative Barr for the loss of his wife, and our friend not on the committee but our good friend, Jim Sensenbrenner, for the loss of his wife. We are living in tough times for everyone but I know that these are particularly difficult times for those mentioned and we just want to wish them strength and peace and know that we are with them during this difficult time.

Today we are discussing how COVID–19 pandemic is exacerbating racial inequalities in education, labor, and health and the steps Congress must take to address these disparities.

A mountain of evidence has made it clear that to effectively respond to this pandemic, we must address the widening existing racial inequities in education, the workforce, and our healthcare system. In the area of education, racial bias, both intentionally and unconscious, and chronic underfunding of schools serving students of color produce persistent achievement gaps.

We know that our Nation's K through 12 public schools entered this pandemic with a $23 billion racial funding gap. That is the difference between the funding in school districts serving predominantly students of color compared to school districts serving predominantly White students.

As schools abruptly closed, this funding gap has positioned students of color to fall even further behind their peers. Black and Latino students who are less likely to attend schools that have the capacity to rapidly establish high-quality distance learning programs. They are also less likely to have the basic technology such as a personal computer, the high-speed internet, and the support at home needed to access virtual learning. As a result, Latino students are expected to lose 9 months of learning and Black students are expected to lose 10 months of learning due to the pandemic. Our White students are expected to lose only 6 months.

In addition to the pandemic's impact on the achievement gap, the Center on Budget and Policy Priorities projects that states will face a $615 billion revenue shortfall over the next three years due to the pandemic. As the committee discussed during a hearing last week, the public education is usually one of the largest expenditures, accounting for an average 40 percent of state budgets. And unless the Federal Government provides immediate relief to State and local governments, it won't matter whether funding for education will be cut. It won't matter whether education funding will be cut but how much those cuts in education will be.

While wealthier districts can fall back on property tax revenue, low-income public school districts will have to continue to rely heavily on state funding. For school districts that predominantly serve students of color, the severe cuts in education and supporting social service programs will come at the time of greatest need. The consequences of these shortfalls are already evident. Nearly 750,000 public school employees have already lost their jobs since March. In Colorado, the State legislature just passed a budget that cuts $1 billion from its schools next year. In the area of the workforce, outlook for workers of color is similarly concerning.

Black and Latino workers that faced significantly higher rates of unemployment and lower wages long before the pandemic have borne a disproportionate share of the layoffs. Although the rate of employment for

White and Latino workers has lowered, rates for Black workers has actually increased in recent weeks.

Among those who remain employed, workers of color are more likely to be employed in occupations such as meatpacking, grocery, healthcare, and transportation with the highest risk of infection. Fewer than 20 percent of Black and Latino workers can work from home, compared to nearly 30 percent of White workers. More than 4 in 10 Black workers lack employment-provided sick days.

Because of these disparities, workers of color have been disproportionately affected by the Department of Labor's refusal to off—to issue enforceable workplace safety standards to protect workers from COVID–19.

In addition to working in sectors with the highest risk of COVID–19 infections, Black and Latino workers disproportionately work in low-wage jobs. Regrettably, Congress has not raised the Federal minimum wage in more than a decade, the longest period of time in its history. Worse still, legal labor laws and hostile courts have eroded labor union membership and workers' collective bargaining rights which have left the very essential workers vulnerable to poverty, unsafe workplaces, and a deadly virus.

The most profound consequence of racial inequality in our society has been the pandemic's devastating impact on the health of people of color. Nationwide, African Americans have been dying from COVID–19 infections at about two and half times the rate of White Americans.

In New York City, the epicenter of COVID–19 infections and deaths, the death rate for Latinos in the months of April was about 22 people per 100,000 adjusted for population size and age. American Indian and Native communities are suffering disproportionately from the COVID–19 infections.

In late May, the Navajo Nation surpassed New York and New Jersey with the most infections per capita. This follows a pattern of past diseases where Native American communities bore the brunt of disease outbreaks due to the chronic, long-term underfunding of healthcare across Indian Country.

As with these challenges in education and workforce issues, the health disparities are rooted in structural inequality. People of color entered the pandemic with health conditions often caused by structural problems including healthcare discrimination, housing instability, food insecurity, and limited access to transportation. Years of statewide budget cuts in public health have led to limited funding of rural health—rural and community hospitals in communities of color, leaving families with few options to receive quality care.

Unfortunately, instead of increasing access to healthcare coverage, the Trump administration has been actively working to take it away in the midst of the public health emergency. The Texas lawsuit threatens the entirety of the Affordable Care Act of all of the law's coverage gains and consumer protections.

These cynical efforts disproportionately impact people of color. If these efforts strike down the law—these efforts to strike down the law are successful, estimates show that the uninsured rate among the African American community would nearly double from 11 percent to 20 percent, and the share of uninsured Hispanic individuals would grow from 21 percent to 31 percent.

But we are not here to talk about the problem or what they call "celebrate" the problem. We are here to discuss solutions. The HEROES Act, which the House passed last month, would take important steps towards addressing racial inequalities that have been exposed and exacerbated through the pandemic.

With respect to education, legislation dedicates nearly $1 trillion in relief for States and localities to help avert painful cuts to public schools. It also goes a step further by proposing more than $100 billion in additional emergency education funding to help cover the costs of cleaning supplies and other expenses required to reopen, purchase educational technology like laptops and hotspots, sustain special education for students with disabilities, and help colleges and universities maintain their institutions.

To support workers, the HEROES Act directs OSHA to rapidly issue an emergency temporary standard that would require employees to implement protections for workers who are at highest risk for contracting COVID–19. It also expands access to emergency paid leave to nearly 140 million—to 140 million workers.

And while paid leave provisions in the Families First Coronavirus Virus Response Act took important steps in the right direction, far too many workers, including many healthcare workers, were excluded from those protections.

So this bill—so the HEROES Act puts family and medical back into family and medical leave by dramatically expanding the circumstances in which workers can take 12 weeks of Emergency Family and Medical Leave Act pay and we should not force workers to choose between a paycheck, their health, and the health of the people around them.

Improved health outcomes, the HEROES Act, expands healthcare insurance coverage for COVID–19 testing and treatment, provides full coverage for the cost of COBRA premiums for laid off and furloughed workers, and increases the investment in health nutrition and community support by including $1 billion for special WIC funding and an additional $1 billion for Community Services Block Grant initiatives to help address poverty.

Finally the HEROES Act invests $75 billion in testing and contact tracing to help contain the virus. This includes $500 million to recruit and train contact workers through the public work case— through the public workforce system and community-based organizations. Collectively these provisions represent a major step taken by Congress to help our Nation get through this global healthcare crisis.

As we confront this unprecedented challenge, we must accept our responsibility to build a recovery that uplifts all communities. But if we fail to act, we will be experiencing a recovery that offers relief to some but leaves many low-income communities and people of color to face long-lasting or even permanent setbacks in education, job opportunities, and access to healthcare.

This systemic problem has stained our country's legacy for too long. I look forward to hearing from our witnesses who will share with us the scope of the challenge and the policy considerations to get us on the right course.

I am now pleased to recognize the distinguished ranking member, Dr. Foxx, for the purpose of her open statement.

Prepared Statement of Hon. Robert C. "Bobby" Scott, Chairman, Committee on Education and Labor

Today, we are discussing how the COVID–19 pandemic is exacerbating racial inequalities in education, labor, and health, and the steps Congress must take to address these disparities.

A mountain of evidence has made it clear that, to effectively respond to the pandemic, we must address the widened existing racial inequities in education, the workforce, and our health care system.

In the area of education, racial bias – both intentional and unconscious – and chronic underfunding of schools serving students of color have produced persistent achievement gaps.

We know that our nation's K–12 public schools entered this pandemic with a $23 billion racial funding gap. That's the difference between the funding in school districts serving predominantly students of color compared to school districts serving predominantly white students.

As schools abruptly closed, this funding gap has positioned students of color to fall even further behind their peers.

Black and Latino students were less likely to attend schools that had the capacity to rapidly establish high-quality distance learning programs. They are also less likely to have the basic technology, such as a personal computer and high-speed internet, and the support at home needed to access virtual learning.

As a result, Latino students are expected to lose 9 months of learning and Black students are expected to lose 10 of learning due to the pandemic, while white students are expected to lose only six months.

In addition to the pandemic's impact on the achievement gap, the Center on Budget and Policy Priorities projects that states will face a $615 billion revenue shortfall over the next three years due to the pandemic.

As the Committee discussed during a hearing last week, public education is usually one of their largest expenditures, accounting for – on average – 40 percent of state budgets. And, unless the federal government provides immediate state and local funding relief, it won't be a matter of whether education funding will be cut, but how much those cuts in education will be.

While wealthier districts can fall back on property tax revenue, low-income public schools district will have to continue to rely heavily on state funding. For school districts that predominantly serve students of color, the severe cuts in education and supporting social service programs will come at a time of greatest need.

The consequences of these shortfalls are already evident. Nearly 750,000 public school employees have lost their jobs since March. In Colorado, the state legislature just passed a budget that cuts $1 billion from its schools for next year.

In the area of the workforce, the outlook for workers of color is similarly concerning. Black and Latino workers, who faced significantly higher rates of unemployment and lower wages long before the pandemic, have borne a disproportionate share of layoffs. Although the rate of unemployment for white and Latino workers has lowered, rates for Black workers have actually increased in recent weeks.

Among those who remained employed, workers of color are more likely to be employed in occupations – such as meatpacking, grocery, health care, and transportation – with the highest risk of infection. Fewer than 20 percent of Black and Latino workers can work from home, compared to nearly 30 percent of white workers. More than 4 in 10 Black workers lack employer-provided paid sick days.

Because of these disparities, workers of color have also been disproportionately affected by the Department of Labor's refusal to issue enforceable workplace safety standards to protect workers from COVID–19.

In addition to working in sectors with the highest risk of COVID–19 infections, Black and Latino workers disproportionately work in low-wage jobs. Regrettably, Congress has not raised the federal minimum wage in more than a decade, the longest period of time in its history. Worse still, weak labor laws and hostile courts have eroded labor union membership and workers' collective bargaining rights, which have left these very essential workers vulnerable to poverty, unsafe workplaces, and a deadly virus.

But the most profound consequence of racial inequality in our society has been the pandemic's devastating impact on the health of people of color.

Nationwide, African Americans have been dying from COVID–19 infections at about two-and-a-half times the rate of white Americans. In New York City, the epicenter of COVID–19 infections and deaths, the death rate for Latinos in the month of April was about 22 people per 100,000, adjusted for population size and age.

American Indian and Alaskan Native communities are suffering disproportionately from COVID–19 infection rates. In late May, the Navajo Nation surpassed New York and New Jersey with the most infections per capita. This follows the pattern of past diseases, where Native American communities bore the brunt of disease outbreaks due to the chronic, long-term underfunding of health care across Indian Country.

As with the challenges in education and workforce issue, the health disparities are rooted in structural inequality. People of color entered the pandemic with health conditions often caused by structural problems, including health care discrimination, housing instability, food insecurity, and limited access to transportation.

Years of statewide budget cuts in public health has led to limited funding for rural and community hospitals in communities of color—leaving families with few options to receive quality care.

Unfortunately, instead of increasing access to health care coverage, the Trump Administration and Republicans are still actively working to take it away in the midst of a public health emergency. The Texas lawsuit threatens the entirety of the Affordable Care Act and all of the law's coverage gains and consumer protections.

These cynical efforts disproportionately impact people of color. If these efforts to strike down the law are successful, estimates show that the uninsured rate among Black people would nearly double from 11 to 20 percent. The share of uninsured Hispanic individuals and families would grow from 21 to 31 percent.

But we are not here to celebrate problems, we are here to discuss solutions.

The Heroes Act, which the House passed last month, would take important steps toward addressing the racial inequities that have been exposed and exacerbated through this pandemic.

With respect to education, the legislation dedicates nearly $1 trillion in relief for states and localities to help avert painful cuts to public schools. It also goes a step further by proposing more than $100 billion in additional emergency educational funding to help cover the cost of cleaning supplies and other expenses required to reopen; purchase educational technology, like laptops and hotspots; sustain special education for students with disabilities; and help colleges and universities maintain their institutions.

To support workers, the Heroes Act directs OSHA to rapidly issue an Emergency Temporary Standard that would require employers to implement protections for workers who are at the highest risk of contracting COVID–19.

It also expands access to emergency paid sick leave to nearly 140 million workers.

While paid leave provisions in the Families First Coronavirus Response Act took important steps in the right direction, far too many workers – including many health care workers – were excluded from these protections.

The Heroes Act also puts “family” and “medical” back into “family and medical leave” by dramatically expanding the circumstances in which workers can take the 12 weeks of emergency F–M-L–A paid leave. We should not force workers to choose between their paycheck, their health, and the health of the people around them.

To improve health outcomes, the Heroes Act expands health insurance coverage for COVID–19 testing and treatment; provides full coverage of the cost of COBRA premiums for laid off and furloughed workers; and, increases investment in health, nutrition, and community support programs, including $1 billion for WIC funding and $1 billion in funding for Community Services Block Grant initiatives to help address poverty.

Finally, the Heroes Act invest $75 billion in testing and contact tracing to contain the virus. This includes $500 million to recruit and train contact tracing workers through public workforce systems and community-based organizations.

Collectively, these provisions represent the immediate next step Congress must take to help our nation get through this global health crisis.

As we confront this unprecedented challenge, we must accept our responsibility to build a recovery that uplifts all communities. But, if we fail to act, we will be experiencing a recovery that offers relief to some but leaves low-income communities and people of color to face long-lasting or even permanent setbacks in education, job opportunities, and access to health care. This systemic problem has stained our country's legacy for too long.

I look forward to hearing from our witnesses who will share with us the scope of this challenge and the policy considerations to right the course.

I now recognize the distinguished Ranking Member, Dr. Foxx, for the purpose of making an opening statement.

Ms. FOXX. Thank you, Mr. Chairman.

Before we begin, I also want to extend my condolences to our colleagues, Andy Barr, Jim Sensenbrenner, Suzanne Bonamici, and Ilhan Omar who suffered the loss of loved ones recently. My prayers go out to them and their families during this difficult time.

Mr. Chairman, you have heard me express my concerns about these virtual committee hearings. But it bears repeating. They fly in the face of 230 years of congressional and legislative precedent. These virtual events undermine what our Founders intended when they created our representative Republic.

Americans are stepping up to help combat this virus while their elected leaders in the House entrusted with the job of representing their constituents stay home. It is shameful, shameful.

A number of my—and, Mr. Chairman, just so you know, you mentioned this was an entirely remote hearing. It is not. A number of my Republican colleagues and I are participating in this hearing today from the committee room in Washington, DC, and I encourage you and all the other Members to return to congressional precedent and hold our hearings in person.

Now turning to the topic of today's virtual hearing, the coronavirus and related State-imposed shutdowns have caused devastating job losses and unemployment rates not seen since the Great Depression. Additionally, schools were forced to close their doors abruptly and switch to remote learning overnight which impacted 97 percent of our country's students.

But let's remember that prior to the COVID–19 pandemic, the U.S. economy and labor market were strong. Real GDP increased 2.3 percent in 2019 and 2.9 percent in 2018. In February, 2020, the unemployment rate was at a historic low of 3.5 percent. Black unemployment was 5.4 percent in August, 2019, the lowest ever recorded.

In September, 2019, the Hispanic unemployment rate was 3.9 percent, also the lowest ever recorded. And in June, 2019, Asian unemployment was a record low 2.1 percent.

Furthermore, at the beginning of 2020, workers in the bottom 10 percent of income had higher average wage growth than those in the top 10 percent. By January, 2020, low income workers—low income earners saw a 15 percent increase in pay since the President took office.

However, we know that Americans, including minority communities, have felt the negative effects of these unprecedented times. The Centers For Disease Control and Prevention, CDC, estimates that Blacks and Hispanics account for nearly 40 percent of COVID–19 deaths in the U.S. Minority communities have also been impacted economically by pandemic-related shutdowns with the rate of Black-owned businesses falling 41 percent, Hispanic-owned businesses falling 32 percent, and Asian-owned businesses falling 26 percent.

We know the pro-growth policies enacted by congressional Republicans and the Trump administration benefited workers, employers, and families before the onset of the COVID–19 pandemic. Reopening the economy responsibly and ensuring public health are not mutually exclusive. We can and we must open America again, while taking into consideration the recommendations from our public health officials.

Look at the May jobs report for proof. Last month 2.5 million jobs were added to the economy, a significant indicator that reopening the economy safely is the best way to help all Americans get back on their feet. Also just last week the Wall Street Journal reported that, quote, new layoffs are being offset by employers hiring or recalling workers their States have allowed more businesses to reopen in recent weeks.

The White House and CDC have issued guidelines for opening up America again. These detailed guidelines which include three phases based on professional guidance from public health officials are intended to help State and local leaders make timely decisions about reopening the economy and getting people back to work, while protecting lives.

And, in fact, every State has started implementing phased reopening plans, allowing nonessential businesses to reopen and operate safely, allowing employees to return to work, and allowing Americans to begin resuming daily activities.

As I previously mentioned, the pre-pandemic economy ushered in under the Republican-led Congress and the Trump administration benefited workers, employers, and families alike. Employment was at record lows including minority unemployment, low-income earners saw a 15 percent increase in pay, and 7 million jobs were available and ready to be filled.

If we hope to achieve pre-pandemic economic conditions that enable Americans to flourish and reach their greatest potential, we must continue forging a forward-looking path to help minority communities to recover and prosper as they were prior to the pandemic.

The Nation's economic recovery and path to prosperity for all Americans is contingent upon reopening our Nation's schools and businesses safely and responsibly. Mandating further topdown Federal laws and policies as proposed by House Democrats will only compound the challenges that all Americans currently face as we continue to combat COVID–19.

I want to thank the witnesses for participating in this hearing, but I hope in the future we can have all our witnesses testify here with us in Washington as we work in person on behalf of hardworking Americans.

I yield back, Mr. Chairman.

Prepared Statement of Hon. Virginia Foxx, Ranking Member, Committee on Education and Labor

Mr. Chairman, you've heard me express my concerns about these virtual Committee hearings, but it bears repeating—they fly in the face of 230 years of congressional and legislative precedent. These virtual events undermine what our Founders intended when they created our representative republic. Americans are stepping up to help combat this virus, while their elected leaders in the House, entrusted with the job of representing their constituents, stay home. It's SHAMEFUL. A number of my Republican colleagues and I are participating in this hearing today from the Committee hearing room in Washington, DC. I encourage you to return to congressional precedent and hold our hearings in person.

Turning to the topic of today's virtual hearing, the coronavirus and related stateimposed shutdowns have caused devastating job losses and unemployment rates not seen since the Great Depression. Additionally, schools were forced to close their doors abruptly and switch to remote learning overnight, which impacted 97 percent of our country's students.

But let's remember that prior to the COVID–19 pandemic, the U.S. economy and labor market were strong. Real GDP increased 2.3 percent in 2019 and 2.9 percent in 2018. In February 2020, the unemployment rate was at a historic low of 3.5 percent. Black unemployment was 5.4 percent in August 2019, the lowest ever recorded. In September 2019, the Hispanic unemployment rate was 3.9 percent, also the lowest ever recorded. And in June 2019, Asian unemployment was a record-low 2.1 percent.

Furthermore, at the beginning of 2020, workers in the bottom 10 percent of income had higher average wage growth than those in the top 10 percent. By January 2020, low-income earners saw a 15 percent increase in pay since the President took office.

However, we know that Americans, including minority communities, have felt the negative effects of these unprecedented times. The Centers for Disease Control and Prevention (CDC) estimates that blacks and Hispanics account for nearly 40 percent of COVID–19 deaths in the U.S. Minority communities have also been impacted economically by pandemic-related shutdowns, with the rate of blackowned businesses falling 41 percent, Hispanic-owned businesses falling 32 percent, and Asian-owned businesses falling 26 percent.

We know the pro-growth policies enacted by congressional Republicans and the Trump administration benefited workers, employers, and families before the onset of the COVID–19 pandemic.

Reopening the economy responsibly and ensuring public health are NOT mutually exclusive. We can, and we must, open America again while taking into consideration the recommendations from our public health officials. Look at the May jobs report for proof. Last month, 2.5 million jobs were added to the economy—a significant indicator that reopening the economy safely is the best way to help all Americans get back on their feet. Also, just last week the Wall Street Journal reported that "new layoffs are being offset by employers hiring or recalling workers as states have allowed more businesses to reopen in recent weeks."

The White House and CDC have issued 'Guidelines for Opening Up America Again.' These detailed guidelines—which include three phases based on professional guidance from public health officials—are intended to help state and local leaders make timely decisions about reopening the economy and getting people back to work while protecting lives.

And in fact, every state has started implementing phased reopening plans, allowing non-essential businesses to reopen and operate safely, allowing employees to return to work, and allowing Americans to begin resuming daily activities.

As I previously mentioned, the pre-pandemic economy—ushered in under the Republican-led Congress and the Trump administration—benefited workers, employers, and families alike. Unemployment was at record lows, including minority unemployment; low-income earners saw a 15 percent increase in pay; and 7 million jobs were available and ready to be filled.

If we hope to achieve pre-pandemic economic conditions that enabled Americans to flourish and reach their greatest potential, we must continue forging a forwardlooking path to help minority communities to recover and prosper as they were prior to the pandemic.

The nation's economic recovery and path to prosperity for all Americans is contingent upon reopening our nation's schools and businesses safely and responsibly. Mandating further top-down federal laws and policies as proposed by House Democrats will only compound the challenges that all Americans currently face as we continue to combat COVID–19.

I want to thank the witnesses for participating in this hearing, but I hope that in the future we can have all our witnesses testifying here with us in Washington as we work in person on behalf of hardworking Americans.

Chairman SCOTT. I thank you, and I look forward to that day myself.

All other Members who wish to insert written statements into the record may do so by submitting them to the Committee Clerk electronically in Microsoft Word format by 5:00 o'clock Sunday, July 5, 2020. I will now briefly introduce our witnesses.

Dr. Camara Jones is an adjunct professor of the Rollins School of Public Health at Emory University, a senior fellow and adjunct associate professor at Morehouse School of Medicine, and past president of the American Public Health Association.

Valerie Wilson is the director of the Program on Race, Ethnicity, and the Economy at the Economic Policy Institute. And I am pleased to note she is an alumni of Hampton University in my district.

Mr. Avik S. A. Roy is president of The Foundation For Research on Equal Opportunity.

And Mr. John King is the president and CEO of the Education Trust and former Secretary of the United States Department of Education.

Instructions to our witnesses. We appreciate the witnesses for participating today and look forward to your testimony. Let me remind the witnesses that we have seen your testimony, and it will appear in full in the hearing record. Pursuant to committee rule 7(d) and committee practice, each of you is asked to limit your oral present tying a five-minute summary of your written statement. Let me remind the witnesses that you are aware that it is illegal to knowingly and willfully falsify any statement to Congress. So we will look forward to your testimony.

During your testimony staff will be keeping track of time and will use a chime to signal when one minute is left, a brief chime when one minute is left. And when time is up entirely, a more obnoxious chime will occur at that time. Please be attentive to time and when your time is over, please wrap up your testimony and remute your microphone.

If anyone is experiencing technical difficulties during your testimony or later in the hearing, you should stay connected on the platform and make sure you are muted with your mute button highlighted in red and use your phone to immediately contact the committee's IT director whose number has been provided.

We will let all witnesses make their presentations before we move to member questions. When answering questions, please remember to unmute your microphone and then remute when you are finished.

We will first recognize Dr. Jones for five minutes.

Statement of Camara P. Jones, MD, MPH, Ph.D., Adjunct Professor, Rollins School of Public Health at Emory University, Senior Fellow and Adjunct Associate Professor, Morehouse School of Medicine, Past President, American Public Health Association Atlanta, GA

Dr. JONES. Thank you, Chairman Scott and Ranking Member Foxx, for inviting my testimony this morning, this afternoon.

And as you outlined, COVID–19 has had a tremendously disproportionate impact on the health and well-being of communities of color. For example, even right now if you compare the death rates from COVID–19 by racial ethnic groups, Black folks are dying at 62 per 100,000, American Indians and Alaska Natives 36 per 100,000, Latinx people 28 per 100,000, Asian folks from 26 per 100,000, and White folks 26 per 100,000. And these racial, especially for Black Americans, the proportion, the 2.3 times that Black Americans are dying compared to White and Asian Americans has never dipped below 2 for the entire course of the pandemic.

And why is this? It is because communities of color are more likely to be infected with the virus. And then once infected, they are more likely to die. They are more likely to be infected because they are more exposed and less protected, and then once infected more likely to die because they are more burdened by chronic diseases with less access to healthcare.

So this doesn't just so happen. You know, we are startled by what we are seeing with COVID–19. But if opportunity were equally distributed across this country and if exposure to risk to equally distributed, there would be no way we could slice and dice our population and see any differences in terms of exposure rates, in terms of, you know, infection, in terms of death.

So what this indicates is that opportunity is not equally distributed by race ethnicity in this country nor is exposure to risk and, in fact, they are differentially distributed by race ethnicity and the name of the system that causes this differential distribution is racism.

Racism is a system for structuring opportunity and assigning value based on so-called race, based on the social interpretations of how one looks, which has three impacts. It unfairly disadvantages some individuals in communities, unfairly advantages other individuals in communities, and saps the strength of the whole society through the waste of human resources.

I know that there are some people who would assert that racism doesn't exist or might assert that, if it did exist, it is systemic. Not, that you know, that it is not systemic, that it is an individual character flaw. I actually use lots of allegories to explain to everybody how racism exists. So if there is one member who wants to ask me in 3 minutes to share an allegory about that, I don't have time in my opening statement. But if somebody was wondering about the dual-reality allegory, I would love that question.

But getting back to what we need to do, first of all, we need to act. Saying that racism is the basis of these differences is not an excuse. It is a call to action because structural racism most often manifests as inaction in the face of need.

So I am providing you all—I have my own ideas for action but you guys are in such a great job. I am providing you with three tools to help guide your future action, to help analyze how you should go, because we need to ask the why—that is racism—in order to get to the what. If you don't have the right answer to why, then the what will never result in improvements that are all the way.

So, the first tool is the question: How is racism operating here? Looking at elements of decision-making in our structures, policies, practices, norms, and values, which are actually, yeah, elements of decision-making structures are the who, what, when, and where of decision-making, especially who is at the table, who is not.

What is on the agenda, what is not. Policies are written hows of decision-making, practices and norms of the unwritten hows of decision-making, values are the why. And after I outline the other two, I am going go back and say how that helps us with COVID– 19.

The second of the three tools are the three principles for achieving health equity, recognizing that health equity is assurance of the conditions for optimal health for all people. It is a governmental function assurance. Three principles for achieving health equity include valuing all individuals and populations equally, recognizing and rectifying historical injustices, and providing resources not equally but according to need. An application of those principles can guide our further actions.

The third tool is something that many of you may not even have heard of, although you are the most erudite and, you know wow, connected folks in the country. That is the International Convention on the Elimination of All Forms of Racial Discrimination, which is an international antiracism treaty that was adopted by the UN General Assembly in 1965, signed by the United States in 1966, ratified by the U.S. Senate in 1994—

So, it took 28 years—but under which we have present-day obligations. One of our obligations is to submit a report about every 6 years to a UN committee, which we do. The last report was submitted in 2013. The committee reviews that report, all of the kinds of reports, and then sends back its concluding observations. And the most recent concluding observations—I hope that was the short one. I never heard the short one.

Chairman SCOTT. You have one minute remaining.

Dr. JONES. Okay. I didn't know that was the short one or the long one. That was pretty obnoxious. Anyway—

So, I will just point out that we have—that the concluding observations provided to us in 2014 highlighted concerns and recommendations around racial profiling, around the disproportionate incarceration of people of color, around health disparities, the achievement gap in education, residential segregation, all of these things.

So, how is racism operating here with regard to COVID–19? In terms of the who, what, when, and where, the structural stuff, the residential segregation leading to educational opportunity segregation, leading to occupational segregation, to we're more on-the-front-line jobs and less—and in terms of the policies, we are less protected in terms of PPE, in terms of paid sick leave, in terms of family and medical leave, all of the things that you are addressing.

In terms of practices, the locations of testing sites and the early policies requiring doctor's orders and the like. In terms of norms, racism denial in this country which then puts the onus of these disproportionate impacts on people's behaviors or whatever, not recognizing that living in chronically disinvested communities, poisoned, no access to fresh fruits and vegetables is related and then, finally, values as reflected in the price and standards of care.

Thank you very much for your attention.

Testimony of Camara Phyllis Jones, MD, MPH, PhD, Adjunct Professor, Rollins School of Public Health at Emory University, Senior Fellow and Adjunct Associate Professor, Morehouse School of Medicine, Past President, American Public Health Association, on behalf of myself, before the U.S. House of Representatives, House Committee on Education and Labor, "Inequities Exposed: How COVID-19 Widened Racial Inequities in Education, Health, and the Workforce," June 22, 2020

Chairman Scott and Members of the Committee, thank you for inviting my testimony.

Racism is foundational in the history of the United States and continues to have profound impacts on the health and well-being of the nation. Today, I will define racism and briefly discuss the impacts of racism on health, especially as manifest through the COVID-19 pandemic, and by extension its impacts on education and labor. I also provide three tools for guiding action in addressing the impacts of racism on health: the question "How is racism operating here?"; three principles for achieving health equity; and the International Convention on the Elimination of all forms of Racial Discrimination.

"Race"-Associated Differences in Health Outcomes Exist

Racial disparities in health outcomes in the United States have been documented across organ systems (heart disease, stroke, cancer, diabetes, asthma, kidney disease), across age groups (infant mortality, maternal mortality, life expectancy at birth), and over time.[1,2,3,4]

In the United States, Black people have higher rates than White people of obesity, high blood pressure, heart disease, kidney disease, diabetes, and asthma. Blacks have the highest age adjusted prevalence of obesity at 49.6% compared to Whites at 42.2%[5]; high blood pressure is most common in Black adults at 54% compared to White adults at 46%[6]; the age-adjusted death rate from heart disease is 208.0 per 100,000 persons for Blacks and 168.9 per 100,000 persons for Whites[7]; prevalence of kidney disease is 3.1% among Blacks and 2.0% among Whites[8]; prevalence of diabetes is 16.4% among Blacks and 11.9% among Whites[9]; prevalence of asthma is 10.7% among

---

[1] National Academy of Sciences, Engineering, and Medicine, *Communities in Action: Pathways To Health Equity* (2017).

[2] Centers for Disease Control and Prevention, CDC Health Disparities and Inequalities Report, 62 *Morbidity and Mortality Weekly Report* 1-187 (Nov. 22, 2013), https://www.cdc.gov/mmwr/pdf/other/su6203.pdf.

[3] U.S. Department of Health and Human Services, Report Of The Secretary's Task Force On Black And Minority Health (1985), https://archive.org/details/reportofsecretar00usde/mode/2up.

[4] WEB DuBois, PHILADELPHIA NEGRO: A SOCIAL STUDY (1899).

[5] Centers for Disease Control and Prevention (CDC), National Center for Health Statistics, Adult Obesity, 2019, https://www.cdc.gov/obesity/data/adult.html.

[6] Centers for Disease Control and Prevention (CDC), National Center for Health Statistics, Hypertension, 2019, https://www.cdc.gov/bloodpressure/facts.htm.

[7] Centers for Disease Control and Prevention (CDC), National Center for Health Statistics, Heart Disease, 2019, https://www.cdc.gov/nchs/hus/spotlight/2019-heart-disease-disparities.htm.

[8] CDC, National Center for Health Statistics, Health United States-Infographics, https://www.cdc.gov/nchs/hus/spotlight/2019-heart-disease-disparities.htm.

[9] Centers for Disease Control and Prevention (CDC), National Center for Health Statistics, National Health Interview Survey 2018, Table A-4a, https://ftp.cdc.gov/pub/Health_Statistics/NCHS/NHIS/SHS/2018_SHS_Table_A-4.pdf.

Blacks and 8.0% among Whites.[10,11,12,13,14,15,16] Racial health disparities are also experienced by American Indian/Alaska Native, Hispanic/Latino, Native Hawaiian and Other Pacific Islander, and some Asian populations.

These racial disparities in health outcomes arise on three levels[12]: differences in quality of health care[13], differences in access to health care[14-16], and differences in underlying exposures and opportunities which make some individuals and communities sicker than others.[17,18,19,20] Mechanisms for differential access to quality health care include insurance, proximity, and representation among physicians.[14]

---

[10] Centers for Disease Control and Prevention (CDC), National Center for Health Statistics, Diabetes, 2020, https://www.cdc.gov/diabetes/pdfs/data/statistics/national-diabetes-statistics report.pdf.

[11] Centers for Disease Control and Prevention (CDC), National Center for Health Statistics, Most Recent National Asthma Data, 2020, https://www.cdc.gov/asthma/most_recent_national_asthma_data.htm.

[12] Jones CP, Jones CY, Perry GS, Barclay G, Jones CA. Addressing the Social Determinants of Children's Health: A Cliff Analogy. Journal of Health Care for the Poor and Underserved 2009;20(4 Suppl):1-12.

[13] Smedley BD, Stith AY, Nelson AR (editors). *Unequal Treatment: Confronting Racial and Ethnic Disparities in Health Care.* Washington, DC: The National Academies Press, 2002.

[14] Agency for Healthcare Research and Quality. Topic: Racial/Ethnic Minorities. https://www.ahrq.gov/topics/racial-ethnic-minorities.html.

[15] Byrd WM, Clayton LA. *An American Health Dilemma: A Medical History of African Americans and the Problem of Race: Beginnings to 1900.* New York, NY: Routledge, 2000.

[16] Byrd WM, Clayton LA. An American Health Dilemma: Race, Medicine, and Health Care in the United States, 1900-2000. New York, NY: Routledge, 2002.

[17] Phelan JC, Link BG, Tehranifar P. Social Conditions as Fundamental Causes of Health Inequalities. *J Health Soc Behav.* 2010;51(S):S28-S40.

[18] Commission on Social Determinants of Health (CSDH) (2008). *Closing the gap in a generation: Health equity through action on the social determinants of health.* Final Report of the Commission on Social Determinants of Health. Geneva, World Health Organization.

[19] Healthy People 2020: Social Determinants of Health. https://www.healthypeople.gov/2020/topics-objectives/topic/social-determinants-of-health.

[20] Jones CP. Systems of Power, Axes of Inequity: Parallels, Intersections, Braiding the Strands. *Medical Care* 2014;52(10 Suppl 3):S71-S75.

Zip Code Is a Much Stronger Predictor of Health Than Is Genetic Code[21,22,23]

Health is not created within the health sector, nor is it primarily determined by genes or individual behaviors. Rather, health outcomes are significantly impacted by social factors. The "social determinants of health" are the determinants of health that are outside of the individual, beyond our genes, and beyond our individual behaviors.[24] They are the contexts of our lives, the conditions in which people are born, grow, live, work and age. They include individual contexts (education, occupation, income, wealth) as well as neighborhood contexts (quality of housing, availability of health foods, availability of green space, air quality, water quality, quality of the schools, availability of work, transportation options, proximity to polluting industries).[25]

The most profound differences between Black people and White people in the United States are in their underlying exposures, opportunities, resources, and risks. Black people have lower average annual income, lower family wealth, poorer housing, live in communities with more environmental degradation, have less access to healthy foods, less access to green space, less access to clean air, and less access to clean water than White people. And this maldistribution of goods, services, and opportunities of society by "race" is not just random.[26]

If the social determinants of health are the contexts of our lives, then the social determinants of equity determine the range of those contexts and which groups live in which contexts.[27] The social determinants of equity include

---

[21] Thomas A. LaVeist, Segregation, Poverty, and Empowerment: Health Consequences for African Americans, 71 The Milbank Quarterly 41-64 (1993).

[22] Thomas A. LaVeist, The Political Empowerment and Health Status of African Americans: Mapping New Territory, 97 American J. Of Sociology 1080-1095 (1992).

[23] Jones CP. "Race," Racism, and the Practice of Epidemiology. *American Journal of Epidemiology* 2001;154(4):299-304.

[24] Jones CP, Truman BI, Elam-Evans LD, Jones CA, Jones CY, Jiles R, Rumisha SF, Perry GS. Using "socially-assigned race" to probe White advantages in health status. *Ethnicity and Disease* 2008;18(4):496-504.

Jones CP. Systems of Power, Axes of Inequity: Parallels, Intersections, Braiding the Strands. *Medical Care* 2014;52(10 Suppl 3):S71-S75.

[25] Jones CP. Confronting Institutionalized Racism. *Phylon* 2003;50(1-2):7-22.

[26] Williams DR, Lawrence JA, Davis BA. Racism and Health: Evidence and Needed Research. *Annu. Rev. Public Health.* 2019;40:105–25.

[27] Yin Paradies, Jehonathan Ben, Nida Denson, Amanuel Elias, Naomi Priest, Alex Pieterse, Arpana Gupta, Margaret Kelaher, Gilbert Gee. Racism as a Determinant of Health: A Systematic Review and Meta-Analysis.

racism, sexism, and other systems of structured inequity. They operate through structures (the "who, "what," "when," and "where" of decision-making); policies (the written "how" of decision-making); practices and norms (the unwritten "how" of decision making); and values (the "why").[28] Of special importance is who is at the decision-making table and who is not, and what is on the agenda and what is not. The health of individuals and communities of color requires unfettered participation of these communities in decision-making processes.[29]

What Does the Variable "Race" Measure?

The variable "race" in the United States is a very rough proxy for socio-economic status, rougher still for culture, and meaningless for genes, so why is it such a good predictor of health outcomes? "Race" precisely captures the social interpretation of how one looks in a "race"-conscious society.[30] Note that the socially-assigned "race" which is noted on a medical record and becomes part of a health statistic is also the same "race" that a taxi driver notices, or a police officer, or a judge in courtroom or a teacher in a classroom. It is the substrate on which racism has operated throughout U.S. history and continues to operate to this day. Indeed, analyses of CDC data reveal that being classified by others as "White" is associated with large and statistically significant advantages in health status, no matter how one self-identifies.[31]

What Is Racism?

Racism is the system of structuring opportunity and assigning value based on the social interpretation of how one looks (which is what we call "race"), that unfairly disadvantages some individuals and communities, unfairly

PLOSONE|DOI:10.1371/journal.pone.0138511, September 23, 2015.

[28] CP. Levels of Racism: A Theoretic Framework and A Gardener's Tale. *American Journal of Public Health* 2000;90(8):1212-1215.

[29] Kendi IX. *Stamped From the Beginning: The Definitive History of Racist Ideas in America.* New York: Bold Type Books, 2016.

[30] Rothstein R. *The Color of Law: A Forgotten History of How Our Government Segregated America.* New York and London: Liveright Publishing Corporation, 2017.

[31] Darity WA, Myers SL. *Persistent Disparity: Race and Economic Inequality in the United States since 1945.* Northampton, MA: Edward Elgar Publishing, 1999.

advantages other individuals and communities, and saps the strength of the whole society through the waste of human resources.[32,33]

Racism Is the Root Cause of "Race"-Associated Differences in Health Outcomes

There is a wealth of empirical research on how racism adversely impacts physical health outcomes and mental health outcomes.[34] There are three levels of racism that impact health: institutionalized (structural), personally-mediated, and internalized.[35] Institutionalized racism results in differential access to the goods, services, and opportunities of society by "race" through a constellation of structures, policies, practices, norms, and values. Personally-mediated racism comprises differential assumptions about the abilities, motives, and intents of others by "race" and differential actions based on those assumptions. Internalized racism is acceptance by members of stigmatized "races" of negative messages about their own abilities and intrinsic worth (and the reciprocal internalization by members of dominant "races" of a sense of entitlement).[36]

Of the three levels of racism, institutionalized racism has the most profound impacts on health.[37] This level of racism does not require an

---

32 Alexander M. *The New Jim Crow: Mass Incarceration in the Age of Colorblindness.* New York: The New Press, 2010.

33 Stevenson B. *Just Mercy: A Story of Justice and Redemption.* New York: Spiegel and Grau, 2014.

34 Williams DR, Lawrence JA, Davis BA. Racism and Health: Evidence and Needed Research. *Annu. Rev. Public Health* 2019;40:105–25.; Yin Paradies, Jehonathan Ben, Nida Denson, Amanuel Elias, Naomi Priest, Alex Pieterse, Arpana Gupta, Margaret Kelaher, Gilbert Gee. Racism as a Determinant of Health: A Systematic Review and Meta-Analysis. PLOSONE|DOI:10.1371/journal.pone.0138511, September 23, 2015.
Jones CP. Coronavirus Disease Discriminates: Our Health Care Doesn't Have To. Newsweek 2020. See https://www.newsweek.com/2020/04/24/coronavirus-disease-discriminates-our-health-care-doesnt-have-opinion-1496405.html (last accessed June 19, 2020).

35 United Nations Office of the High Commissioner for Human Rights. International Convention on the Elimination of all forms of Racial Discrimination. See https://www.ohchr.org/en/professionalinterest/pages/cerd.aspx (last accessed June 7, 2020).

36 United Nations Office of the High Commissioner for Human Rights. Committee on the Elimination of Racial Discrimination. See https://www.ohchr.org/EN/HRBodies/CERD/Pages/CERDIndex.aspx (last accessed June 7, 2020).

37 Committee on the Elimination of Racial Discrimination. Concluding observations on the combined seventh to ninth periodic reports of the United States of America. Download at https://tbinternet.ohchr.org/_layouts/15/treatybodyexternal/Download.aspx?symbolno=CERD%2fC%2fUSA%2fCO%2f7-9&Lang=en (last accessed June 7, 2020).

identifiable perpetrator since it has been institutionalized in our laws, customs, and background norms. Rather, it often manifests as inherited disadvantage or its reciprocal inherited advantage. Institutionalized racism can operate through acts of commission (*doing*) as well as through acts of omission (*not doing*), and it very often manifests as inaction in the face of need.[38]

Institutionalized racism impacts both material conditions and access to power. With regard to material conditions, examples include differential access to quality education, sound housing, gainful employment, appropriate medical facilities, and a clean environment.

With regard to access to power, examples include differential access to information (including one's own history), resources (including wealth and organizational infrastructure), and voice (including civic and political participation, voting rights, representation in government, and control of the media).[39]

Racism is foundational in our nation's history and continues to have profound impacts on the health and well-being of the nation.[40] The association between socioeconomic status and "race" in the United States has its origins in discrete historical events, but persists because of contemporary structural factors that perpetuate those historical injustices. Structural racism is manifest in legal segregation of housing and schools, discrimination in the labor market, disproportionate incarceration, and unequal justice.[41,42,43,44,45]

Present day practices and policies rooted in institutionalized racism, which include ongoing discrimination in housing and lending markets, redlining, and divestment from poor communities, continue to plague "Black," Indigenous, and other People of Color in the United States and are evidenced by disproportionately high levels of poverty and unemployment, substandard

---

38 *Ibid, paragraph 25.*

39 *Ibid, paragraph 32.*

40 Jones CP. Launching an APHA presidential initiative on racism and health (in "Vital Signs," the President's Column of the American Public Health Association). *The Nation's Health* 2016;45(January):3.

41 American Public Health Association. Racism and Health. See https://apha.org/racism (last accessed June 7, 2020).

42 Milwaukee County, Wisconsin. See https://county.milwaukee.gov/EN/County-Executive/Off-Nav/News/Press-Releases/Milwaukee-County-Executive-Chris-Abele-Signs-Resolution-Declaring-Racism-as-a-Public-Health-Crisis (last accessed June 7, 2020).

43 Dane County, Wisconsin. See https://madison365.com/dane-county-health-council-commits-to-action-on-racism-a-public-health-crisis/ (last accessed June 7, 2020).

44 Allegheny County, Pennsylvania. See https://www.wesa.fm/post/county-council-deems-racism-public-health-crisis-party-line-vote#stream/0 (last accessed June 7, 2020).

45 Franklin County, Ohio. See https://www.cnn.com/2020/05/21/us/franklin-county-ohio-race-public-health-crisis-trnd/index.html (last accessed June 7, 2020).

educational settings and opportunities, concentration in poor neighborhoods with unsafe, and under-resourced living environments, overall economic instability, and limited access to quality healthcare.[46]

Racism Is the Root Cause of the Disproportionate Impact of COVID-19 on Communities of Color in the United States

The disproportionate Black COVID-19 infection and death rates that are being documented across the United States are due to the ways that racism has structured our opportunities so that Black people are more likely to be infected by the virus (SARS-CoV-2), and the ways that racism has impacted our underlying health status so that Black people are more likely to experience severe forms of the disease (COVID-19) once infected. It is important to recognize that the disproportionate impact is NOT due to some inherent biological weakness nor some reluctance to comply with public health advisories. Black people are getting more infected with SARS-CoV-2 because they are more exposed and less protected. Black people are dying from COVID-19 at higher rates because they are more burdened by chronic diseases with less access to health care.[47]

Black People Are More Likely to Get Infected with COVID-19 Because They Are More Exposed and Less Protected

Black people are more exposed because they are overrepresented in low-paid frontline jobs (e.g., home health aides, transit drivers, postal workers, sanitation workers, hospital orderlies and custodians, grocery workers, meat packers, and warehouse workers). Black people are also more exposed because they are disproportionately impacted by housing instability, more reliant on public transportation, and live in more crowded home settings and more densely populated communities.[48] Communities of color do not have

---

[46] San Bernardino County, California. See http://www.hidesertstar.com/news/article_e6a854d4-ad1c-11ea-90d7-ff2e468c052b.html (last accessed June 13, 2020).

[47] Montgomery County, Maryland. See https://www.localdvm.com/news/i-270/montgomery-county-passes-resolution-to-make-racism-a-public-health-emergency/ (last accessed June 13, 2020).

[48] Genesee County, Michigan. See https://www.abc12.com/content/news/Genesee-County-declares-racism-a-public-health-emergency--571169991.html (last accessed June 15, 2020).

many opportunities to work from home nor the savings nor paid sick leave to be off the job to preserve their health. Black workers are also overrepresented in low-income, frontline jobs, and more affected by residential, educational, and occupational segregation.[49]

People of color are less protected when doing their low-income frontline work – which has only recently been lauded as "essential" – because they are not provided adequate personal protective equipment to prevent their contracting the virus on the job.

Once Infected, Black People Are More Likely to Die from COVID-19 Because They Are More Burdened by Chronic Diseases and Have Less Access to Health Care

Black people are more burdened by chronic disease because Black communities are more likely to be disinvested and actively neglected communities of concentrated poverty with poor access to healthy foods including fresh fruits and vegetables; poor access to green space and healthy environments for active living; increased likelihood of proximity to polluting industries which poison the air, soil, or water; and crowded and unhealthy living spaces. These conditions greatly constrain residents from making healthy behavioral choices, resulting in higher prevalence of obesity, high blood pressure, diabetes, asthma, heart disease, and kidney disease (among many other health outcomes), all of which make COVID-19 more severe and potentially deadly.[50]

Black people have less access to timely, responsive, and physically proximate health care services compared to the rest of the United States. During the COVID-19 pandemic, testing sites were first located in affluent communities (with lower proportions of Black residents) and people seeking a COVID-19 test were required to have an order from a primary care physician, which Black residents are more likely to lack. In rural parts of many states, recent hospital closures associated with the failure to expand Medicaid under the Affordable Care Act have exacerbated the lack of ready access to

---

[49] King County, Washington. See https://publichealthinsider.com/2020/06/11/racism-is-a-public-health-crisis/ (last accessed June 15, 2020). See also https://southseattleemerald.com/2020/06/11/king-county-officially-declares-racism-a-public-health-crisis/(last accessed June 15, 2020).

[50] Pittsburgh, Pennsylvania. See https://www.citylab.com/equity/2020/01/pittsburgh-racism-health-pollution-environmental-justice/603775/ (last accessed June 7, 2020).

health care.[51] Finally, Black adults in the United States are substantially more likely than White adults to express high levels of concern over the possibility that they will contract COVID-19 or transmit it to others. Those fears are well-founded.

Racism Is Foundational in the History of the United States and Continues to Have Profound Impacts on the Health and Well-Being of the Nation

At least eight U.S. counties (Milwaukee County, WI; Dane County, WI; Allegheny County, PA; Franklin County, OH; Genesee County, MI; San Bernardino County, CA; Montgomery County, MD; and King County, WA) and nine U.S. cities (Pittsburgh, PA; Columbus, OH; Somerville, MA; Medford, MA; Boston, MA; Cleveland, OH; Denver, CO; Indianapolis, IN; and Flint, MI) have declared that racism is a public health crisis.[52,53]

During this COVID-19 pandemic, the unfair disadvantage that racism has structured for communities of color is even more life-threatening than during "normal" times. It is noteworthy that the most profound impacts of racism occur without bias. They manifest instead as inaction in the face of need.

How Is Racism Operating Here?

The question "How is racism operating here?" provides a useful tool for identifying targets for action by examining the elements of decision-making in our structures, policies, practices, norms, and values, where structures are the "Who?," "What?," "When?," and "Where?" of decision-making (especially "Who is at the table and who is not?," and "What is on the agenda and what is not?"); policies are the written "How?" of decision-making; practices and norms are the unwritten "How?" of decision-making; and values

---

[51] Somerville, Massachusetts. See https://www.somervillema.gov/policereform (last accessed June 7, 2020).

[52] Medford, Massachusetts. See https://patch.com/massachusetts/medford/medford-council-declares-racism-health-crisis-calls-action (last accessed June 13, 2020).

[53] Boston, Massachusetts. See https://www.bostonglobe.com/2020/06/12/metro/mayor-walsh-declares-racism-be-public-health-crisis-bostonholding-press-confernece/ (last accessed June 13, 2020).

are the "Why?." Following is a brief application of this question with regard to the disproportionate impact of COVID-19 on communities of color.

Structures

The racial segregation of housing structured into our society (see Rothstein R, The Color of Law) results in racial segregation of education (public school funding tied to local property taxes, with poor funding often leading to poor educational outcomes and another generation lost) which then results in racial segregation of occupational opportunities. This accounts for the disproportionate representation of Black and Brown people in frontline jobs (home health aides, sanitation, postal work, drivers, warehouse workers, meat and poultry plant workers, many others).

Another structural mechanism is the well-described school to prison pipeline (unequal administration of discipline in schools, disproportionate suspensions, poorly administered foster care, disproportionately harsh adjudication in juvenile justice systems, over-policing of communities of color, unequal sentencing guidelines, and others) lead to disproportionate incarceration of Black and Brown men and women. Even the limited decarceration of older prisoners and those with pre-existing health conditions during the COVID-19 pandemic has been unevenly applied because of structural barriers to attorney access.

Policies

Many frontline workers in jobs which are now recognized as "essential" are poorly paid with limited paid sick leave and inadequate protection from exposure to the virus (crowded work conditions, inadequate personal protective equipment, limited testing at the workplace). Both Congress and the Occupational Safety and Health Administration can assume stronger roles in addressing these issues.

Practices

The widespread practice (especially early on in the pandemic) of locating testing centers in affluent areas or as drive-up centers or requiring doctor's orders systematically disadvantaged residents in poor areas, with access to cars, and with access to a primary care physician. As a nation, our testing strategies for the virus are still narrowly focused on the individual in a medical care model, confirming diagnoses for those with symptoms, and as such are only useful for documenting the course of the pandemic, and then only partially. A population-based public health approach to testing would enable us to not only document the course of the pandemic but also to CHANGE the course of the pandemic by implementing public health surveillance approaches to testing probability samples of both symptomatic and asymptomatic persons, followed by community endorsed isolation strategies, contact tracing, and quarantine. These public health approaches to managing the pandemic will benefit all United States residents, but especially those communities that are being most adversely affected by the pandemic.

Norms

Several cultural norms in the United States inhibit widespread acknowledgement that racism exists. Among these:

- Our narrow focus on the individual makes systems and structure invisible or seemingly irrelevant.
- Our a-historical stance acts as if the present were disconnected from the past, and as if the current distribution of advantage and disadvantage were just a happenstance.
- Our widespread endorsement of the myth of meritocracy, that "If you work hard you will make it," acknowledges that most (although not all) people who have made it have worked hard, but ignores the reality that there are many, many other people working just as hard or harder who will never make it because of an uneven playing field (which has been structured and is being maintained by racism, sexism, heterosexism, and other systems of structured inequity).

Values

COVID-19 is a public health problem which has been treated in this country as if it were instead a medical care problem, and as a result it is manifesting as a tremendous challenge to the medical care system. We are at risk of experiencing local scarcities of life-saving interventions including ventilators, intensive care unit beds, and emergency dialysis. When "Crisis Standards of Care" are promulgated by states and by health care systems, they have often reflected a hierarchy of valuation by work role (medical care worker over other essential workers), age (younger people over older people), and existence of chronic diseases (which systematically disadvantages communities of color who bear a greater burden of chronic diseases from living in segregated, chronically disinvested, actively neglected, and environmentally poisoned communities). Suggestions to implement a lottery for the rationing of scarce life-saving resources are often met with skepticism, reflecting a deep-seated commitment to the differential valuation of human life in this country.

Principles for Achieving Health Equity

Health equity is the assurance of the conditions for optimal health for all people. Achieving health equity requires valuing all individuals and populations equally, recognizing and rectifying historical injustices, and providing resources according to need. Health disparities will be eliminated when health equity is achieved. The three principles for achieving health equity can provide a framework for addressing the short-term and long-term challenges posed by the COVID-19 pandemic.

The "pre-existing health conditions" that put a person at risk of severe disease and death from COVID-19 are overrepresented in communities of color and poor communities as a result of long-term disinvestment and neglect.[54] Delayed responses to the COVID-19 pandemic have resulted in unprecedented and under-resourced demands on our health care system. With limited medical equipment and fewer resources, health care providers have had to make decisions about COVID-19 treatment in real time at the bedside, regarding which patients will receive life-saving treatment and which patients will not. These decisions used to be made from a distance by our health insurance companies, our economic system, and by residential segregation. During this pandemic, the decisions have become more personal in a whole new way.

Health equity is the assurance of the conditions for optimal health for all people. It is a process, not a magical outcome. The Affordable Care Act (ACA) has been one of the most important steps toward reducing racial inequities in health insurance coverage in the past decade.[55] In the first few years of its implementation, the ACA improved access to health care coverage for low-income communities of color in both states that did expand eligibility for

---

[54] Cleveland, Ohio. See https://www.cleveland.com/cityhall/2020/06/cleveland-city-council-declares-racism-a-public-health-crisis-launching-community-wide-effort-to-tackle-inequities.html (last accessed June 13, 2020).

[55] Denver, Colorado. See https://www.thedenverchannel.com/news/front-range/denver/denver-city-council-approves-proclamation-calling-racism-a-public-health-crisis (last accessed June 13, 2020).

Medicaid under the ACA and states that did not expand Medicaid.[56] However, these health care coverage gains were larger in states that expanded Medicaid. Socioeconomic disparities in health care access narrowed significantly under the ACA. The gap in insurance coverage between people in households with annual incomes below $25,000 and those in households with incomes above $75,000 fell from by 46 percent in states that expanded Medicaid and by 23 percent in non-expansion states.[57]

In Medicaid expansion states, more than 74% of Black adults and 58% of Hispanic adults reported having a regular health care provider in 2018 compared to 71% and 55% in 2013. Gaps in health insurance coverage among racial and ethnic groups narrowed the most in states that expanded Medicaid, and supporting Medicaid expansion in additional states has the potential to improve racial equity in health insurance coverage. The Affordable Care Act also resulted in proportionate declines in uninsured rates among all racial and ethnic groups in the United States. Because uninsured rates in Hispanic communities started off much higher, the health insurance coverage gap between Black people and non-Hispanic white people declined from 11.0 percentage points in 2013 to 5.3 percentage points in 2017. The health care coverage gap between Hispanic people and non-Hispanic white people dropped from 25.4 points to 16.6 points.[58,59]

As we navigate through the immediate health, economic, and social demands of the COVID-19 pandemic, three principles for achieving health equity can provide us with both a moral and practical compass: valuing all individuals and populations equally, recognizing and rectifying historical injustices, and providing resources according to need. These principles can serve as a framework for evaluating current and proposed policy solutions, as well as a checklist for identifying gaps in policy where no solutions have yet been suggested. They can also be the basis for decision-making at the health care provider level. There are ways we can operationalize these principles for response to the COVID-19 pandemic.

---

[56] Indianapolis, Indiana. See https://www.indystar.com/story/news/local/indianapolis/2020/06/08/indianapolis-declares-racism-public-health-crisis/5323769002/ (last accessed June 13, 2020).

[57] Flint, Michigan. See https://www.mlive.com/news/flint/2020/06/flint-city-council-denounces-illegal-police-restraints-declares-racism-a-public-health-crisis.html (last accessed June 15, 2020).

[58] Ajay Chaudry, Adlan Jackson, and Sherry A. Glied, *Did the Affordable Care Act Reduce Racial and Ethnic Disparities in Health Insurance Coverage?* (Commonwealth Fund, Aug. 2019). https://doi.org/10.26099/d8hs-cm53.

[59] Griffith, Kevin, Leigh Evans, and Jacob Bor. "The Affordable Care Act reduced socioeconomic disparities in health care access." Health Affairs 36.8 (2017): 1503-1510.

Valuing All Individuals and Populations Equally

Valuing all individuals and populations equally. We need to consider how to reach all communities with our life-saving messages of social distancing, frequent handwashing, stay-at-home orders and symptoms of COVID-19. We need to enable all individuals to take up these practices. We have to be bold in imagining solutions to the issues raised when we decide to value all individuals and populations equally. These solutions include connections to community resources to provide housing of previously unhoused individuals in available vacant properties, or, at least, provide hand-washing stations and opening public restrooms for their use.

At the policy level, the most important way to value all individuals and populations equally is by looking at who is at the decision-making table and who is not, what is on the agenda and what is not. When any of us is at a decision-making table, we must look around and ask, "Who is not here who has an interest in this proceeding?" Our job is not just to represent the interests of the missing parties, although that may be a necessary short-term strategy. Our job is to create space for them at the table.

Even now, when Congress is working on the fourth COVID-19 legislative package for the nation, we need to ensure that all voices from communities of color are heard throughout the legislative process. In the short term, that may require active constituent engagement by our elected representatives. In the long term, that may require a more vigorous defense of voting rights and deep reforms of campaign financing to make sure all voices are heard in our democracy.

Communities of color should not be "sacrifice zones" with regard to the COVID-19 response. The decision to disembark infected persons from the Diamond Princess cruise ship in Oakland Bay rather than in San Francisco Bay, given that Oakland has a much larger Black population, is a decision that requires closer examination. The decision to convert Carney Hospital in the Dorchester neighborhood of Boston to be the nation's first hospital solely devoted to the care of COVID-19 patients deprived that predominantly Black neighborhood of access to other medical services and possibly increasing the risk of infection in the area.

At the bedside, decisions about the allocation of life-saving treatments should not be done by the medical professionals directly involved in the patient's care. It is too easy for implicit bias about relative worth based on race or ethnicity, class, gender, language, disability or other characteristic to manifest itself in decision-making when a provider is tired or stressed. If patient prioritization will instead be done by a hospital ethics board, the composition of that board also needs to be examined for balance along axes of difference and power, and community input into the criteria and processes for decision-making should be rapidly sought.

If we really want to value all individuals and populations equally, should we use a lottery system for allocation of scarce resources? At least structured inequity and subjective valuation would be taken out of the decision-making. This is a provocative suggestion. But perhaps the threat of a fair system in which all people would have equal chances at life would stimulate a more rapid production and distribution of life-saving health resources, solving the issue of scarcity.

Recognizing and Rectifying Historical Injustices

The principle manifestation of historical injustices during the crisis of the COVID-19 pandemic is in how segregation of resources and risks, societal devaluation, and environmental hazards and degradation are written into the bodies of people of color and poor people. The greater health burden borne by these people may not only predispose them to more severe manifestations of COVID-19 itself, but may also disadvantage them in any ethical protocol established for the rationing of scarce health resources. That would be wrong. It would be counter to the health equity principle of recognizing and rectifying historical injustices, putting at double jeopardy those who already bear the brunt of chronic assaults to health. Instead, this principle should lead to the provision of more ventilators, COVID-19 treatment, and health care services in populations with higher pre-existing health burdens.

Recognizing and rectifying historical injustices also requires the collection and disaggregation of data on COVID-19 testing, diagnosis, treatment, and outcome by "race" and ethnicity so that the impacts of those historical injustices can be recognized and addressed.

In the longer term, attention from policymakers to the history of each problem to be solved will always provide useful insight into effective solutions. Understanding how a knot was tied will always help in untying the knot. Our nation is notoriously ahistorical, thinking that the present is disconnected from the past and that the current distribution of advantage and disadvantage is just a happenstance. The long-term application of this principle will involve the large-scale teaching of our full histories as a nation and a commitment to apologize and make reparations for past injustices, recognizing that they continue to have present-day impacts.

Providing Resources According to Need

This principle is perhaps the easiest of the three principles to understand, but often the hardest to implement because it takes a tremendous amount of political will. The first step is to establish a metric of need on which there is wide consensus. In the context of the COVID-19 pandemic, this metric might be the number of diagnosed COVID-19 patients, or indicators of the trajectory of the epidemic (e.g., the doubling time and basic reproduction number of SARS-CoV-2, the virus that causes COVID-19) in a given jurisdiction. It might include projected number of deaths, projected demands on the health care system, current health system capacity, or current levels of resources in an area.

Once a metric of need is established and agreed upon, it would then seem simple to take all available resources and distribute them according to that metric of need. However, even in the clear current situation of New York City, topping off these measures of need all around, there is not a rapid deployment of national resources to the city. Other jurisdictions are holding on to their resources because of the anticipated changes to projected need in a few weeks. The federal government is slow in using its full power to rapidly commission and deploy resources to areas of need. Instead of conducting targeted and fluid mobilization as the pandemic moves across the nation, there appears to be a stance of disbelief and paralysis at the scope of the need.

As often happens, people (and political jurisdictions) never compare themselves to those who have less than what they have. They always compare themselves to those who have more, so they always feel needy. A pre-established metric of need should solve that. But perhaps strong community pressure is also required.

The COVID-19 pandemic will not end in days or weeks. It could be a year, maybe 18 months. By then, the world will have faced immeasurable loss of life. The economy will improve, but it is my hope that these three principles for achieving health equity will be useful in guiding decision-making during these treacherous times. Looking forward, I also hope that they will provide a guide for how we value and treat one another as we build a better, new normal after this devastating pandemic.

Recommendations for Action

The Following Are Specific Recommendations for Action in the Short-Term

- Make it more feasible for more people to safely shelter in place
  - Mandate that all employers provide at least four weeks of paid leave
  - Increase the federal minimum wage to $15 an hour
- Make workplaces safer
  - Fund the Occupational Health and Safety Administration (OSHA) to investigate all workplaces where COVID-19 transmission has occurred
  - Mandate that OSHA promulgate safety guidelines for meatpacking and poultry plants, warehouses, nursing homes and other congregate living communities for seniors, and other workplaces that have already experienced widespread COVID-19 transmission
  - The COVID-19 transmission in these workplaces is not just a labor concern, it is a public health concern because workers return to their homes and communities and where they could further spread the virus
  - Require weekly COVID-19 testing of all workers and residents in these settings, not just COVID-19 testing for those exhibiting symptoms, since it has been estimated that at least 25 percent of persons infected with COVID-19 show no symptoms but can still transmit the virus
- Make communities safer
  - Mandate mask-wearing in all public indoor and outdoor spaces
  - Ensure that states accurately collect and report data on COVID-19 antigen testing, hospitalization, morbidity, and mortality to allow phased re-openings to be informed by public health experts using scientific data
  - Ensure that states report all COVID-19 testing, hospitalization, and death data stratified by "race"/ethnicity as well as by zip code
  - Ensure adherence to CDC guidelines in the phased re-opening and re-closing of states, counties, and cities

- Fully fund the U.S. Postal Service to enable continued delivery of mail and medicines
- Fund and equip local public health departments to be able to do weekly public health surveillance testing of probability samples of their populations to enable real-time assessment of the current level of COVID-19 infection in their jurisdictions (both symptomatic and asymptomatic), as opposed to using positive test results from symptomatic persons (which lag COVID-19 infection rates by 1 to 2 weeks), hospitalization rates (which lag infection rates by 2 to 3 weeks), or death rates (which lag infection rates by 3 to 4 weeks)
- Fund free-standing isolation centers for those who test positive for COVID-19 and cannot safely return to their homes (e.g., older people, and vulnerable groups who do not have safe housing options) where their body temperatures and oxygen saturation levels can be monitored twice a day by health care providers who can also make timely transfers to hospitals as needed
- Invest in the hiring, training, and deployment of local community members to build a diverse contact tracer workforce for their communities

- Strengthen health care financing and the health care system
  - Strengthen the Affordable Care Act
  - Expand access to Special Enrollment Periods (SEP) and Open Enrollment periods for the ACA Marketplace plans during the COVID-19 pandemic to all who need access to health care, especially those formerly covered by employer-sponsored health insurance who are now unemployed
  - Hire, train, and deploy more ACA Navigators to enable seamless access to health care coverage through the Affordable Care Act
  - Invest in minority-serving institutions at all levels to increase the number of Black, Latinx, and Indigenous health care providers coming through the pipelines
  - Increase investment in the National Health Service Corps to increase the number of providers in medically underserved areas and make medical education more accessible to students from low-income communities
  - Provide incentives to states that have not yet expanded Medicaid under the Affordable Care Act to do so now, so that all states expand Medicaid during this public health and health care crisis.

- Protect civic and political participation in the time of COVID-19
  - Fund states to enable the safe and secure receipt of mail-in ballots from all voters who desire to vote from home in elections at least through the end of 2021
- Increase the protection of essential workers
  - Provide N95 masks and protective gowns to all workers upon request
  - This might be more easily achieved if the Defense Production Act is activated with regard to the production of N95 masks
  - Provide hazard pay for all workers providing essential labor during the COVID-19 pandemic
  - Provide at least 4 weeks of paid leave for all workers

The Following Recommendations Include More Long-Term Solutions

- Value all individuals and populations equally
  - Provide for equal protection of voting rights by strengthening the Voting Rights Act and instating provisions for review of changes in voting procedures by all states.
- Recognize and rectify historical injustices
  - Apologize for the enslavement of African people and their progeny for generations, acknowledging the role of their coerced unpaid labor to build this country
  - Provide reparations for Descendants of Africans Enslaved in the United States.
- Provide resources according to need
  - Massively invest in communities of color that have been historically segregated and disinvested by strengthening investments in quality housing options and schools, employment opportunities, green space and environmental clean-up services for the removal of polluting industries, healthy food access, beautiful recreation spaces, business investment, cooperative land ownership
  - Massively invest in programs to support all families with particular attention to families of color, including one year of paid maternal and paid paternal leave at the birth of each child and strong financial support for children and their families

- These efforts will be deemed successful when the phrase "disadvantaged child" will have no meaning because it will be unthinkable that any child will be born into disadvantage

- Measure the impacts of racism on the health and well-being of the nation
    - Restore the CDC's Racism and Health Workgroup,[60] an official CDC scientific working group
    - Restore the 6-question "Reactions to Race" module as an optional module on the Behavioral Risk Factor Surveillance System (BRFSS) and consider moving the first two questions of the module to the BRFSS Core Questionnaire
    - Include the six reactions to "race" questions on the National Health and Nutrition Examination Survey, the National Health Interview Survey, and other national data collection efforts
- Launch a National Campaign Against Racism
    - In 2016, the American Public Health Association launched a National Campaign Against Racism with three tasks: Name racism, ask "How is racism operating here?," Organize, and Strategize to act[61]
    - At least eight U.S. counties – Milwaukee County and Dane County, Wisconsin; Allegheny County, Pennsylvania; Franklin County, Ohio; Genesee County, Michigan; San Bernardino County, California; Montgomery County, Maryland; King County, Washington – and nine U.S. cities – Pittsburgh, Pennsylvania; Columbus, Ohio; Somerville, Massachusetts; Medford, Massachusetts; Boston, Massachusetts; Cleveland, Ohio; Denver, Colorado; Indianapolis, Indiana; Flint, Michigan – have declared that racism is a public health crisis
- Adhere to the United Nations International Convention on the Elimination of all forms of Racial Discrimination
    - The International Convention on the Elimination of all forms of Racial Discrimination (ICERD) is an international anti-racism treaty adopted by the United Nations General Assembly in 1965

---

[60] MacIntosh, Tracy, et al. "Socially-assigned race, healthcare discrimination and preventive healthcare services." *PloS one* 8.5 (2013).

[61] Buchmueller, Thomas C., and Helen G. Levy. "The ACA's Impact On Racial And Ethnic Disparities In Health Insurance Coverage And Access To Care: An examination of how the insurance coverage expansions of the Affordable Care Act have affected disparities related to race and ethnicity." *Health Affairs* 39.3 (2020): 395-402.

- The United States signed ICERD in 1966 and the United States Senate ratified ICERD in 1994, so that our country has obligations to comply with this international anti-racism treaty, including submission of periodic reports to the United Nations Committee on the Elimination of Racial Discrimination (CERD)
- In its 2014 Concluding Observations to the third periodic report submitted by the United States government, the UN CERD thanked for the United States for its report and then noted many "Concerns and Recommendations," including those related to disproportionate incarceration, the achievement gap in education, differential access to health care, and residential segregation
- The UN CERD also "recommends that the State party adopt a national action plan to combat structural racial discrimination"
- The UN CERD further "recommends that the State party increase its efforts to raise public awareness and knowledge of the Convention throughout its territory"

- Support an Anti-Racism Collaborative with eight Collective Action teams: Following are guiding questions and opportunities for action for each of the Collective Action Teams
    - Communication and Dissemination
      Guiding questions: How can we support the naming of racism in all public and private spaces? What tools and strategies are needed to start community conversations on racism?
      Opportunities for action: Develop a communication toolbox: allegories, billboards, films, podcasts, songs, tweets, webinars. Put racism and anti-racism on community agendas: Anti-Racism Conversation, Civic Dinners, Town Hall Meetings.
    - Education and Development
      Guiding questions: How can we support training around issues of "race," racism, and anti-racism at educational institutions of all levels? What does effective anti-racism curriculum look like?
      Opportunities for action: Convene anti-racism scholars and activists. Develop curricula for schools of public health, medicine, social work, law. Develop curricula for K-12 education. Publish allegories as children's books.
    - History
      Guiding questions: What is the history of successful anti-racism struggle in the United States and around the world? How can this history guide our anti-racism work today? How can we

institutionalize attention to history in all decision-making processes?

Opportunities for action: Teach our full histories: The 1619 Project from The New York Times, textbooks, museums, school curricula, after-school programs. Hire historians to staff City Councils, State Legislatures, U.S. Congress.

- Liaison and Partnership

  Guiding questions: What anti-racism work is happening at the community level? What anti-racism work is happening in other sectors? How can we create linkages?

  Opportunities for action: Catalog and connect local anti-racism efforts throughout the nation and the world. Draft an anti-racism commitment agreement for communities, businesses, and organizations across sectors.

- Organizational Excellence

  Guiding questions: We must consider the ways in which we should answer the following question in each of our environments: "How is racism operating here?" in each of our settings? How do we examine structures, policies, practices, norms, and values?

  Opportunities for action: For example, identify policies that: allow segregation of resources and risks; create inherited group disadvantages and advantages; favor the differential valuation of human life by "race"; and limit self-determination.

- Policy and Legislation

  Guiding questions: What are current policy and legislative strategies to address and dismantle racism? What new strategies should we propose?

  Opportunities for action: Catalog formal anti-racism policies adopted by U.S. jurisdictions, including the state of Maryland, Milwaukee County, the state of New Mexico, and Seattle and King Counties in the state of Washington. Develop and disseminate model legislation addressing the many mechanisms of structural racism.

- Science and Publications

  Guiding questions: What research has been done to examine the impacts of racism on the health and well-being of the nation and the world? What intersection strategies have been evaluated? What new measures and methods are needed?

Opportunities for action: Put measures of racism on population-based surveys: the Behavioral Risk Factor Surveillance System (BRFSS), the National Health and Nutrition Examination Survey (NHANES), the Youth Risk Behavior Surveillance Survey (YRBSS); Develop the science and practice of anti-racism.

Toward the Science and Practice of Anti-Racism: Launching a National Campaign against Racism

Camara Phyllis Jones

Setting the Agenda for Anti-racism

As president of the American Public Health Association (APHA) from 2015-2016, I launched a National Campaign Against Racism as a key agenda of my APHA presidency.[62,63] I set this agenda for the nation's flagship professional society for public health practitioners and researchers because I identified racism as the root cause of "race"-associated differences in health outcomes.[64] We must now set this agenda for our nation. Although some in this country will acknowledge that racism is foundational in our nation's history, many in this country are in denial about the continued existence of racism and its profound impacts on the health and well-being of the nation. Indeed, it is because of this widespread denial of racism that we must launch a National Campaign against Racism with three tasks: 1) naming racism; 2) asking "how is racism operating here?" and 3) organizing and strategizing to act. Following are brief descriptions of each of these tasks, including a framework for an Anti-Racism Collaborative as a platform for organizing our work going forward.

---

[62] Jones CP. Launching an APHA presidential initiative on racism and health. Nations Health. 2016;45:3. [Google Scholar].

[63] American Public Health Association Racism and Health. Last accessed July 3, 2018 from https://www.apha.org/racism.

[64] Jones CP. Invited commentary: "race," racism, and the practice of epidemiology. Am J Epidemiol. 2001;154(4):299-304. 10.1093/aje/154.4.299 [PubMed] [CrossRef] [Google Scholar].

Naming Racism

Racism is a system of structuring opportunity and assigning value based on the social interpretation of how one looks (which is what we call "race"), that unfairly disadvantages some individuals and communities, unfairly advantages other individuals and communities, and saps the strength of the whole society through the waste of human resources.[65,66] This definition of racism as a system (rather than an individual character flaw, personal moral failing, or psychiatric illness) helps start conversations because we are no longer trying to divide the room into who is racist and who is not. By acknowledging that racism saps the strength of the whole society, we recognize that we all have "skin" in the game to dismantle this system and put in its place a system in which all people can know and develop to their full potentials.

My use of allegory to illustrate different aspects of "race" and racism has been effective in naming racism to people who have been raised in denial and taught not to see. My Gardener's Tale[67,68] illustrates three levels of racism (institutionalized, personally mediated, and internalized) and strongly suggests that we must address institutionalized/structural racism if we are to set things right in our garden. The story also illustrates the importance of addressing both how racism structures opportunity and how it assigns value. Even if we could compel the gardener in that allegory to enrich the poor, rocky soil until it was as rich as the rich, fertile soil, if she continues to prefer the red flowers over the pink flowers, she will continue to privilege red over pink going forward. This story highlights that we must address both the opportunity structures (differential access to the goods, services, and opportunities of society by "race") and the value assignment (White supremacist ideology) in our anti-racism work.

---

[65] Jones CP. Confronting institutionalized racism. Phylon. 2003;50(1-2):7-22. [Google Scholar].

[66] Jones CP, Truman BI, Elam-Evans LD, et al. Using "socially assigned race" to probe white advantages in health status. Ethn Dis. 2008;18(4):496-504. [PubMed] [Google Scholar].

[67] Jones CP. Levels of racism: a theoretic framework and a gardener's tale. Am J Public Health. 2000;90(8):1212-1215. 10.2105/AJPH.90.8.1212 [PMC free article] [PubMed] [CrossRef] [Google Scholar].

[68] CityMatCH Annual Urban MCH Leadership Conference, 2002. A Discussion with Camara P. Jones, MD, MPH, PhD. Last accessed July 3, 2018 from: https://www.youtube.com/watch?v=1QFCcChCSMU.

Among my other published allegories, my Cliff Analogy[69,70] illustrates that to eliminate health disparities and achieve social justice, health interventions must address racism and other systems of structured inequity. My Japanese Lanterns[71] allegory illustrates how easy it is to be beguiled by the illusion of "race" as a fixed biological trait. My Dual Reality Restaurant Saga[71,72] illustrates how easy it is for those who are privileged by systems of structured inequity to be blind to the existence of those systems. My Conveyor Belt[71,73] allegory illustrates the three tasks of becoming actively anti-racist against the backdrop of societal indifference and complicity in racism.

Asking "How Is Racism Operating Here?"

The mechanisms of racism are in our structures, policies, practices, norms, and values, which are different elements of decision-making.[65] Structures are the "who?," "what?," "when?," and "where?" of decision-making; policies are the written "how?" of decision-making; practices and norms are the unwritten "how?" of decision-making; and values are the "why?" In evaluating these mechanisms of racism, we need to be especially attentive to the "absence of." Who is at the table, and who is not? What is on the agenda, and what is not? And when we note the "absence of," we need to take action to fill in the gaps. We need to become vigilant in identifying and addressing inaction in the face of need.

Answering the question, "How is racism operating here?" can be a powerful approach to identifying levers for potential intervention. Following is a thought exercise asking, "How is racism operating here?" with regard to police killings of unarmed Black and Brown men and women. Structures: the presence or absence of Citizen Review Boards to hold police departments accountable. Policies: reliance on the Grand Jury system to bring indictments against police officers. Practices: the over-policing of communities of color, which causes more "accidental" interaction. Norms: the Blue Code of Silence,

---

[69] Jones CP, Jones CY, Perry GS, Barclay G, Jones CA. Addressing the social determinants of children's health: a cliff analogy. J Health Care Poor Underserved. 2009;20(4)(suppl):1-12. 10.1353/hpu.0.0228 [PubMed] [CrossRef] [Google Scholar].

[70] The Urban Institute, 2018. Dr. Camara Jones Explains the Cliff of Good Health. Last accessed July 3, 2018 from https://www.youtube.com/watch?v=to7Yrl50iHI.

[71] TEDx Emory, 2014. Allegories on "Race" and Racism. Last accessed July 3, from https://www.youtube.com/watch?v=GNhcY6fTyBM.

[72] Jones CP. How understanding of racism can move public health to action: allegory highlights dual reality of privilege. Nations Health. 2016;46(1):3. [Google Scholar].

[73] Jones CP. Life on a conveyor belt: making a choice to take action on racism. Nations Health. 2016;46(8):3. [Google Scholar].

which constrains reporting of and punishment for police misconduct by other police officers. Values: the widely held societal view of Black men as inherently threatening, which leads to justifying the excessive use of force. Any one of these mechanisms could be a fruitful focus for action. Better yet, we could organize to address several of these mechanisms at the same time.

Organizing and Strategizing to Act

During my term as president of APHA, I proposed an Anti-Racism Collaborative with eight Collective Action Teams as a structure for harnessing the wisdom and energy of anti-racism activists across the country and around the world. I envisioned much of the early work of the Anti-Racism Collaborative happening within social networking spaces, with later work extending into local geographies. I imagined the Anti-Racism Collaborative as the structure that would survive my presidency as APHA members and many other partners in communities across the country engaged in a sustained National Campaign against Racism.

Because the APHA social networking infrastructure was insufficient for hosting the Anti-Racism Collaborative, it was never launched by APHA. However, both the Center for the Study of Racism, Social Justice, and Health at UCLA[74] and the Social Medicine Consortium[75] have since embraced the National Campaign Against Racism as part of their work and are using the Anti-Racism Collaborative as a framework. Following are the initial guiding questions for each of the eight proposed Collective Action Teams:

1. Communication and Dissemination: How can we support the naming of racism in all public and private spaces? What tools and strategies are needed to start community conversations on racism?
2. Education and Development: How can we support the training of public health professionals and researchers around issues of "race," racism, and anti-racism at educational institutions of all levels? How does an effective anti-racism curriculum look?

[74] Center for the Study of Racism, Social Justice, and Health. National Anti-Racism Collaborative. Last accessed July 3, 2018 from https://www.racialhealthequity.org/projects/.

[75] Social Medicine Consortium Campaign Against Racism. Last accessed July 3, 2018 from http://www.socialmedicineconsortium.org/campaign-against-racism/.

3. Global Matters: How can we use the International Convention on the Elimination of all forms of Racial Discrimination[76] to support anti-racism work in the United States? What can we learn from anti-racism work in other nations?
4. History: What is the history of successful anti-racism struggle in the United States and around the world? How can this history guide our anti-racism work today? How can we institutionalize attention to history in all decision-making processes?
5. Liaison and Partnership: What anti-racism work is happening at the community level? What anti-racism work is happening in other sectors? How can we create linkages?
6. Organizational Excellence: How do we answer the question "How is racism operating here?" in each of our settings? How do we examine structures, policies, practices, norms, and values?
7. Policy and Legislation: What are current policy and legislative strategies to address and dismantle racism? What new strategies should we propose?
8. Science and Publications: What research has been done to examine the impacts of racism on the health and well-being of the nation and world? What intervention strategies have been evaluated? What are next steps?

Through this Anti-Racism Collaborative, we aim to develop the science and practice of anti-racism, a science and practice complementary to, but quite distinct from, the efforts to document the adverse impacts of racism on the health and well-being of the nation and world. The science and practice of anti-racism will equip us to anticipate and respond to resistance and roadblocks that are thrown up as progress toward social equity is being made.

Barriers to Achieving Health Equity

Health equity has been defined as assurance of the conditions for optimal health for all people.[76] Achieving health equity requires valuing all individuals and populations equally, recognizing and rectifying historical injustices, and providing resources according to need.[76] Health disparities will be eliminated when health equity is achieved.[76]

---

[76] Jones CP. Systems of power, axes of inequity: parallels, intersections, braiding the strands. Med Care. 2014;52(10)(suppl 3):S71-S75. 10.1097/MLR.0000000000000216 10.1097/MLR.0000000000000216 [PubMed] [CrossRef] [CrossRef] [Google Scholar].

In addition to economic and political barriers, there are at least three major cultural barriers to achieving health equity in the United States. The first cultural barrier is our narrow focus on the individual, which makes the systems and structures that drive inequities either invisible or irrelevant.[65,77] Self-interest becomes narrowly defined, sometimes not even encompassing extended family. There is a limited sense of inter-dependence and a limited sense of collective efficacy.

The second cultural barrier is our a-historical stance. The present is viewed as disconnected from the past, and the current distribution of advantage and disadvantage is routinely viewed as happenstance despite the legacy of racism and its current manifestations.[78] Systems and structures are accepted as givens and treated as immutable.[79]

The third cultural barrier is our endorsement of the myth of meritocracy. This is the story-line that if you work hard in this country, you will make it. Certainly many (perhaps most) of the people who have made it in this country have worked hard. But there are many, many other people who are working just as hard or harder who will never make it in this country because, as research[80] has shown, an uneven playing field exists—one created and perpetuated by racism and other systems of structured inequity. Therefore, when we deny racism, we support the myth of meritocracy. And we can deny racism in at least two ways. We can say "I don't believe that racism exists." Or we can simply never say the word "racism." When we refuse to say the word "racism" in the context of its widespread denial, we are complicit with that denial.

---

[77] Gee GC, Ford CL. Structural racism and health inequities: old issues, new directions. Du Bois Rev. 2011;8(1):115-132. 10.1017/S1742058X11000130 [PMC free article] [PubMed] [CrossRef] [Google Scholar].

[78] Gamble VN. A legacy of distrust: african Americans and medical research. Am J Prev Med. 1993;9(6)(suppl):35-38. 10.1016/S0749-3797(18)30664-0 [PubMed] [CrossRef] [Google Scholar].

[79] Bonilla-Silva E. Rethinking racism: toward a structural interpretation. Am Sociol Rev. 1997;62(3):465-480. 10.2307/2657316 [CrossRef] [Google Scholar].

[80] Bertrand M, Mullainathan S. Are Emily and Greg more employable than Lakisha and Jamal? A field experiment on labor market discrimination. Am Econ Rev. 2004;94(4):991-1013. 10.1257/0002828042002561 [CrossRef] [Google Scholar].

One Last Thing: Treaty Obligations

The *International Convention on the Elimination of all Forms of Racial Discrimination*[81] is an international anti-racism treaty that was adopted by the United Nations General Assembly in 1965. It was signed by the United States in 1966. The US Senate ratified the treaty 28 years later in 1994. We have international treaty obligations to "do right" under this nine-page treaty.

One of our obligations is to submit periodic reports to the United Nations Committee on the Elimination of Racial Discrimination (UN CERD). The US Department of State submits reports roughly every six years, with the most recent report having been submitted in 2013.[82] The UN CERD reviewed this official US report, along with 82 parallel reports submitted by non-governmental organizations, and returned to the US government its Concluding Observations[82] in 2014. Among the Concerns and Recommendations expressed by the UN CERD were racial profiling (paras 8 and 18), residential segregation (para 13), the achievement gap in education (para 14), differential access to health care (para 15), and disproportionate incarceration (para 20).[82] In addition to recommendations in those areas, the UN CERD also "recommends that the State party adopt a national action plan to combat structural racial discrimination" (para 25).[82]

Conclusion

So here we are, recognizing the importance of launching a National Campaign Against Racism, and now also recognizing the international mandate for our government to do so. But a successful struggle against racism will require strong efforts and effective organization outside of the government. I hope that the nascent efforts to launch a National Campaign Against Racism that I made during my APHA presidency will bloom with the continued support and involvement of the Center for the Study of Racism, Social Justice, and Health at UCLA,74 the Social Medicine Consortium,[75] and others. I hope that you, the reader, will get involved by naming racism, asking "How is racism

---

[81] United Nations, Office of the High Commissioner for Human Rights International Convention on the Elimination of All Forms of Racial Discrimination. Last accessed July 3, 2018 from http://www.ohchr.org/EN/ProfessionalInterest/Pages/CERD.aspx.

[82] United Nations, Office of the High Commissioner for Human Rights Reports submitted by States parties under Article 9 of the Convention: Seventh to ninth periodic reports of States parties due in 2011. United States of America. CERD/C/ USA/7-9, 3 October 2013. Last accessed July 3, 2018 from http://tbinternet.ohchr.org/_layouts/treatybody external/Download. aspx?symbolno=CERD%2fC%2fUSA%2f7-9&Lang=en.

operating here?," and organizing and strategizing to act. We need all of us, with our wisdom, energy, passion, questions, and gifts. I am convinced that together, we can dismantle this system that structures opportunity and assigns value based on "race,"[65,66] and put in its place a system in which all people can know and develop to their full potentials. Let's go!

Achieving Health Equity: The Crisis in Flint, and What Should Be Done Next

Creating health equity is one of APHA's three guiding priorities, and achieving health equity is a goal that many of us share. But what is health equity? And how can a definition help guide our response to the public water supply in Flint, Michigan?

I published this definition of health equity in 2014: "Health equity is assurance of the conditions for optimal health for all people. Achieving health equity requires valuing all individuals and populations equally, recognizing and rectifying historical injustices and providing resources according to need. Health disparities will be eliminated when health equity is achieved."

Understanding the assurance aspect of health equity may have prevented the neglect, inattention and inaction in the face of need that are poisoning our children and elders in Flint.

What happened in Flint was the opposite of assurance of the conditions for optimal health for all people. Municipal decision-making power was wrested from the democratically elected City Council and mayor and turned over to an emergency manager appointed by the governor under a 2012 state law. The source of the public water supply was changed to the Flint River to save money. The corrosive water from the Flint River was not properly treated, causing lead to leach into the water from the city's aging pipes.

When the citizens of Flint noticed that their water was now smelly and discolored, causing rashes and hair loss, their complaints were ignored. When pediatricians in Flint documented increasing numbers of children with elevated blood lead levels, their alarm was disregarded. Even warnings from a scientist at the Environmental Protection Agency went unheeded. Only in October 2015, after 19 months, was the Flint water supply switched back to Lake Huron. But to this day, the water remains poisoned because it continues to flow through the city's badly-damaged pipes.

Achieving health equity requires valuing all individuals and populations equally. Michigan's emergency manager law must be repealed so that democracy can return to Flint. The people of Flint must have central seats and powerful voices at all decision-making tables to redress this dreadful wrong.

Achieving health equity requires recognizing and rectifying historical injustices. The people of Flint must have their medical, social and civic needs addressed for at least the next 70 years. Investment in the infrastructure and the people of Flint must reflect the profound injury sustained across generations.

Achieving health equity requires providing resources according to need. Not only clean bottled water now, or even vitamins, fresh fruits and vegetables, lead chelation and health monitoring over the next few years. The people of Flint need aggressive investment in their neighborhoods, assurance of excellent educational and employment opportunities, affirmative protection of their environment and the cherishing of their full humanity in all the ways that a government can cherish its people.

We who strive for health equity are incredulous at the poisoning of Flint. We are heartbroken. We are angry. We are strong, Flint on steel igniting.

Chairman SCOTT. Thank you very much, Ms. Jones. Dr. Wilson.

Statement of Valerie Rawlston Wilson, Ph.D., Director, Program on Race, Ethnicity, and the Economy, Economic Policy Institute, Silver Spring, MD

Ms. WILSON. Thank you, Chairman Scott, Ranking Member Foxx, and distinguished Members of this committee for the opportunity to testify.

I am going to discuss evidence to date of the racially disparate economic impact of COVID–19, the large and persistent inequities that were predictive of the needlessly heavy burden borne by communities of color, and solutions that will avoid prolonged effects of the pandemic, while helping to narrow persistent racial disparities in the economy.

There are three main groups of workers in the COVID–19 recession: One, those who have lost their jobs and face economic insecurity; two, those who are essential workers and face health insecurity; and, three, those who are able to continue working from the safety of their home.

Black, Latinx, Native American, and low-income workers are least likely to be in that last group to have few good options to protect both their help and economic well-being. The first group of workers in the COVID–19 recession includes the tens of millions who have lost jobs during the pandemic. The national unemployment rate declined to 13.3 percent in May, but this masks huge disparities by race.

As of May, the Hispanic unemployment rate was highest at 17.6 percent, followed by the Black unemployment rate at 16.8 percent, the Asian unemployment rate at 15 percent, and the White unemployment rate at 12.4 percent.

Black and Asian workers were the only racial or ethnic group whose unemployment rates did not improve over the last month. Still, the unemployment rate of all groups remains higher than the previous overall high of 10 percent in 2009.

The second group of workers in the COVID–19 recession are essential frontline workers. While in the near term these workers have been protected from job loss, they face greater likelihood of contracting COVID–19 while performing their jobs. Black workers are overrepresented among this group, making up about 1 in 9 workers overall but about 1 in 6 frontline industry workers. They are also more likely to be uninsured and less likely to have paid sick leave.

Prior economic insecurity magnifies the current economic damage to workers and their families but in the United States a long history of government-sanctioned racial exclusion, discrimination, oppression, and exploitation have inextricably linked economic inequality and race.

For example, the Black unemployment rate is typically double the White unemployment rate. This difference cannot be explained away by differences in educational attainment. Even for workers with college or advanced degrees, Black unemployment rate is significantly higher than the White unemployment rate, including at the record low rates of unemployment reached prior to the pandemic.

Among the employed, Black workers face significant pay challenges at all pay levels and at every level of education. Research has shown that these pay gaps have grown over the last several decades and have grown most among college-educated workers.

Significant racial gaps in employment opportunities and wage levels translate into lower income, less savings, and higher poverty rates among Black and other people of color relative to White households. These disparities have changed little over the last 50 years, making job losses during the pandemic especially devastating.

Such longstanding racially stratified social and economic structures require that we center the needs of those who face the greatest economic insecurity, thus improving the overall incepitus of any policy response, while narrowing the disparities by race, ethnicity, gender, and class.

Many of the policies needed to address the immediate needs raised by the pandemic are included in the HEROES Act and other legislation that has been introduced since. I will mention a few as I conclude.

First, a robust economic recovery is directly tied to our ability to secure the health and safety of communities and workplaces across the country. OSHA must exercise its authority to protect workers by issuing an enforceable emergency temporary standard that addresses the specific workplace health and safety risks associated with COVID–19. And workers who voice their concerns must be free of employer retaliation.

Second, we must develop a national system of testing and contact tracing with targeted efforts in underserved communities to provide employment, adequate access to testing, and other services necessary for healthy communities.

Third, since the loss of employment also means loss of health insurance, federally funded comprehensive health insurance with full coverage for COVID–19 testing and treatment, as well as paid sick leave and paid family leave, are essential to the economic and health securities.

Fourth, continuing crucial unemployment insurance provisions will help avoid far more serious and persistent damage to the economy. The expiration of expanded UI and other critical support provisions should be tied to automatic triggers that are measurable and reliable indicators of labor market recovery across all communities as opposed to arbitrary expiration dates.

This and more will be needed to rebuild a better-than-normal economy with more widely shared prosperity.

Thank you for your attention, and I will be happy to answer any questions.

Inequities Exposed: How COVID-19 Widened Racial Inequities in Education, Health, and the Workforce, Testimony before the U.S. House of Representatives, Committee on Education and Labor, Valerie Rawlston Wilson, Ph.D., Economist and Director of the Program on Race, Ethnicity and the Economy Economic Policy Institute, June 22, 2020

Chairman Scott, Ranking Member Foxx and distinguished members of the Committee on Education and Labor, thank you for the opportunity to testify today. My name is Valerie Wilson and I am a labor economist and director of the Program on Race, Ethnicity and the Economy (PREE) at the Economic Policy Institute (EPI) in Washington, DC. EPI is a nonprofit, nonpartisan think tank created in 1986 to include the needs of low-and middle-wage workers in economic policy discussions. EPI conducts research and analysis on the economic status of working America, proposes public policies that protect and improve the economic conditions of low-and middle-wage workers, and assesses policies with respect to how well they further those goals. In 2008, EPI launched PREE to provide a more focused and integrated approach to exploring and explaining how race, ethnicity, gender and class intersect to affect economic outcomes in the United States.

My testimony draws from a recent report I co-authored with my EPI colleague, Elise Gould, titled "Black Workers Face Two of the Most Lethal Pre-existing Conditions for COVID-19: Racism and Economic Inequality" as well as over 20 years of experience in conducting research on racial and economic inequality. I will discuss evidence to date of the racially disparate impact of COVID-19 on the economic and health insecurity of American workers, and the large and persistent inequities that were predictive of the needlessly heavy burden born by Black workers, in particular. I will conclude by recommending solutions for avoiding prolonged effects of the pandemic long after the immediate crisis is over while helping to narrow persistent racial disparities in the labor market.

"We're all in this together" has become a rallying cry during the coronavirus pandemic. While it is true that COVID-19 has affected everyone in some way, the magnitude and nature of the impact has been anything but universal. Evidence to date suggests that Black and Hispanic workers face much more economic and health insecurity from COVID-19 than white workers.

Although the current strain of the coronavirus is one that humans have never experienced before, the disparate racial impact of the virus is deeply rooted in historic and ongoing social and economic injustices. Persistent racial disparities in health status, access to health care, wealth, employment, wages, housing, income, and poverty all contribute to greater susceptibility to the virus—both economically and physically.

There are three main groups of workers in the COVID-19 economy: those who have lost their jobs and face economic insecurity, those who are classified as essential workers and face health insecurity as a result, and those who are able to continue working from the safety of their homes. Unfortunately, Black, Latinx, Native American, and low-income workers are least likely to be in that last group, leaving them with few good options to protect both their health and economic well-being.

While each of the groups I just named share similar experiences that make them more susceptible to death and economic devastation as a result of COVID-19, my research is primarily centered on Black workers, as my testimony will reflect. I want to make clear that this in no way minimizes the challenges and struggles of other racial and ethnic groups. Rather, history has shown that progress made toward equal rights and equal opportunity for Black Americans has also expanded opportunity and opened doors for all marginalized communities.

Spiking Unemployment Rates

Black workers have suffered record numbers of job losses during the COVID-19 recession, along with the ensuing related economic devastation. They also are disproportionately found among the essential workers in the economy today---continuing to go to their workplaces, risking their health and that of their families because they are unable to sustain adequate social distance from their co-workers and customers.

The latest national data available to assess the impact of job losses is the Current Population Survey for May 2020. After falling by 22.1 million between February (the official start of the COVID-19 recession) and April, payroll employment rose by 2.5 million in May. This is likely due to the fact that 31 states started lifting stay-at-home orders, or easing restrictions, within the reference period. In spite of this modest improvement, jobs losses since

February still total 19.6 million, and payroll employment is currently 13% below its February level[83].

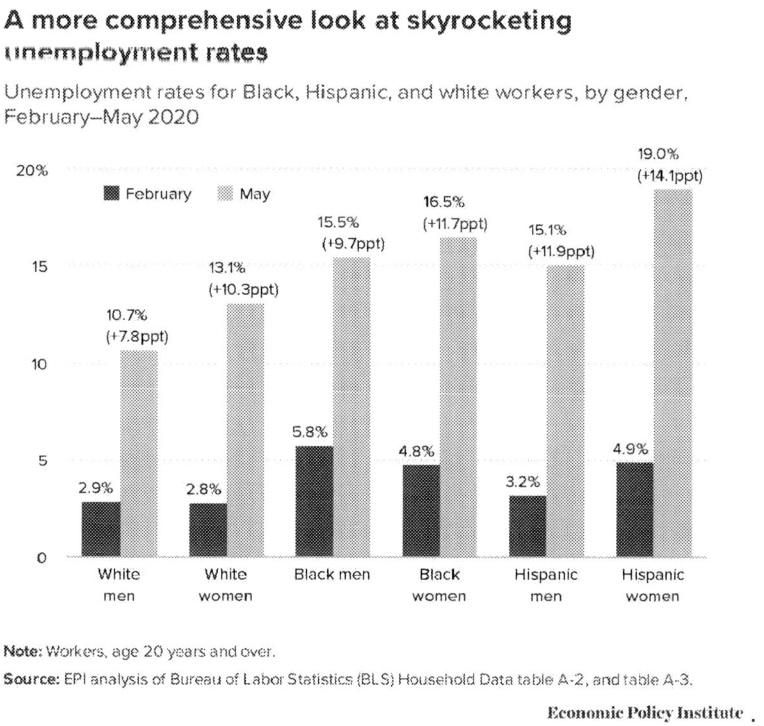

Figure A.

The national unemployment rate declined to 13.3% in May (down from 14.7% in April), but this rate is still up nearly 10 percentage points since February[84]. This overall rate of unemployment also masks huge disparities by race and gender. As of May 2020, the Hispanic unemployment rate was highest at 17.6%, followed by the black unemployment rate at 16.8%, the

---

[83] Economic Policy Institute (EPI). 2020. *Economic Indicators: Jobs and Unemployment*. Last updated June 5, 2020.

[84] The Bureau of Labor Statistics has published guidance acknowledging that official unemployment rate likely understates the extent of job loss and economic pain. Based on this guidance, an "adjusted" unemployment rate of 19.7% in May can be calculated, which includes those who are officially unemployed, the misclassified (the excess number of those who reported that they were employed but not at work for other reasons), and those who had been employed but left the labor force when the virus hit but would otherwise have been counted as unemployed if they were actively seeking work.

Asian unemployment rate at 15.0% and the white unemployment rate at 12.4%. Women have been hit especially hard during this recession. As shown in Figure A, across all racial and ethnic groups reported by BLS, women's unemployment rates were higher than those of men. In May, Hispanic women had the highest unemployment rate at 19.0%, followed by black women at 16.5% and white women at 13.1%. It is also important to note that the unemployment rate of women and men in all racial and ethnic groups remains higher than the previous overall high of the Great Recession - 10.0% in 2009.

Falling Employment-to-Population Ratios

The unemployment rate is a commonly used measure of labor market slack. One limitation, however, is that it relies on would-be workers to either be on temporary layoff or have looked for work in the last four weeks to be counted as unemployed. In this economy, with the health requirements to stay home and with sectors being completely decimated, it is likely that many would-be workers are not actively looking for work and therefore would not be counted in the official unemployment rate. Given these unique circumstances, policymakers should consider additional measures for evaluating labor market slack, including the employment-to-population ratio (EPOP), or the share of the population with a job.

Employment losses were stark across racial lines between February and May. Hispanic and Black workers saw greater losses in employment than white workers (12.3, 9.8 and 7.9 percentage-point losses, respectively). Approximately one in six black workers and nearly one in five Hispanic workers lost their jobs between February and May.

Black-Owned Businesses Are More Concentrated in Industries Hardest Hit by COVID-19

Providing support to small businesses has been a top priority of legislation designed to lessen the harmful economic effects of the pandemic. While less than 10% (9.4%) of all U.S. business owners are Black, Black-owned businesses are more concentrated in industries hardest hit by reduced demand during the pandemic. According to a recent analysis of government data, more than 40% of Black business owners reported they were not working in April, compared to only 17% of white business owners[85] Given that the overwhelming majority of Black-owned businesses (95.8%) are self-employed individuals and the sole employee of the business, this represents yet another dimension of disproportionate job losses experienced by Black workers during the pandemic.

According to the Bureau of Labor Statistics, the industries with the largest total job losses in April, and therefore most immediately affected by reduced demand, were in accommodation and food services, retail, and health care and social assistance. 27.6% of black-owned businesses are in those three sectors, compared with 19.7% of white-owned businesses. The large number of job losses in these industries is due in part to the fact that they employ many more people than other industries.

Another way of measuring the impact of losses is to consider job losses as a percentage of the previous month's payroll employment. This will capture industries that include many more small employers that experienced a sharp decline in employment. Based on this measure, the largest percentage losses in payroll employment were in arts, entertainment and recreation; accommodation and food services; and other services. These three industries account for almost a third of black-owned businesses (32.3%), but just 18.8% of white-owned businesses.

Black Workers Are More Likely to Be in Front-Line Jobs That Are Categorized as 'Essential' - Forcing Them to Risk Their Own and Their Families' Health to Earn a Living

Not only are black workers losing their jobs at an incredible pace, those who aren't losing their jobs are more likely to be found on the front lines of the economy in essential jobs. Rho, Brown, and Fremstad (2020) conducted an important and useful study of six sectors of the economy that are considered essential and in which most workers are on the front lines of the COVID-19 labor market[86]. Their results show that black workers make up a disproportionate share of these essential workers who are forced to put

---

[85] Fairlie, Robert. 2020. "The Impact of Covid-19 on Small Business Owners: Evidence of Early-Stage Losses from the April 2020 Current Population Survey." Stanford Institute for Economic Policy Research Working Paper No. 20-022, May 2020. https://siepr.stanford.edu/sites/default/files/publications/20-022.pdf.

[86] Rho, Hye Jin, Haley Brown, and Shawn Fremstad. 2020. *A Basic Demographic Profile of Workers in Frontline Industries.* Center for Economic and Policy Research, April 2020.

themselves and their family members at additional risk of contracting and spreading COVID-19 in order to put food on the table.

Black workers make up about one in nine workers overall; they represent 11.9% of the workforce. However, black workers make up about one in six of all front-line-industry workers. They are disproportionately represented in employment in grocery, convenience, and drug stores (14.2%); public transit (26.0%); trucking, warehouse, and postal service (18.2%); health care (17.5%); and child care and social services (19.3%). While, in the near term, this protects them from job loss, it exposes them to greater likelihood of contracting COVID-19 while performing their jobs.

Underlying Economic Factors Exacerbate the Effect of the COVID-19 Recession on Black Workers and Their Families

Black workers and their families were economically insecure before the pandemic tore through the United States. The pandemic and related job losses have been especially devastating for black households because they have historically suffered from higher unemployment rates, lower wages, lower incomes, and much less savings to fall back on, as well as significantly higher poverty rates than their white counterparts. This prior insecurity has magnified the current economic damage to these workers and their families.

Higher Unemployment Rates

Historically, black workers have faced unemployment rates twice as high as those of their white counterparts. When the overall unemployment rate averaged 3.7% in 2019, the white non-Hispanic unemployment rate was 3.0% and the black unemployment rate was twice as high, coming in at an average of 6.1% over the year. This difference cannot be explained away by differences in educational attainment. Figure B shows that at every level of education, the black unemployment rate is significantly higher than the white unemployment rate, even for those workers with college or advanced degrees.

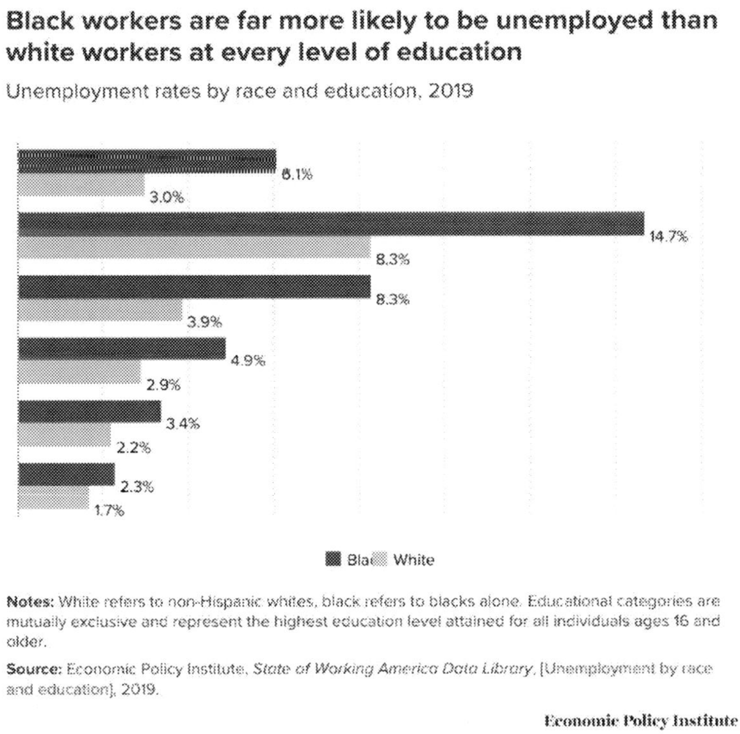

Figure B.

Significant Wage Gaps

Among the employed, black workers face significant pay penalties. No matter how you cut the data, black workers face significant pay gaps in the labor market, and research has shown that these pay gaps have grown since 2000 and in the decades before[87]. On average, black workers are paid 73 cents on the white dollar. We know from a host of economic research that a person's wages are not a simple function of individual ability. Instead, workers' ability to claim higher wages rests on a host of social, political, and institutional factors outside their control[88]. Because of historic and current privilege in the

---

[87] Gould, Elise. 2020. *State of Working America Wages 2019: A Story of Slow, Uneven, and Unequal Wage Growth Over the Last 40 Years*. Economic Policy Institute, February 2020. Wilson, Valerie, and William M. Rodgers III. 2016. *Black–White Wage Gaps Expand with Rising Wage Inequality*. Economic Policy Institute, September 2016.

[88] Manning, Alan. 2003. *Monopsony in Motion: Imperfect Competition in Labor Markets*. Princeton, N.J.: Princeton Univ. Press.

labor market[89], white men enjoy exceptionally high wages. Therefore, the gap between white men and black men is particularly stark. Black men are paid only 71 cents on the white male dollar. Black women, who face both gender and race discrimination, are paid even less—64 cents on the white male dollar.

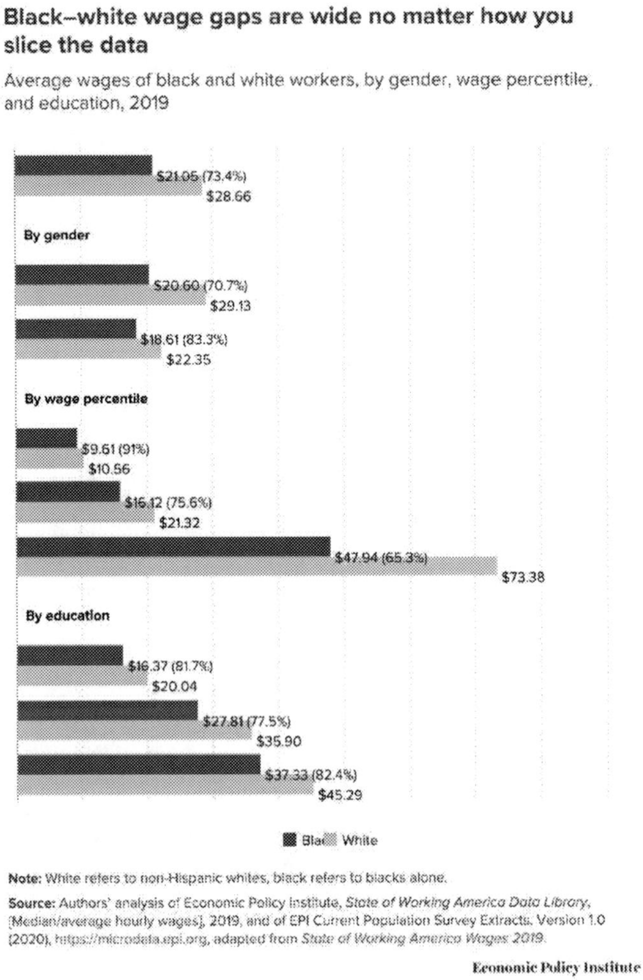

Figure C.

Card, David, Francesco Devicienti, and Agata Maida. 2011. *Rent-Sharing, Hold-Up, and Wages: Evidence from Matched Panel Data*. IZA (Institute for the Study of Labor) Discussion Paper no. 6086, October 2011.

[89] National Advisory Commission on Civil Disorders. 2016. *The Kerner Report*. Princeton, N.J.: Princeton Univ. Press.

As Figure C shows, black--white wage gaps persist across the wage distribution as well as at different levels of education in the pre-pandemic economy. The black–white wage gap is smallest at the bottom of the wage distribution, where a wage floor---otherwise known as the minimum wage---keeps the lowest-wage black workers from being paid even lower wages. The largest black–white wage gaps are found at the top of the wage distribution and are explained in part by occupational segregation---the underrepresentation of black workers in the highest-wage professions and overrepresentation in lower-wage professions – and the pulling away of the top more generally.

Similarly, across various levels of education, a significant black–white wage gap remains. Black workers can't simply educate their way out of the gap. Even black workers with an advanced degree experience a significant wage gap compared with their white counterparts.

Benefits Gaps

Not only is black worker pay significantly less than that of their white counterparts, but their benefits are as well. Along with health insurance, two benefits are acutely important at this particular time: paid sick days and the ability to work from home. These two workplace benefits help shield workers from economic losses by allowing them to take paid time off to care for themselves or family members and allowing them to stay out of harm's way and still earn a paycheck by working from home.

Given what we know about job losses and essential workers, it's not surprising that significantly fewer black workers can telework than white workers. Fewer than one in five black workers in the pre-pandemic economy were able to work from home, compared to 30% of white workers. Black workers were also less likely than white workers to have paid sick leave (58.7% vs. 66.6%). This inability to keep their jobs and stay safe makes it even harder for black workers to maintain economic and health security during this difficult time.

Lower Household Incomes and Higher Poverty Rates

Significant gaps in both employment opportunities and wage levels translate into lower incomes and higher poverty rates in the pre-pandemic economy, as shown in Figure D.

In 2018, median household income for white households was 70% higher than for black households ($70,642 vs. $41,692). On top of decades of preferential wealth accumulation for white families versus black families[90], lower incomes are one of the reasons that black families haven't been able to build up savings to weather storms such as the one our country finds itself in today.

At the bottom of the income distribution, the black poverty rate is two-and-a-half times the white poverty rate. One in five black people in this country live below the poverty line---that's below about $26,000 annual income for a family of four. Job loss for those living at such low incomes is absolutely shattering.

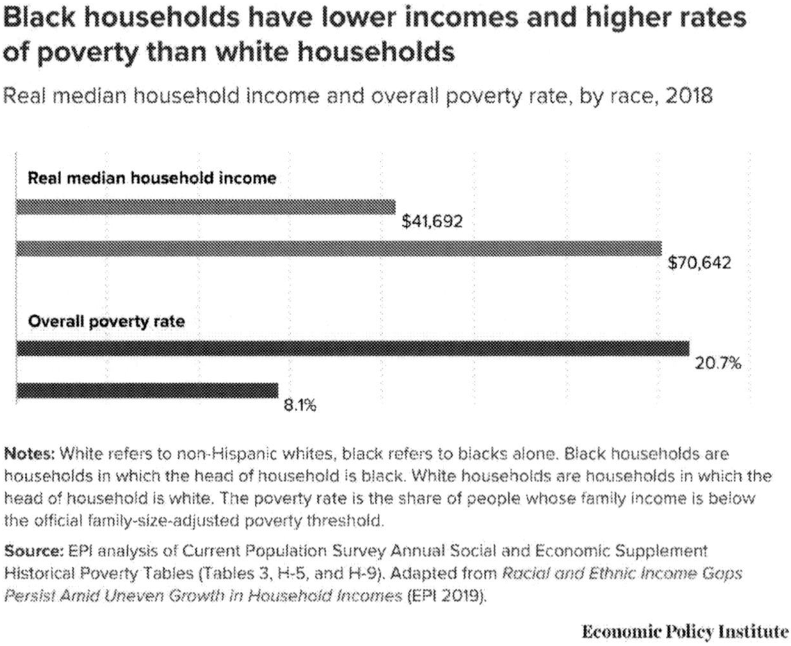

Figure D.

---

[90] Rothstein, Richard. 2017. *The Color of Law: A Forgotten History of How Our Government Segregated America.* New York: Liveright.

Darity Jr., William, Darrick Hamilton, Mark Paul, Alan Aja, Anne Price, Antonio Moore, and Caterina Chiopris. 2018. *What We Get Wrong About Closing the Racial Wealth Gap.* Samuel DuBois Cook Center on Social Equity and Insight Center for Community Economic Development, April 2018.

Less Cash Reserves

On top of lower wages and incomes and higher poverty rates, black families have significantly less access to liquid assets than white families. It's been long established that black families face a large and persistent wealth gap. Economist William Darity Jr. and others have shown that no matter how it's measured, the racial wealth gap is large and persistent[91]. To weather a financial loss, families often must dip into their liquid assets to pay for their living expenses. If they lose their job or experience a serious health shock, their only hope of making ends meet and continuing to pay their rent or mortgage and put food on the table is to rely on their savings. Wealth is often tied up in housing assets, particularly for black families, and therefore is inaccessible when dealing with sudden and large losses in income.

Figure E below displays one component of wealth, the total value of all transaction accounts for black and white families. Transaction accounts include checking or savings accounts, cash, prepaid cards, and directly held stocks, bonds, and mutual funds. These are assets that can quickly be used to purchase goods and services, unlike less liquid sources of wealth like homeownership or assets in 401(k)s. Overall, white families hold, on average, more than five times as much liquid assets as black families do, $49,529 versus $8,762. This makes white families far more capable of weathering the storm of COVID-19, whether it be job loss or another financial hit.

The attainment of higher education does not bridge this divide. This gap remains large when we compare white and black families whose heads of household have the same level of education. In fact, the absolute gap in liquid assets between black and white families is far larger among those *with* a college degree or more versus those with less than a college degree. White families headed by a college-degree holder have nearly five times the access to money in transaction accounts as similarly degreed black families. The gap persists whether the black family owns a home or not. The gaps in liquid assets differ by what sector the family head works in, but no matter how the data are cut, white families have far more access to liquid wealth.

It is not surprising then that research by Ganong et al. finds that income volatility has a much greater impact on the spending of black households than white households. They report that these differences in ability to smooth consumption leads to a 50% reduction in black families' ability to spend on

---

[91] Darity Jr., William, Darrick Hamilton, Mark Paul, Alan Aja, Anne Price, Antonio Moore, and Caterina Chiopris. 2018. *What We Get Wrong About Closing the Racial Wealth Gap*. Samuel DuBois Cook Center on Social Equity and Insight Center for Community Economic Development, April 2018.

essential goods and services as compared with white families when they are faced with similar income losses[92].

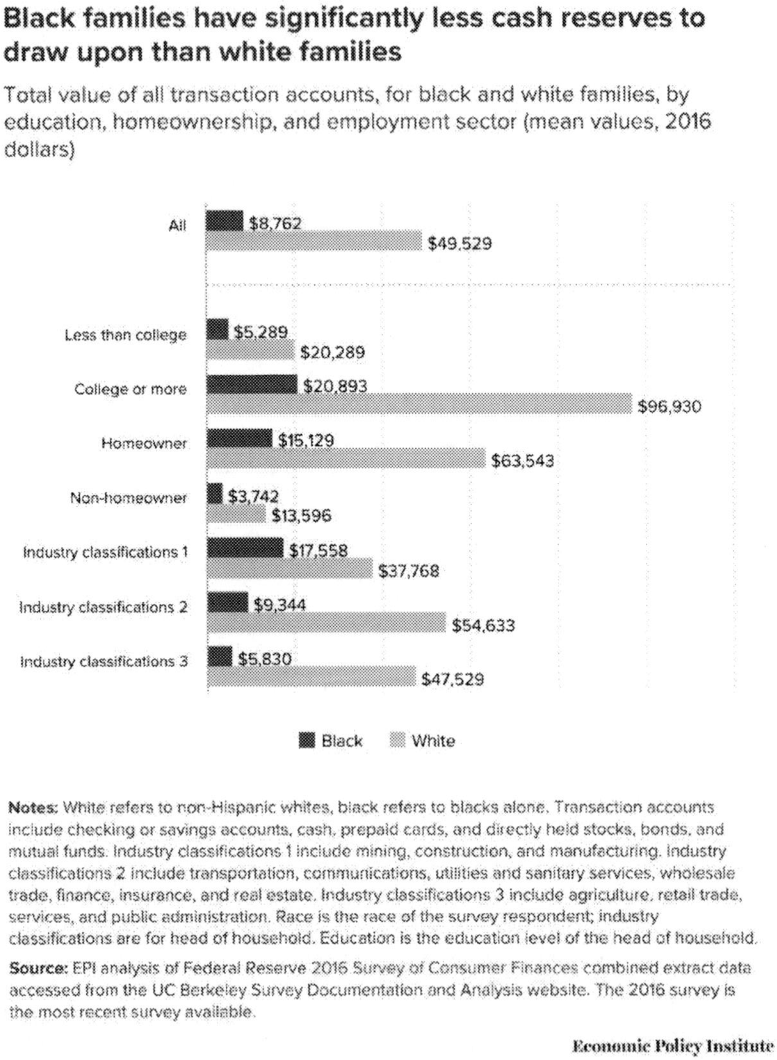

Figure E.

---

[92] Ganong, Peter, Damon Jones, Pascal Noel, Diana Farrell, Fiona Greig, and Chris Wheat. 2020. "Wealth, Race, and Consumption Smoothing of Typical Income Shock." University of Chicago, Becker Friedman Institute for Economics Working Paper no. 2020–49. http://dx.doi.org/10.2139/ssrn.3583707.

Policy Divides: The Fallacy of Race-Neutral Policy Is Further Exposed by COVID-19

The once-in-a-generation challenges presented by the coronavirus have required leaders in government and private industry to respond quickly in order to minimize the threat to public health as well as the economic harm. Consistent with the scale of the crisis, many of the actions taken have been widespread in terms of the number of people helped, and the magnitude of the interventions has been unprecedented. Still, even such a broad-reaching response can yield uneven results for many of the reasons I have laid out in my testimony.

The first step, therefore, is for policymakers to recognize that no policy is truly race-neutral. Even when a policy is race neutral on its face, the implementation of that policy often is not because it is being applied to racially stratified social and economic structures. All policy essentially shapes how the nation's income and wealth will flow, and as a result, how access and opportunity will flow. Equitably shared opportunity and prosperity starts with a careful assessment of social and economic conditions across all affected communities prior to policy development, but it doesn't end there. You must also closely monitor whether that policy is having the intended effects post-implementation.

By centering the needs of those who face the greatest economic harm, the overall effectiveness of any policy response is likely improved as it serves to minimize disparities by race, ethnicity, gender and class. This requires the consistent collection of reliable data on economic and social conditions by race, ethnicity and gender, among other important demographic categories, that can be used to inform and improve upon the federal response.

Second, a robust economic recovery is directly tied to our ability to secure the health and safety of communities and workplaces across the country. A recent Washington Post--Ipsos poll found that nearly 60% of workers who are working outside of their homes were concerned about the possibility of exposure to COVID-19 while on the job[93]. For Black and Hispanic workers, the concern was even greater (68% and 72%, respectively)[94]. Even more troubling are the findings of a National Employment Law Project (NELP) survey indicating that Black workers were more than twice as likely as white

[93] Craig, Tim, and Emily Guskin. 2020. "A Majority of Americans Going to Work Fear Exposing Their Household to the Coronavirus." *Washington Post*, May 15, 2020.

[94] Ibid.

workers to have seen possible retaliation by their employer when concerns were voiced about safety at work[95]. OSHA must step in and exercise its authority to protect these workers by issuing an emergency temporary standard that addresses the specific workplace health and safety risks associated with COVID-19, as directed in the COVID-19 Every Worker Protection Act included in the Heroes Act (H.R. 6800) which also prohibits employers from retaliating against workers who voice their concerns.

The pandemic has exposed clear shortcomings in our public health infrastructure, but these are also opportunities for creating good jobs that meet many of our most immediate public health needs. Provisions in the Heroes Act to expand testing capacity in underserved communities, and develop a national system of testing and contact tracing seize upon these opportunities.

Targeting these efforts in high unemployment and high poverty communities serves the dual purpose of providing employment as well as adequate access to testing and other critical health services necessary for healthy communities.

Third, provisions in the CARES Act that temporarily expanded eligibility and enhanced Unemployment Insurance (UI) benefits have been a critical lifeline for unemployed workers. Money spent on continuing crucial unemployment insurance provisions will help avoid far more serious and persistent damage to the economy resulting from prolonged high unemployment. According to an economic impact analysis by economist Mark Zandi, under the *Heroes Act,* spending on UI benefits has one of the largest bang for the buck effects on the national economy – a dollar provided in UI benefits will generate $1.46 in GDP one year later[96]. This bang for the buck is second only to spending on food assistance, estimated at $1.67[97].

The expiration of expanded UI and other critical support provisions, however, should be tied to automatic triggers that are measurable and reliable indicators of labor market strength.

Decisions about the best and most accurate measure of the nation's progress toward recovery should also take account of disparate rates of recovery by race, ethnicity and gender.

Prior to the pandemic, workers of color were already more likely to be uninsured than white workers. But, the loss of employment means loss of health insurance for many more workers. As of May 9, an estimated 16.2

---

[95] Tung, Irene, and Laura Padin. 2020. *Silenced About COVID-19 in the Workplace*. National Employment Law Project, June 2020.

[96] Zandi, Mark. 2020. "HEROES Act to the Rescue." Moody's Analytics, June 2020.

[97] Ibid.

million workers likely lost their employer provided health insurance as a result of unemployment[98]. The *Heroes Act* and the recently introduced *Medicare Crisis Program Act* help to address the need for comprehensive health insurance with full coverage for COVID-19 testing & treatment, as well as paid sick leave and paid family leave.

This includes federal funding for extensions of Medicare and Medicaid to all those suffering job losses during the pandemic period, federal funding to pay for all of COBRA coverage so that workers who are laid off or furloughed may continue their employer-provided coverage, and eliminating exemptions in the *Family First Coronavirus Response Act* that left millions of private sector workers without access to vital paid sick days[99].

Finally, worker power is about expanding the set of options available to workers so that they are in a position to exert their right to earn a decent living by having a job with good pay and benefits (including equal pay and equal opportunity), decent hours, and safe working conditions. At a minimum, that means creating a stronger, more stable labor market through consistent full employment, and strengthening worker voice and enforcement of existing protections.

The policies mentioned above contribute to these aims in light of the current situation and immediate needs raised by the pandemic. But in looking toward rebuilding a "better than normal" economy with more widely shared prosperity, the following are pillars for establishing a solid foundation:

- The Fed should prioritize low unemployment
- As a complement to monetary policy, fiscal policy should prioritize investments that create jobs in high unemployment and high poverty communities
- Strengthen the rights of workers to organize, join unions and collectively bargain, as directed in the *PRO Act*, passed by the House of Representatives in February 2020
- Strengthen enforcement of anti-discrimination laws and policies through banning the use of forced arbitration agreements as a condition of employment, prohibiting employers from asking

98 Zipperer, Ben and Josh Bivens. 2020. "16.2 million workers have likely lost employer-provided health insurance since the coronavirus shock began." *Working Economics Blog* (Economic Policy Institute), May 14, 2020.

99 Gould, Elise, and Heidi Shierholz. 2020. "Senate Coronavirus Bill Is Crucial—But It's a Fraction of What's Needed." *Working Economics Blog* (Economic Policy Institute), March 18, 2020.

potential employees about pay history, and requiring employers to provide greater pay transparency

- Update existing labor standards so that they continue to provide a robust floor for job quality, including increases to the minimum wage, as provided in the Raise the Wage Act of 2019, preventing further erosion of the federal overtime salary threshold, and elimination of exclusions to basic labor standards that are historically rooted in racial exclusion and discrimination

Conclusion

The global impact of COVID-19, both in lives lost and economic devastation, is likely to leave a lasting mark for years to come. The best path forward includes making sure that we use the painful lessons learned during this crisis to better prepare ourselves for the next one. The disparate racial impact of COVID-19 should come as no surprise given the ongoing legacy of racism that continues to produce unequal outcomes affecting nearly every aspect of life in the United States. If we are to protect Black, Latinx, and Native American communities from suffering under the same needlessly heavy burden during the next economic or public health crisis that they are suffering under now, we must work diligently to address long-standing underlying racial disparities in economic and health outcomes.

Chairman SCOTT. Thank you very much. Mr. Roy.

Statement of Avik Roy, Co-Founder and President, the Foundation for Research on Equal Opportunity, Austin, TX

Mr. ROY. Chairman Scott, Ranking Member Foxx, Members of the committee, thanks for inviting me here today.

The Foundation For Research on Equal Opportunity, or FREOPP for short, is a nonpartisan think tank that focuses exclusively on ideas that can improve the lives of Americans on the bottom half of the economic ladder.

I welcome the opportunity to discuss our work on how COVID–19 economic lockdowns have widened racial inequities in education, health, and the workforce.

My written statement contains a more detailed discussion of our findings. In my oral remarks, I will focus on three topics. First, I will discuss how economic lockdowns imposed by States and localities, have disproportionately harmed minority employment and minority-owned businesses.

Second, I will touch on how school closures disproportionately harm minority students and their parents.

Third, I will discuss COVID–19 mortality by race and ethnicity and how States' failure to protect nursing homes has harmed vulnerable seniors of all races.

In late 2019, Black unemployment reached its lowest rate in history, 5.4 percent. Today the Black unemployment rate is 16.8 percent. Hispanic unemployment rate reached 3.9 percent in late 2019. Today it is 17.6 percent.

In my written testimony I detail how disparities between White and non-White unemployment rates also reached their lowest levels in history prior to the pandemic, but the economic lockdowns have brought those disparities back to levels seen a decade ago.

Compared to Whites and Asians, Blacks and Latinos are less likely to work in white-collar occupations where working from home is feasible. Instead they are seeing their jobs and hours slashed. Hourly wage work is down 50 percent on average and even more in places with the most stringent lockdowns.

But Black-owned businesses have also been hit far harder than White-owned businesses. As Ms. Foxx noted it is estimated that Black-owned businesses have experienced losses of 41 percent between February and April versus 32 percent for Hispanic-owned businesses and 17 percent for White-owned companies. Put simply, racial and ethnic disparities are worse when the economy is worse and especially during the government-mandated shutdowns of the economy that we are experiencing today.

As you noted, Mr. Chairman, this brings school closures disproportionately harmed children from lower-income families. That is because wealthy families are far better equipped than low-income ones to provide their kids with opportunities to learn outside of school. Poor children are also less likely to be able to take advantage of virtual learning because they often lack high-speed internet access.

Nearly 30 million low-income children receive free or reducedprice lunch through the National School Lunch Program. School closures also affect parents, especially single parents, who are unable to work if work means leaving their children at home, unattended.

The good news is that it is possible to safely reopen schools as a forthcoming paper from FREOPP will show. Other countries have done it while protecting public health because children are at extremely low risk of death or severe illness from COVID–19.

One rising concern is how COVID–19 is affecting different racial and ethnic populations overall. The latest data from CDC indicates that Blacks represent a greater share of COVID deaths then they do of the general population, even when adjusted for the fact COVID–19 is more prevalent in cities where minorities live disproportionately.

Mortality rates are also higher in Native American communities especially in Arizona and new New Mexico. What may be surprising is that Whites are also dying of COVID at higher-than-predict rates. On the other hand, Hispanics and Asians represent a lower share of COVID deaths than would be implied by their geographically adjusted share of the U.S. population.

The likely reason for these differences is that morbidity and mortality from COVID–19 is most common among the elderly. Eightyone percent of all COVID deaths in the U.S. have occurred in people aged 65 or older, and Whites are the oldest racial group in the U.S. with a median age of 44. Asians have a median age of 37, Blacks, 34, Hispanics, 30. Hence, we should expect to see higher fatality rates in Whites relative Asians and Hispanics due to their age, and indeed we do. On the other hand, African Americans are relatively young but we are still seeing higher mortality among Blacks.

Some of you are familiar with our research on the tragedy taking place in our nursing homes and assisted living facilities. Zero point six percent of Americans live in long-term care facilities, and yet within this 0.6 percent of the population lies 43 percent of all U.S. deaths from the novel coronavirus, 43 percent.

Communal nursing homes or residential facilities for medically vulnerable seniors who have challenges with activities of daily living such as taking a shower or getting dressed. Nursing home residents are disproportionately poor, non-White, and enrolled in Medicaid. The nursing home tragedy has a bronze lining, we could say, because it means that the risk of death for COVID–19 for the rest of the population is considerably lower than we may have thought.

We can use that information to reopen the economy safely and reduce the harm that we are imposing on hundreds of millions of Americans of all colors.

Thank you.

Testimony before the United States Congress, House Education & Labor Committee, Inequities Exposed, How COVID-19 Economic Lockdowns Widened Racial Inequities in Education, Health, and the Workforce, AVIK S. A. ROY, President, the Foundation for Research on Equal Opportunity, June 22, 2020

The Foundation for Research on Equal Opportunity (FREOPP) is a non-partisan, non-profit, 501(c)(3) organization dedicated to expanding economic opportunity to those who least have it. FREOPP does not take institutional positions on any issues. The views expressed in this testimony are solely those of the author.

Introduction

Broadly speaking, there are two key sources of racial disparities with regards to the COVID-19 pandemic. The first is the differential impact of the coronavirus disease on different ethnic and racial populations. The second is the differential economic and health impact of governments' *policy response* to the pandemic: specifically, the mandatory school and business closures that have dramatically increased unemployment.

Racial Disparities in Covid-19 Mortality Are Mixed

On a population level, both whites' and blacks' shares of COVID-19 deaths are higher than one would expect if deaths were evenly racially distributed. On the other hand, Asians' and Hispanics' shares of COVID-19 deaths are lower than one would expect. For example, whites represent 53 percent of all COVID-19 deaths, but only 42 percent of a geographically adjusted population. 23 percent of fatalities are among blacks, while blacks represent 18 percent of the geographically adjusted population.[100]

---

[100] Centers for Disease Control and Prevention. Weekly Updates by Select Demographic and Geographic Characteristics. https://www.cdc.gov/nchs/nvss/vsrr/covid_weekly/; accessed June 3, 2020.

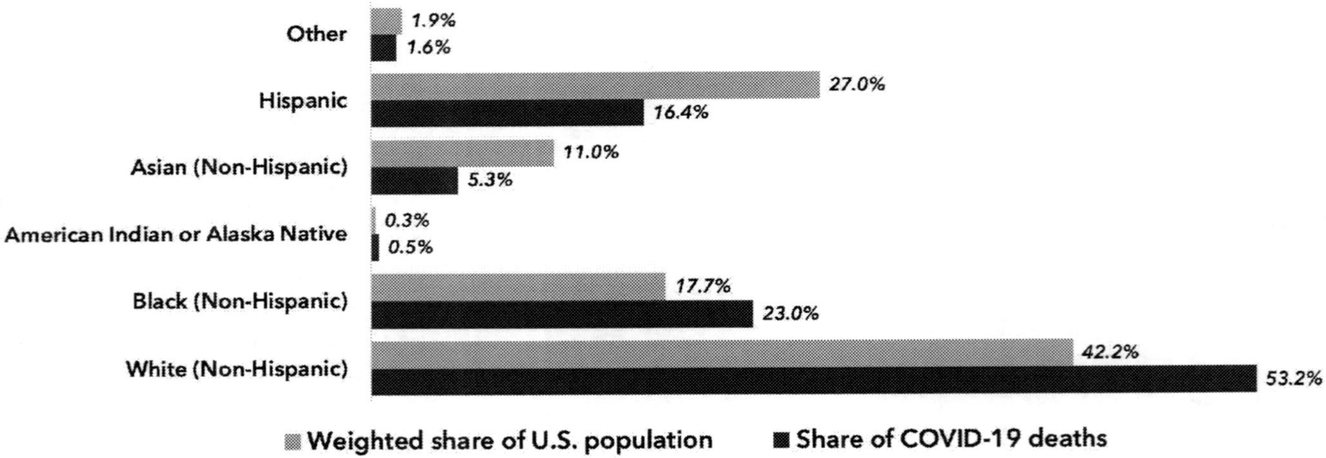

Racial and ethnic distribution of COVID-19 fatalities is mixed. Whites and blacks are both overrepresented in their share of COVID-19 deaths, relative to their geographically adjusted share of the U.S. population. In contrast, Asians and Hispanics are underrepresented in their share of COVID-19 fatalities.
(Source: Centers for Disease Control and Prevention).

Figure 1. CDC: Share of COVID-19 Fatalities by Race & Ethnicity, vs. Geographically Weighted Share of U.S. Population.

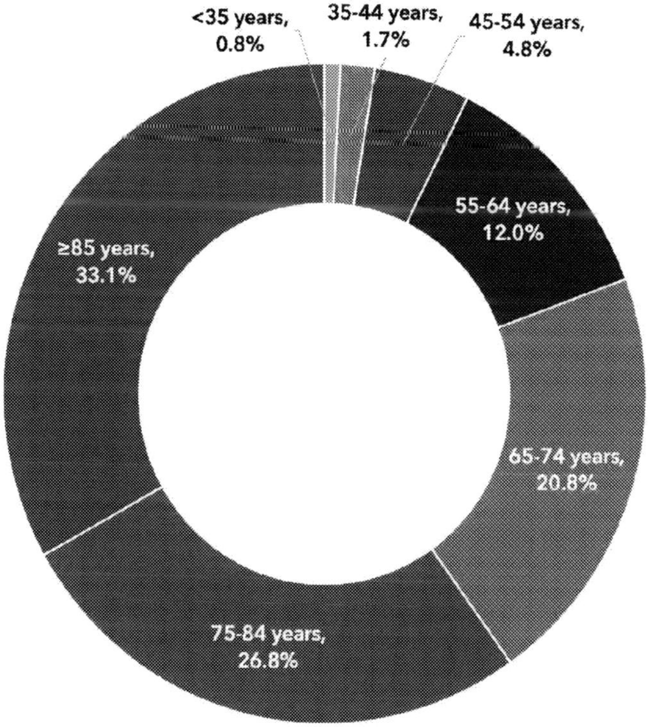

COVID-19 mortality is heavily skewed toward those over 65. 81 percent of all deaths from COVID-19 have occurred among those 65 and older. Those under 35 years of age represent 0.8 percent of deaths.
(Sources: CDC, FREOPP analysis).

Figure 2. Share of COVID-19 Fatalities by Age Bracket.

(The Centers for Disease Control and Prevention geographically adjust racial and ethnic groups' shares of the U.S. population in order to take into account the fact that COVID-19 fatalities are concentrated in cities, where a higher percentage of the population is non-white).

The most probable explanation for most of these differences is related to age. Serious illness and death from COVID-19 are highly concentrated among the elderly. 81 percent of all U.S. COVID-19 deaths have taken place among those aged 65 or older; by contrast, only 0.8 percent of U.S. COVID-19 deaths have taken place among U.S. residents younger than 35. This is important to account for, because while the median age of white Americans is 44, for

Asians it is 37, and for Hispanics it is 30. In other words, the disparity in share of deaths relative to whites, Hispanics, and Asians may turn out to be mostly explained by age differences.

The same explanation does not fully apply to blacks. The median age of African-Americans is 34–somewhere in between that of Hispanics and Asians–but blacks suffer from a disproportionate share of COVID-19 mortality.

Further data from the CDC, breaking out racial and ethnic shares by age bracket, should help us learn more about these differences.

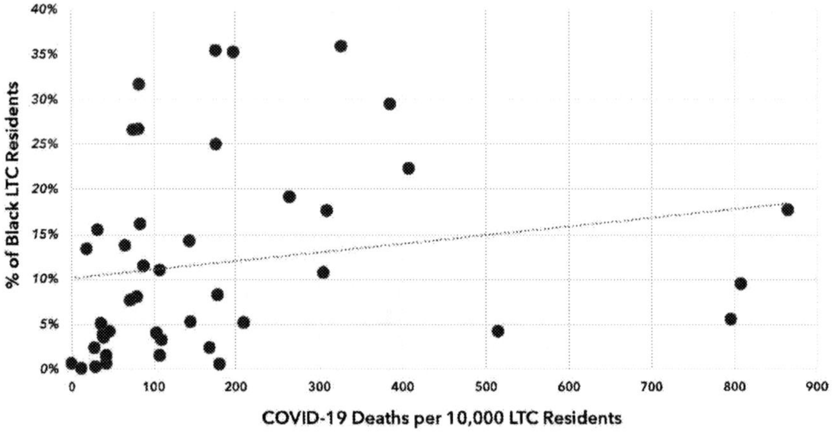

At the state level, there is no correlation between African-American race and mortality in nursing homes and assisted living facilities. States with high black population shares in nursing homes and assisted living facilities were not correlated to those with high levels of black mortality. The r2—the probability of a linear correlation—was only 3.5%.
(Sources: Brown University, FREOPP analysis).

Figure 3. No Correlation Between Long-Term Care COVID-19 Fatality Rates and State-Level African-American LTC Resident Share.

LTC Facilities: 42% of COVID-19 Deaths, but 0.6% of the Population

Another source of racial disparities in COVID-19 health outcomes may come from nursing homes and assisted living facilities. Nursing homes, in particular, serve disproportionately poor individuals, with a large number of Medicaid enrollees. Vulnerable seniors residing in such long-term care facilities represent 42 percent of U.S. COVID-19 fatalities, while residents of such facilities only account for 0.6 percent of the total U.S. population.[1]

In part this is due to disastrous decisions taken by some state governors to force nursing homes to accept COVID-infected patients who had been discharged from a hospital, including New York, New Jersey, and Michigan.[2] This catastrophic policy helped spread COVID-19 in long-term care facilities, leading to needless deaths and additional hospitalizations that we then asked our health care personnel to take on.

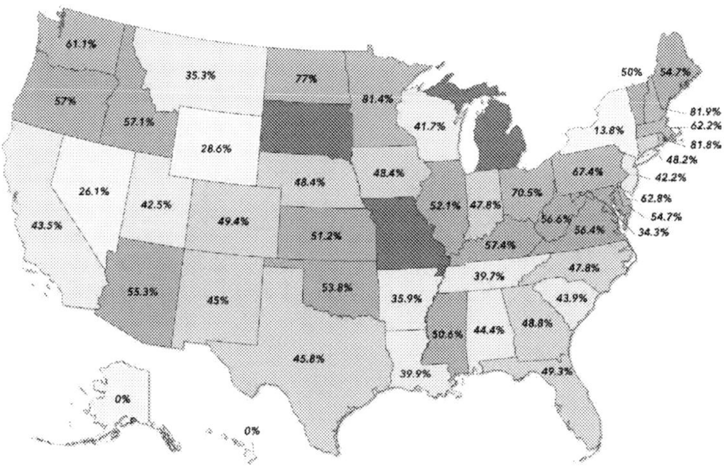

0.6% of Americans live in long-term care facilities that account for 42% of all COVID-19 deaths. In some states, this tragedy was compounded by policies that forced nursing homes to accept patients infected with the novel coronavirus SARS-CoV-2.
(Source: G. Girvan and A. Roy, FREOPP.org).

Figure 4. COVID-19 Deaths in Long-Term Care Facilities as a Share of Total COVID-19 Deaths (as of June 1, 2020).

[1] G. Girvan and A. Roy, Nursing Homes & Assisted Living Facilities Account for 42% of COVID-19 Deaths. The Foundation for Research on Equal Opportunity. 2020 May 7: https://freopp.org/the-covid-19-nursing-home-crisis-by-the-numbers-3a47433c3f70?source=collection_home---1------0; accessed June 3, 2020.

[2] A. Roy, The Most Important Coronavirus Statistic: 42% of U.S. Deaths Are From 0.6% Of The Population. *Forbes*. 2020 May 26: https://www.forbes.com/sites/theapothecary/2020/05/26/nursing-homes-assisted-living-facilities-0-6-of-the-u-s-population-43-of-u-s-covid-19-deaths/#232a01f074cd; accessed June 3, 2020.

In order to examine racial disparities in COVID-19 deaths in nursing homes, I and my FREOPP colleagues Gregg Girvan and Mark Dornauer looked at state-level long-term care facility mortality rates, and compared them to the percentage of blacks living in long-term care facilities, and also the relationship between nursing home mortality and Medicaid eligibility.

There was no correlation between black race and state-level long-term care fatalities. The r^2–the probability of a linear relationship between high black population and high longterm care death rates–was only 3.5 percent. Similarly, there was no correlation between states with high Medicaid enrollment and those with high COVID-19 mortality rates in their assisted living facilities; the probability of a linear correlation was only 2.3 percent.

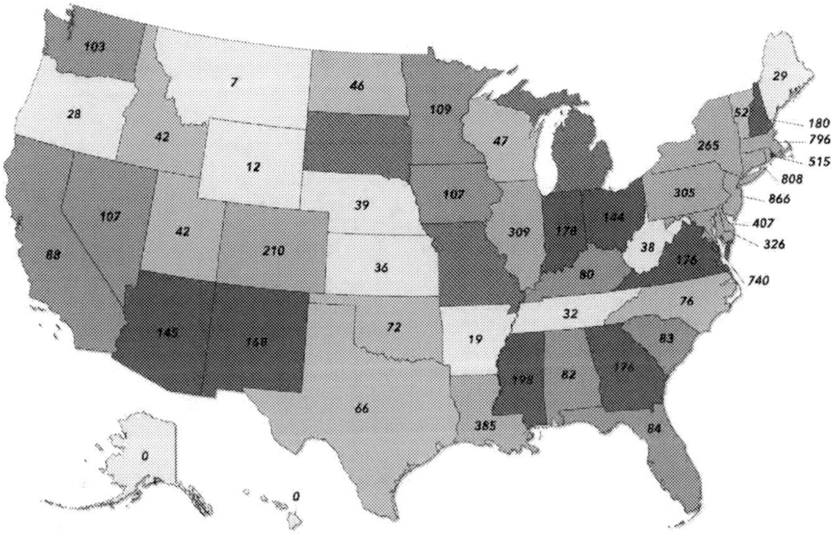

COVID-19 deaths in nursing home and assisted living facilities are concentrated in the Northeast. In New Jersey, nearly one in ten long-term care facility residents have died of the novel coronavirus.
(Source: G. Girvan and A. Roy, FREOPP.org).

Figure 5. COVID-19 Deaths in Long-Term Care Facilities per 10,000 Long-Term Care Residents (as of June 1, 2020).

This finding was surprising, because we would expect to see that nursing homes with a high volume of low-income patients would fare worse under COVID-19. We aim to investigate this question further, at the county level, in order to determine if the correlations are stronger within states.

One explanation for this finding could be that nursing home and assisted living facility residents are, as a group, vulnerable to the coronavirus pandemic, and that therefore African-American resident share is less impactful on overall long-term care mortality statistics.

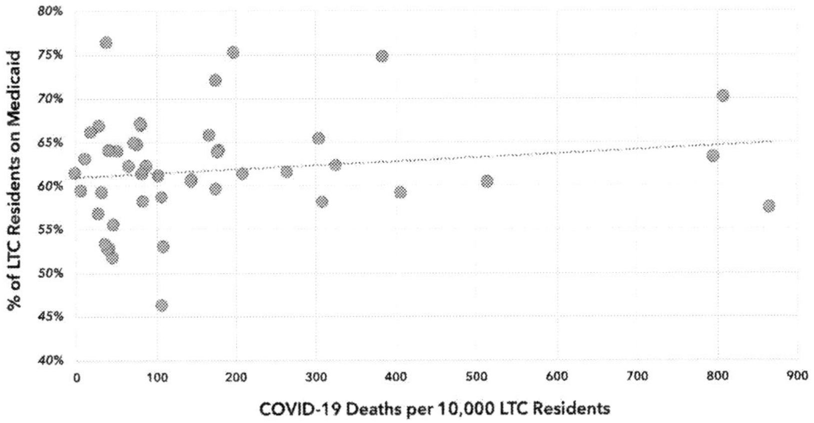

At the state level, there is no correlation between enrollment in Medicaid and COVID-19 mortality in nursing homes and assisted living facilities. States with high Medicaid enrollment in nursing homes and assisted living facilities were not correlated to those with high levels of COVID-19 mortality. The r2—the probability of a linear correlation—was only 2.3%.
(Sources: Brown University, FREOPP analysis).

Figure 6. No Correlation Between Long-Term Care COVID-19 Fatality Rates and State-Level Medicaid LTC Resident Share.

Economic Lockdowns Have Harmed Minorities

Prior to the pandemic, unemployment rates for all racial and ethnic groups reached record lows. In August of last year, black unemployment fell to 5.4 percent: the lowest rate ever recorded. The following month, Hispanic unemployment hit a record low of 3.9 percent. And in June of that year, Asian unemployment hit a record low of 2.1 percent.

The economic lockdowns have destroyed those gains. Today, the unemployment rates for whites, blacks, Hispanics, and Asians are 12.4, 16.8, 17.6, and 15.0 percent, respectively.

Notably, last fall, the disparities between white and black unemployment, and between white and Hispanic unemployment, also fell to record lows. Over the last five decades, the association is clear: a strong economy most benefits minorities, and a worsening economy most harms them.

For most of the 21st century, Asian-Americans have enjoyed a lower unemployment rate than whites. But since the lockdown, Asians have faced record unemployment.

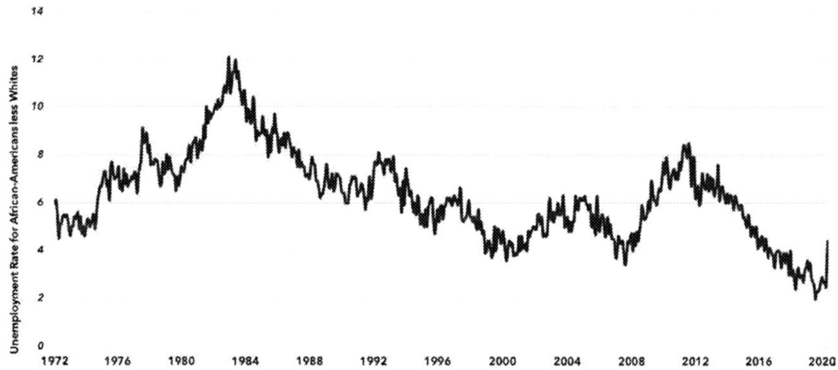

Figure 7a. Black Unemployment Rate Minus White Unemployment Rate, 1972–2020.

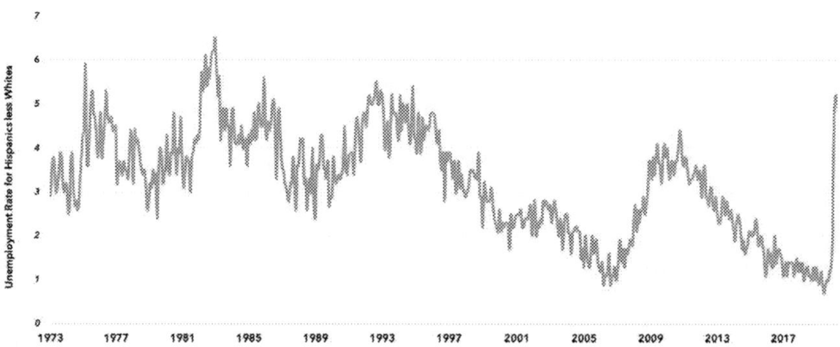

Lockdowns have widened the disparities between white vs. black and Hispanic unemployment. Hourly-wage workers, who are disproportionately non-white, were most harmed by economic lockdowns that forced small businesses to close. (Source: Bureau of Labor Statistics; Graphics: A. Roy/FREOPP).

Figure 7b. Hispanic Unemployment Rate Minus White Unemployment Rate, 1973–2020.

These disparities are in part caused by the fact that racial and ethnic minorities make up a disproportionate share of hourly wage earners; 25% are Hispanic, 15% are black, and 5% are Asian. In contrast, for the overall workforce, 17% are Hispanic, 13% are black, and 6% are Asian.[3] [4]

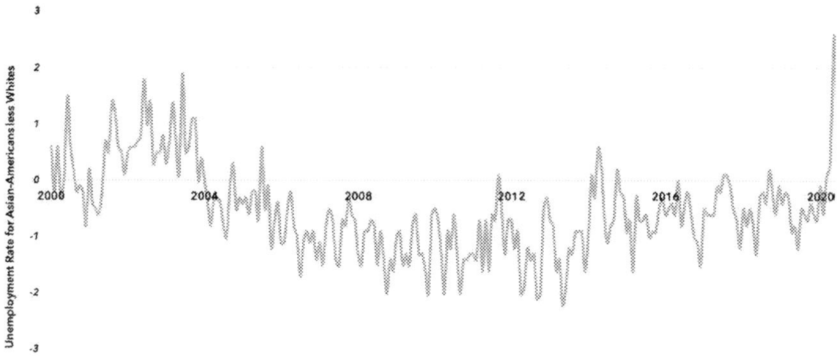

The disparity between the Asian and white unemployment rates has reached a record high. For most of the 21st century, Asians have enjoyed a lower unemployment rate than whites. That changed during the COVID-19 pandemic.
(Source: Bureau of Labor Statistics; Graphics: A. Roy / FREOPP).

Figure 8. Asian Unemployment Rate Minus White Unemployment Rate, 2000–2020.

While many white workers are in white collar professions in which remote work is possible, blacks and Hispanics often work in hourly-wage jobs where in-person attendance is essential. Researchers at the University of Chicago's Rustandy Center for Social Sector Innovation have found that hourly-wage workers have seen their hours cut by 50 percent in states that have continued to lock down their economies. In states that have reopened their economies, by contrast, hourly work is recovering.[5] Racial and ethnic minorities, unfortunately, live in many states where lockdowns have continued.

---

[3] M. Ross and N. Bateman, Meet the Low-Wage Workforce. The Brookings Institution. 2019 Nov: https://www.brookings.edu/wp-content/uploads/2019/11/201911_Brookings-Metro_low-wage-workforce_Ross-Bateman.pdf; accessed June 9, 2020.

[4] Bureau of Labor Statistics, Labor force characteristics by race and ethnicity, 2018. 2019 Oct: https://www.bls.gov/opub/reports/race-and-ethnicity/2018/home.htm; accessed June 9, 2020.

[5] A. Bartik, M. Bertrand, F. Lin, J. Rothstein, & M. Unrath, Week 7 and 8: Labor Market Impacts of COVID-19 on Businesses: Update with Homebase Data through May 23. University of Chicago: https://www.chicagobooth.edu/research/rustandy/blog/2020/week-7-labor-market-impacts-from-covid19; accessed June 3, 2020.

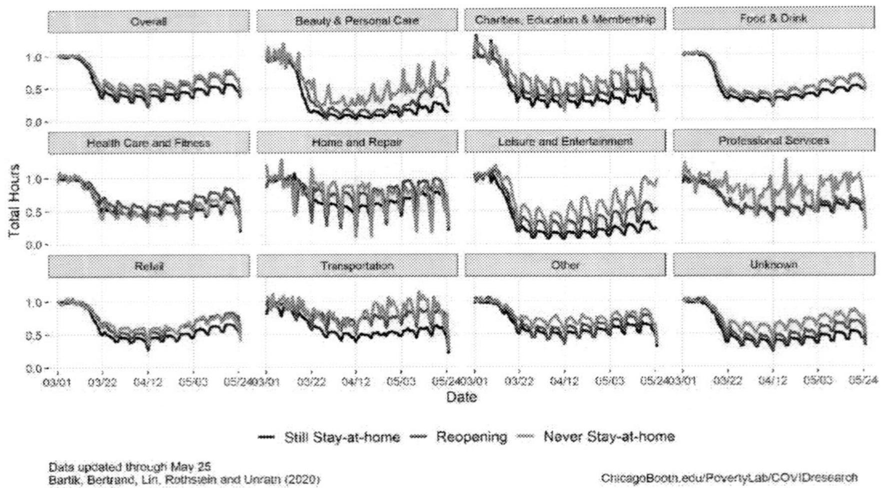

Racial and ethnic minorities have been disproportionately harmed by economic lockdowns. Blue-shaded curves represent work reductions for those in lockdown states; red and orange curves represent reopening and open states, respectively. (Source: A. Bartik et al., University of Chicago).

Figure 9. Hourly Wage Reductions by Industry and Economic Lockdown Policies.

Small businesses have also been hammered by the policy response to COVID-19. A new working paper by Robert Fairlie of the University of California, Santa Cruz, estimates that "the number of active business owners in the United States plummeted by 3.3 million or 22 percent over the crucial two-month window from February to April 2020." Black-owned businesses fell 41 percent, Hispanic-owned businesses 32, percent, and Asian-owned businesses 26 percent. Immigrant-owned businesses dropped by 36 percent.[1]

Economic Lockdowns Impact Public Health

Economic lockdowns do not merely have a financial impact on racial and ethnic minorities who lose their jobs or have their hours cut. Economic dislocation also worsens health outcomes in myriad ways, whether by deaths of despair, inability to access or afford physicians, or disruption in health insurance coverage.

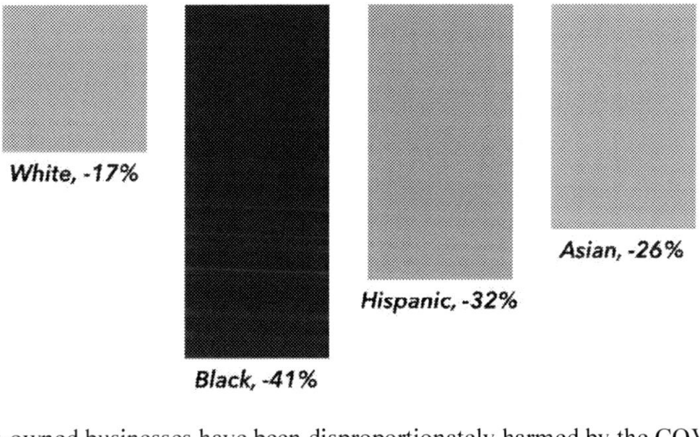

Minority-owned businesses have been disproportionately harmed by the COVID-19 lockdowns. In particular, businesses owned by African-Americans have seen substantial losses.
(Source: R. Fairlie, National Bureau of Economic Research).

Figure 10. Reduction in Small Business Activity, by Ownership, February–April 2020.

[1] R. Fairlie, The Impact of Covid-19 on Small Business Owners: Evidence of Early-Stage Losses from the April 2020 Current Population Survey. National Bureau of Economic Research. 2020 Jun: https://www.nber.org/papers/w27309.pdf; accessed June 9, 2020.

Hence, it is essential and urgent that states and localities do everything possible to responsibly reopen their economies.[2]

Lockdowns Widen Educational Disparities

A necessary step to allow the nation to go back to work is to reopen K-12 schools, preschools, and child care centers. Beyond their mission of providing learning opportunities, K-12 schools, preschools and child care centers allow their parents to work.

Reopening the nation's education and child care programs is also important to ensure that American children continue to learn, and particularly to help children from lower-income families who often have fewer opportunities to learn outside of school. Researchers have found that differences in outside of school learning opportunities contribute to the academic achievement gap between rich and poor children.[3] The current situation is likely exacerbating this opportunity gap, particularly since poor children are less likely to have internet access at home.[4]

Widespread school closures have other negative consequences for the nation's children, and particularly those from low-socioeconomic backgrounds. For example, American schools provide food to more than half of the school aged population. Nearly 30 million children receive free or reduced-price lunch through the National School Lunch Program. (While most children will not go hungry without free or subsidized meals, children from the poorest families could be affected by the lack of regular access to these services.) Schools and child care centers also play a critical role in state child welfare systems and supporting children's health.

---

[2] L. Chen, B. Kocher, A. Roy, & B. Wachter, A New Strategy for Bringing People Back to Work During COVID-19. The Foundation for Research on Equal Opportunity. 2020 Apr 14: https://freopp.org/a-new-strategy-for-bringing-people-back-to-work-during-covid-19-a912247f1ab5; accessed June 3, 2020.

[3] J. McCombs et al., Making Summer Count. RAND Corporation: 2011: https://www.rand.org/content/dam/rand/pubs/monographs/2011/RAND_MG1120.pdf; accessed June 19, 2020.

[4] National Center for Education Statistics. Table 218.70: Number and percentage distribution of 5- to 17-year-old students, by home internet access, poverty status, and locale: 2017. https://nces.ed.gov/programs/digest/d18/tables/dt18_218.70.asp?current=yes; accessed June 19, 2020.

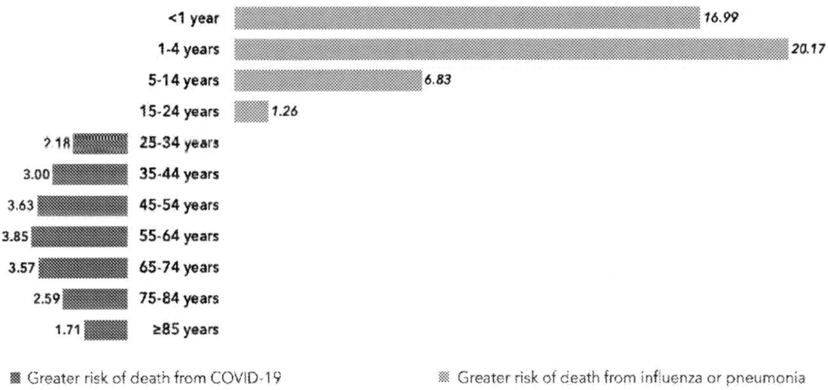

Those under aged 25 are at the lowest risk of death from COVID-19. A clear pattern emerges from what we know, in which those under aged 25 are at the lowest risk of death from COVID-19, relative to influenza or pneumonia.
(Source: A. Roy, FREOPP.org).

Figure 11. Estimated Relative Risk of Death from Influenza vs. COVID-19. (Assuming 150,000 Total COVID-19 Deaths).

In addition, other student populations, including children with special needs and English language learners, suffer from school closures and the lack of specialized instruction outside of school.

Beyond these direct educational effects, widespread closures are having significant impacts on school systems. For example, dozens of private schools are closing due to the loss of revenue and families' inability to afford tuition after the pandemic. These closures may increase the burdens on traditional public school systems as private school students enroll in public schools. (A coalition of organizations that support choice in education estimated that public schooling costs will increase by $15 billion if 20 percent of private school students enroll in public schools.) Moreover, many states are projecting revenue shortfalls due to the pandemic and economic downturn.

American policymakers and school leaders have an opportunity to study and learn from international examples, particularly as several nations have already reopened and are operating their school systems. Schools in other countries are applying a range of tactics to protect public health, such as modifying school calendars and schedules, promoting social distancing, keeping windows open to improve ventilation, and checking students' temperatures.

The good news is that children and young adults are at extremely low risk of dying of COVID-19, as detailed in Figures 2 and 11.

State and local policymakers must quickly work to develop two distinct but aligned education systems: (1) a physical school system for in-person learning consistent with public health guidance, and (2) a virtual or distance learning that supports all children's options to learn at-home or outside of the traditional school setting. A forthcoming paper from the Foundation for Research on Equal Opportunity, co-authored by Dan Lips, Preston Cooper, and Avik Roy, among others, will explore these questions in detail.

https://www.wsj.com/articles/reopening-the-u-s-economy-even-if-the-pandemic-endures-11587740529

THE SATURDAY ESSAY

Reopening the U.S. Economy Even if the Pandemic Endures

It's not true that the only way to improve public health is by shutting down the economy and the only way to improve the economy is by sacrificing public health.

By Avik Roy
April 24, 2020 11:02 am ET

As the Covid-19 shutdown enters its second month, policy makers and commentators have emphasized that we're not yet out of the woods. Deaths and hospitalizations are continuing to rise, albeit more slowly than before. The flattening curves have encouraged some people to talk about reopening the economy, and others to rise in protest against ongoing restrictions, but most Americans remain cautious. We've been willing to endure the staggering economic damage because we're convinced that it's necessary for public health—and that the lockdowns won't last too long.

Indeed, a kind of conventional wisdom has emerged among public health officials and policy experts. We're told that life will go back to normal just as soon as we've reached a series of public health milestones: near-universal testing, the development of effective treatments, the emergence of herd immunity and, ultimately, approval of a vaccine.

But this conventional wisdom has a critical flaw. We've taken for granted that our ingenuity can solve almost any problem. But what if, in this case, it can't? What if we can't scale up coronavirus testing as quickly as we need to? What if it takes us six or 12 months, instead of three, to identify an effective treatment for Covid-19? What if those who recover from the disease fail to gain immunity and are therefore susceptible to getting reinfected? And what if it takes us years to develop a vaccine?

Once we start asking these questions, a terrible truth becomes clear: The scenario in which we meet all the public health milestones, and then return to our regularly scheduled economic programming, is highly optimistic. A more realistic scenario is that we will fail to reach one or more of the milestones. If that happens, do we prolong the economic shutdown for six months or longer? Do we impose a series of on-and-off stay-at-home orders that could go on for years?

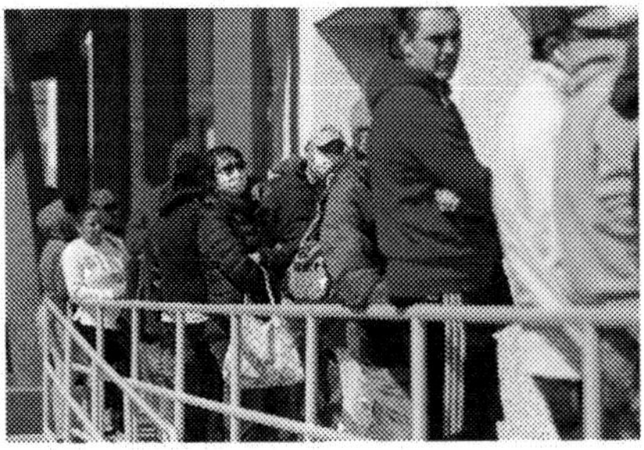

People wait on line for help with unemployment benefits in Las Vegas, March 17.
PHOTO: JOHN LOCHER/ASSOCIATED PRESS

The damage from a prolonged economic shutdown is difficult to contemplate. Tens of millions of Americans have already lost their jobs. Countless small businesses have closed—many for good. Two months ago, 20% unemployment seemed unthinkable. Two months from now, 20% unemployment might seem like the good old days.

Americans are optimistic by nature, and the public is right to hope for the best. But policy makers must prepare for the worst. And that means we must consider options for reopening the economy in a world in which we have not completely controlled the Covid-19 pandemic.

Cash Crunch

Some businesses can last longer than others without money coming in.

Days of bills a typical business could pay from its cash balance, without inflows.

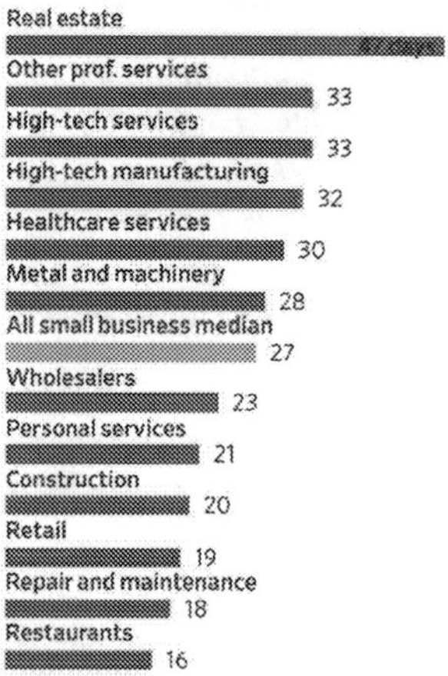

Note: Estimates cash buffer days for a business by computing the ratio of its average daily cash balance to its average daily cash outflows
Source: J.P. Morgan Chase Institute

Time is of the essence. Every week matters. A 2016 study by the JPMorgan Chase Institute found that the median small business holds just 27 days' worth of cash in reserve. For restaurants, retail shops and construction firms, the buffer is even thinner.

The good news is that there are ways to get America back to work while we control the spread of SARS-CoV-2, the novel coronavirus that causes Covid-19. We need to escape from the false dichotomy which insists that the only way to improve public health is by shutting down the economy and the only way to improve the economy is by sacrificing public health.

How hard will it be to achieve the conventional public health milestones? Harder than it looks.

Consider testing. There are two principal kinds of tests: those that detect if a patient has developed antibodies to the virus and those that measure viral RNA levels in a patient's nasal secretions. Both have significant technical limitations. Antibody tests often suffer from accuracy problems and can fail to detect an active infection. Viral RNA tests are highly accurate, but most versions must be administered in a clinical setting like a doctor's office or a hospital, making them difficult to scale up.

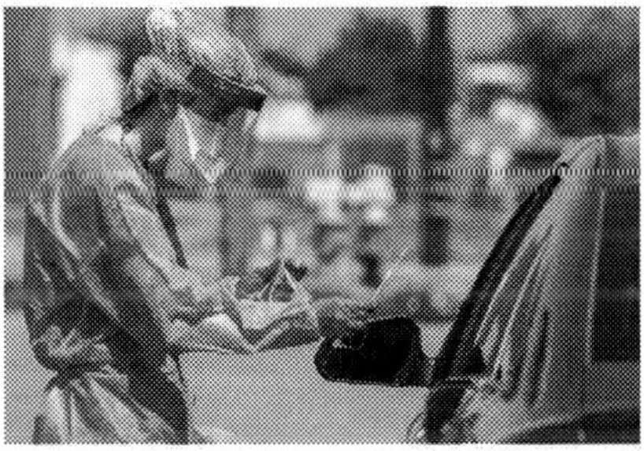

A drive-through testing site for Covid-19 in Santa Ana, Calif., April 21.
PHOTO: LEONARD ORTIZ/ORANGE COUNTY REGISTER/ZUMA PRESS

To match the modestly high level of coronavirus testing for which South Korea has been praised, the U.S. would need to administer 7 million tests a week. We'll be fortunate if we reach half that number by September.

There's good reason to be confident that we'll eventually find an effective treatment against Covid-19. According to the Milken Institute, there are more than 150 drugs being actively tested against the disease. Some of them are likely to work. But when will we know?

The first drug to get some positive buzz was hydroxychloroquine, but in the latest published clinical trial, more patients on the drug died relative to those taking a placebo. Over the past week, remdesivir, a failed Ebola drug, was generating excitement because of positive anecdotal data out of Chicago. On Thursday, however, the World Health Organization inadvertently posted preliminary findings from a larger, randomized study, in which patients on remdesivir actually fared worse than those on a placebo.

Gilead Sciences, remdesivir's manufacturer, insists that "trends in the data suggest a potential benefit." But if future studies produce similarly negative results, we may be waiting several more months to find an effective therapy.

We'd be less dependent on treatments if more Americans could become immune to SARS-CoV-2. Most people who recover from Covid-19 develop antibodies to the virus; epidemiologists hope that these antibodies will confer protection from

MORE SATURDAY ESSAYS

- What Makes a Summer Movie? June 26, 2020
- Bolton Savages Trump's China Policy June 17, 2020
- It's Not Too Late to Save the 2020 Election June 12, 2020
- The Long Reach of Racism in the U.S. June 5, 2020

future reinfection. If more people can gain immunity, the virus will have a harder time spreading, eventually dying out.

But what if antibodies don't confer immunity or if the protection doesn't last very long? This is a very real possibility, based on our experience with other coronaviruses, like the original SARS from 2003 and even the common cold.

The same issue may make it hard for biotech companies to develop an effective vaccine. Vaccines are hard enough to develop in normal circumstances. After decades of trying, we still don't have vaccines against HIV or hepatitis C. The fastest vaccine ever developed for a viral infection is the Ebola vaccine, which took five years. And yet many commentators talk about developing a SARS-CoV-2 vaccine within 12 to 18 months, as if it were a piece of cake.

For these reasons, it's essential for the U.S. to move rapidly away from an unrealistic checklist of public health milestones and to focus instead on the specific biology of the new coronavirus and specific evidence of how Covid-19 spreads. If we do that, we'll find that we have better options to reopen the economy than we once believed.

The starting point for a more realistic strategy is the key fact that not everyone is equally susceptible to hospitalization and death due to Covid-19. There is considerable evidence that younger people largely avoid the worst health outcomes. According to the Centers for Disease Control and Prevention, those over the age of 65 are 22 times more likely to die of Covid-19 than those under 55.

That is not to say that younger people are invulnerable. We've seen significant numbers of deaths among those of middle age and above who suffer from chronic diseases like high blood pressure, cardiovascular disease, diabetes and kidney failure. Men appear to have nearly twice the fatality rate of women.

Age Discrimination

The novel coronavirus has hit the elderly the hardest.

U.S. deaths involving Covid-19, by age group

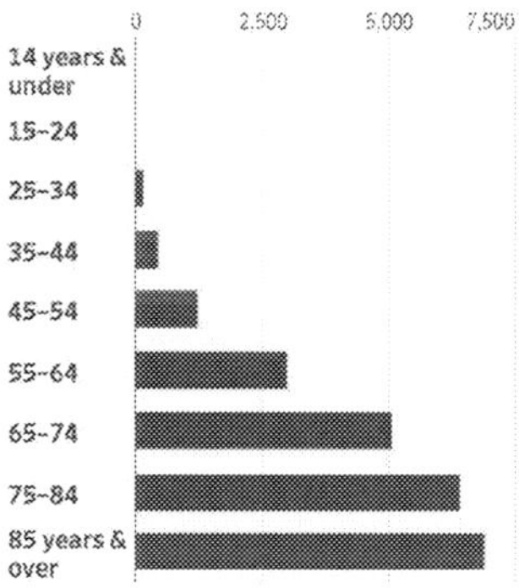

Note: Deaths recorded and causes attributed as of April 23, date is incomplete because of lag times in reporting.
Source: National Center for Health Statistics

Still, the much lower incidence of death among younger people warrants a reconsideration of our one-size-fits-all approach to stay-at-home policies, especially outside the hard-hit tri-state region of New York, New Jersey and Connecticut.

To start, states and localities should work as quickly as possible to reopen pre-K and K-12 schools. Children have a very low risk of falling seriously ill due to Covid-19, and the majority can and should return to school this academic year. Switzerland, for example, is planning to reopen schools on May 11, based on research showing that school closures were among the least effective measures at reducing European Covid-19 cases.

Children who live with the elderly or other at-risk individuals should continue to stay home. Teachers and staff from vulnerable populations should stay home as well, with paid leave. School districts should immediately begin to develop virtual lesson plans for those who must remain home.

Similarly, we should reopen workplaces to healthy, non-elderly individuals who don't live with vulnerable people. At-risk individuals with jobs should continue to have opportunities to work from home or to receive paid medical leave.

SHARE YOUR THOUGHTS

What steps do you think the country should take to reopen the economy? Join the conversation below.

And we should reopen businesses that may not be "essential" but can be safely operated while maintaining appropriate physical distance between workers and customers. We should offer a fixed-dollar per-worker tax credit to employers who test their employees, thereby giving businesses an incentive to scale up testing and increase consumer confidence.

Nursing homes are at especially high risk for Covid-19. Indeed, in many European countries, roughly half of all deaths due to Covid-19 have taken place in assisted living facilities. In the U.S., the share of nursing home deaths is lower. But, disastrously, New York state has forced nursing home operators to accept previously hospitalized Covid-19 patients, exacerbating the outbreak.

We must ensure that nursing homes get all the help that they need to protect their residents, including regular testing for residents and staff. Jails and prisons will also need additional resources to manage their most crowded facilities.

While we're reopening the schools and the economy to lower-risk individuals, and protecting the vulnerable, we should make sure that we're using modern public health techniques to help slow the spread of the virus. The most important of these is contact tracing.

If we succeed in encouraging people to use contact tracing apps in the U.S., we may be able to control the spread of Covid-19 with the modest levels of testing we already have.

Once someone tests positive for Covid-19, local officials should interview the patient to see who he or she has spent time with in previous weeks. The officials can then work backward to talk to those contacts—and their contacts, and so on—to ensure that those at risk get tested and treated.

In recent months, East Asian countries like Singapore, Taiwan and South Korea have deployed a much more sophisticated version of contact tracing, in which Bluetooth or GPS-enabled smartphones help officials automatically alert those who have recently been in close contact with an infected individual. U.S. companies are working on versions of the technology, including some with robust privacy protections.

A key virtue of contact tracing is that it can work in an environment where testing for SARS-CoV-2 is far from universal. Indeed, if we succeed in encouraging people to use contact tracing apps in the U.S., we may be able to control the spread of Covid-19 with the modest levels of testing we already have.

On April 16, President Trump unveiled his plan for reopening the economy. It improves on the conventional wisdom by setting aside comprehensive testing, effective treatment and herd immunity as absolute prerequisites for action. Still, the Trump plan is overly cautious about reopening the economy and especially schools. The president's team recommends that schools only reopen in "states and regions with no evidence of a rebound" in infections and hospitalizations.

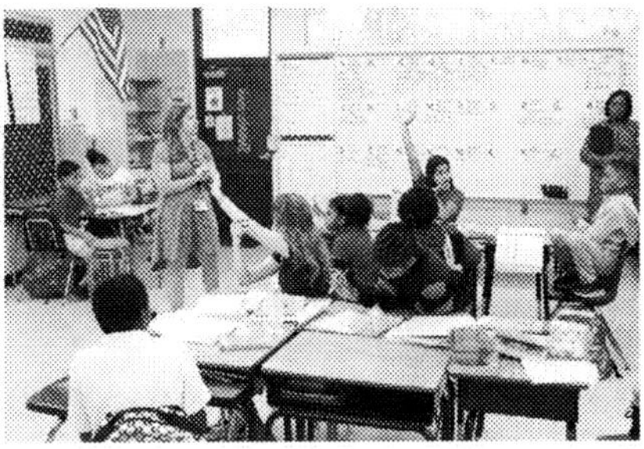

Reopening the schools is important for the welfare of children, especially those in low-income communities.
PHOTO: OCTAVIO JONES/TAMPA BAY TIMES/ZUMA PRESS

Reopening the schools is important for the welfare of children, especially those in low-income communities, but it's also important for their parents. Think of the pharmacist single mother who can't go to work because the schools are closed and her children would be left alone at home. We might even consider extending school into the summer, so that children and parents can make up for lost time, and camps and summer programs also should be released from lockdown restrictions.

There are more things that we can do to help improve our economy. We should expand the role of telemedicine for those who cannot see their physicians in person. We should accelerate highway construction projects while road traffic is meaningfully reduced. And we should do more to restore consumer confidence in air travel.

But most of all, we have to completely change our mind-set. Instead of thinking up creative ways to force people to stay home, we should think hard every day about how to bring more people back to work.

That doesn't mean the choices are easy. Minority communities are the ones most harmed by school closures, because they often lack the resources and opportunities to educate their children in other ways. At the same time, however, a larger share of African-Americans are at high risk from Covid-19, so under a partial reopening, more black children may need to stay home to protect their families.

Similarly, a faster reopening of workplaces will require vulnerable individuals of working age to remain home. While that may feel like an inequity, getting many more Americans back to work will have beneficial effects even for those who aren't among the first to return.

Reopening the economy is not merely about livelihoods, but also about lives. All of us can see the mounting mental and emotional toll of our ongoing lockdowns, and we've learned a great deal in recent years about how high unemployment increases deaths of despair. If we keep these urgent problems in mind—and not just infection rates and case fatality ratios—we may yet find our way out of this crisis.

Mr. Roy is president of the Foundation for Research on Equal Opportunity and the co-author (with Lanhee Chen, Bob Kocher and Bob Wachter) of the foundation's "A New Strategy for Bringing People Back to Work During Covid-19," from which this essay is partially adapted.

* * *

Chairman SCOTT. Thank you very much, Mr. Roy.
Secretary King.

Statement of John B. King, Jr., President and Ceo, the Education Trust, Washington, DC

Mr. KING. Thank you so much.

Chairman Scott, Ranking Member Foxx, and Members of the committee, thank you for the opportunity to testify.

This hearing takes place in the shadow of massive global protests against police violence, seeking to ensure that #BlackLivesMatter is more than just a hash tag. The murders of George Floyd, Breonna Taylor, Ahmad Aubrey, and Rayshard Brooks remind us yet again that systemic racism, antiblackness and the legacy of slavery still infect our institutions, public discourse, and daily interactions.

Our education system is fraught with racial inequities that existed before COVID–19. Far too few Black and Latino children have access to affordable, high-quality preschool. Black children, especially Black boys, are disproportionately suspended and expelled from early learning.

The pandemic has pushed our early childhood education sector toward collapse which could have dire consequences for families of color and early child and workforce disproportionately made up of women of color.

Over 65 years after Brown versus Board of Education, district lines and school assignment policies still segregate K-12 students by race and class. Districts with the most Black, Latino, and Native Americans students spend almost $2,000 less per student per year than districts with mostly White students.

Students of color are less likely to be assigned to the strongest teachers, less likely to have access to school counselors, less likely to be enrolled in advanced course work, and more likely to be subjected to exclusionary discipline. These opportunity gaps, in turn, generate gaps in learning, high school graduation, and college matriculation.

The higher ed sector still doesn't reflect America's diversity. Not one State's public colleges enroll or graduate a representative share of Black and Latino students relative to the State population. Meanwhile the burden of student debt falls disproportionately on Black students who are more likely than their White peers to have to borrow and are also more likely to default.

COVID–19 has exacerbated these educational disparities. During the necessary school closures, Black, Latino, and Native American students disproportionately had less access to devices and home internet services, teachers with less support to execute online learning, parents unable to telework and assist with schoolwork, and more socio-emotional stressors.

In response, we urge Congress to take the following actions. First, Congress must act boldly to support and strengthen P-12 education. To address devastating budget shortfalls, over 70 stakeholders have called on Congress to allocate at least $500 billion for State and local governments, including at least $175 billion for K-12 education and 50 billion for higher ed.

This Federal stabilization funding must include a strong maintenance of effort provision and add a maintenance of equity provision so States and districts can ensure that the most vulnerable students retain critical support.

Congress must allocate dedicated funding for broadband expansion to support distance learning, for extended learning time to tackle significant learning loss from the pandemic, and resources to address students' and educators' nutritional, social, emotional, and mental health needs.

Congress should refrain from permitting blanket waivers to key civil rights laws like ESSA and IDEA and protect the historic interpretation of the Title 1 equitable services provision. Additionally, the Federal Government must promote diverse schools, require data to be desegregated by race, and uphold student civil rights.

Second, Congress must enact equitable reforms to higher education. Congress should extend the student loan relief provisions included in the CARES Act into next year and offer equitable, targeted debt forgiveness in recognition that the recession will make repaying student debt impossible for millions of borrowers.

To counter widespread losses of financial assistance and employment, Congress should double the Pell Grant and simplify the FAFSA process. Implementing those policies would increase enrollment and limit debt for students of color.

But there is more Congress could do including expanding Pell access to incarcerated students and undocumented students, increasing investments in HBCUs and MSIs, supporting diversity in educator preparation programs, investing in evidence-based strategies to improve outcomes for low-income students and students of color, reigning in predatory for-profit institutions, and collecting better data to monitor progress.

Finally, the Federal government should never waver in its commitment to protect the civil rights and safety of all students. The racial inequities we face in education are significant, but not insurmountable. The Education Trust stands ready to assist you in the work ahead.

Thank you again, for the opportunity to speak with you today, and I look forward to taking your questions.

United States House Committee on Education and Labor, "Inequities Exposed: How COVID-19 Widened Racial Inequities in Education, Health, and the Workforce," June 22, 2020, Written Testimony Dr. John B. King Jr., President and Ceo of the Education Trust

Dr. John B. King Jr. – Biography

John B. King Jr. is the president and CEO of The Education Trust, a national nonprofit organization that seeks to identify and close opportunity and achievement gaps, from preschool through college. King served in President Barack Obama's cabinet as the 10th U.S. Secretary of Education. In tapping him to lead the U.S. Department of Education (ED), President Obama called King "an exceptionally talented educator," citing his commitment to "preparing every child for success" and his lifelong dedication to education as a teacher, principal, and leader of schools and school systems.

Before becoming the Secretary of Education, King carried out the duties of the U.S. Deputy Secretary of Education, overseeing all policies and programs related to P-12 education, English learners, special education, and innovation. In this role, King also oversaw the agency's operations. King joined the department following his tenure as the first African American and Puerto Rican to serve as New York State Education Commissioner.

King began his career in education as a high school social studies teacher in Puerto Rico and Boston, Mass., and as a middle school principal.

King's life story is an extraordinary testament to the transformative power of education. Both of King's parents were career New York City public school educators, whose example serves as an enduring inspiration. Both of King's parents passed away from illness by the time he was 12 years old. He credits New York City public school teachers — particularly educators at P.S. 276 in Canarsie and Mark Twain Junior High School in Coney Island — for saving his life by providing him with rich and engaging educational experiences and giving him hope for the future.

King holds a Bachelor of Arts in government from Harvard University, a J.D. from Yale Law School, as well as a Master of Arts in the teaching of social studies and a doctorate in education from Teachers College at Columbia University. King serves as Professor of Practice at the University of Maryland's College of Education and is a member of several boards, including those of The Century Foundation, The Robin Hood Foundation, Teach Plus, MDRC, and the American Museum of Natural History. He was elected to Harvard University's Board of Overseers and serves on several advisory boards, including Former First Lady Michelle Obama's Reach Higher Initiative, the Rework America Task Force, the GOOD+ Foundation's Fatherhood Leadership Council, the National Center for Free Speech and Civic Engagement at the University of California, the National Center for Learning Disabilities, and the National Advisory Council for the Prenatal-to-Three Policy Impact Center at the University of Texas at Austin.

King lives in Silver Spring, Md., with his wife (a former kindergarten and first-grade teacher) and his two daughters, who attend local public schools.

Summary of Testimony

Chairman Scott, Ranking Member Foxx, and members of the Committee, thank you for the opportunity to testify on racial equity and COVID-19.

This hearing takes place in the shadow of massive global protests against police violence seeking to ensure that "Black Lives Matter" is more than just a hashtag. The murders of George Floyd, Breonna Taylor, Ahmaud Arbery, and Rayshard Brooks remind us yet again that systemic racism, anti-Blackness, and the legacy of slavery still infect our institutions, public discourse, and daily interactions. Now is the time to transform the lofty rhetoric of statements about solidarity into concrete action toward achieving justice.

Our education system is fraught with racial inequities that existed before COVID-19. Far too few Black and Latino children have access to affordable, high-quality preschool. Black children, especially Black boys, are disproportionately suspended and expelled from early learning programs. The pandemic has pushed our early childhood education sector toward collapse, which could have dire consequences for families of color and an early childhood workforce disproportionately made up of women of color.

Over 65 years after *Brown v. Board of Education*, district lines and school assignment policies still segregate K-12 students by race and class. Districts with the most Black, Latino, and Native American students spend almost $2,000 less per student per year than districts with mostly White students. Students of color are less likely to be assigned to the strongest teachers, less likely to have access to school counselors, less likely to be enrolled in advanced coursework, and more likely to be subjected to exclusionary discipline. These opportunity gaps in turn generate gaps in learning, high school graduation, and college matriculation.

The higher education sector still doesn't reflect America's diversity: Not one state's public colleges enroll or graduate a representative share of Black and Latino students relative to the state population. Meanwhile, the burden of student debt falls disproportionately on Black students, who are more likely than their White peers to have to borrow and also more likely to default.

COVID-19 has exacerbated these educational disparities. During the necessary school closures, Black, Latino, and Native American students disproportionately had less access to devices and home internet service; teachers with less support to execute online learning; parents unable to telework and assist with schoolwork; and more socioemotional stressors. As noted in my recent Senate HELP Committee testimony: "Our nation's students of color and their families find themselves enduring a pandemic that disproportionately impacts their health and safety, mired in an economic crisis that disproportionately affects their financial well-being, and living in a country that too often still struggles to recognize their humanity."

In response, we urge Congress to take the following actions:

First: Congress Must Act Boldly to Support and Strengthen P-12 Education

To address devastating budget shortfalls, over 70 stakeholders have called on Congress to allocate at least $500 billion for state and local governments, including at least $175 billion for K-12 education, and $50 billion for higher education. This federal stabilization funding must include a strong maintenance of effort provision, and add a maintenance of equity provision so states and districts can ensure that the most vulnerable students retain critical supports. Congress must allocate dedicated funding for broadband expansion to enable distance learning for millions of low-income students, for extended learning time to tackle the significant learning loss resulting from the pandemic, and for resources to address students' and educators' nutritional, social, emotional, and mental health needs. Congress should refrain from permitting blanket waivers to key civil rights laws like ESSA and IDEA, and protect the historic interpretation of the Title I equitable services provision in administering the CARES Act and future funds. Additionally, the federal government must promote diverse schools, require data to be disaggregated by race, and uphold students' civil rights.

Second: Congress Must Enact Equitable Reforms to Higher Education

Congress should extend the student loan relief provisions included in the CARES Act into next year and offer equitable, targeted debt forgiveness in recognition that the recession will make repaying student debt impossible for millions of borrowers. To counter widespread losses of financial assistance and employment, which may keep millions of students from enrolling or staying enrolled, Congress should double the Pell Grant and simplify the FAFSA process.

Implementing those policies would increase enrollment and limit debt for students of color, but there is more Congress can do, including: expanding Pell access to incarcerated students and undocumented students, increasing investments in HBCUs and MSIs, supporting diversity in educator preparation programs, investing in evidence-based strategies to improve outcomes for low-income students and students of color, reigning in predatory for-profit institutions, and collecting better data to monitor progress. Finally, the federal government should never waver in its commitment to protect the civil rights and safety of all students.

The racial inequities we face in education are significant, but not insurmountable. The Education Trust stands ready to assist you in the work ahead.

Thank you for the opportunity to speak with you today. I look forward to taking your questions.

Written Testimony

Chairman Scott, Ranking Member Foxx, and members of the Committee, thank you for the opportunity to testify on the structural racial inequities in our nation's educational systems that are being exacerbated by the COVID-19 pandemic and how best to address them going forward.

As I had the opportunity to share with the Senate HELP Committee earlier this month, this hearing takes place in the shadow of massive demonstrations across the globe by millions protesting the continued toll of systemic racism in America. The murders of George Floyd, Breonna Taylor, Ahmaud Arbery, and Rayshard Brooks remind us that the legacies of slavery and Jim Crow, racial discrimination, and anti-Blackness still infect many of our institutions, our public discourse, and our daily interactions. Students of color, their families, and millions of others are risking their own lives amid an ongoing public health crisis to ensure that "Black Lives Matter" is more than just a hashtag. Now is the time to transform the lofty rhetoric of solidarity into concrete action toward achieving educational justice.

Our nation's education system is fraught with racial inequities, some of which manifest before students of color even enter kindergarten. Young children of color face particularly challenging barriers to high-quality early care and education, while disproportionately living in poverty. Infant care can cost up to 116% of a low-income family's total income, yet far too few families receive financial assistance to access it: for instance, Early Head Start provides access to only 7% of eligible infants and toddlers. Child care subsidies through the Child Care and Development Block Grant (CCDBG) serve a very small portion of potentially federally eligible children of color: only 15% of Black children and 6% of Latino children. Accessing any type of child care is challenging for many families of color: 57% of Latino families and 60% of American Indian and Alaskan Native families live in child care deserts. And when states do fund high-quality preschool programs, access is often lower for Black and Latino children, who are underrepresented in several such programs. Young children of color who do have access to early childhood education are pushed out of the classroom at alarming rates: Black children, and especially Black boys, are disproportionately suspended and expelled from early learning settings. The COVID-19 crisis has compounded these inequities, and has pushed early care and learning toward collapse, which has potentially deleterious consequences for families of color with young children and an early childhood workforce disproportionately made up of women of color.

As students enter our K-12 systems, the inequities persist. School districts with the most Black, Latino, and Native American students receive roughly $1,800, or 13%, less per student in state and local funding than those serving mostly White students. Students of color and students from low-income backgrounds are less likely to have access to strong, consistent teaching than their White and higher-income peers. Furthermore, only 20 percent of teachers are teachers of color compared to half of all students in the United States being students of color. Beyond ensuring that the teacher workforce is representative of the country, there are proven benefits of having a diverse teacher workforce. Students of color who have had teachers of the same race do better academically and are more likely to graduate from high school and attend a four-year college. Research suggests that Black teachers are also more likely than White teachers to have high expectations for Black students, and less likely to use exclusionary discipline on them. Furthermore, schools staffed by leaders and teachers of color expose all students to positive role models of different races, and counteract negative stereotypes.

In 38 states, the schools that serve more students of color and students from low-income backgrounds have fewer counselors per student than schools that serve fewer of these students, which puts underrepresented students at a disadvantage when social, emotional, and academic supports are needed beyond the classroom. Additionally, despite studies showing that Black students do not misbehave more than other students, Black students are disproportionately suspended, expelled and arrested at school. According to the Civil Rights Data Collection, Black students comprise only 15% of school enrollment, but account for 40% of students who receive an out-of-school suspension, 35% of those expelled, and 36% of students who were arrested at school.

Racial disparities exist in relation to coursework, as well. Based on The Education Trust's analysis of data from the Civil Rights Data Collection and the Common Core of Data, Black and Latino students are locked out of advanced coursework at every critical stage of their education – they are denied these opportunities in elementary school, middle school and high school. We know students of color can be and are successful in eighth grade Algebra I courses, yet students who attend schools with the lowest percentages of students of color are about 1.5 times as likely to be enrolled in eighth grade algebra as students attending schools with the highest percentages of students of color.

Given these inequities in opportunity and access, it is not surprising that we see different outcomes when we look at measures of student learning and graduation rates. On the National Assessment of Educational Progress (NAEP), Black and Latino students are more likely to score at the basic and below basic levels than their White peers. For example, in 2019, 18% of students from low-income backgrounds, 14% of Black students, and 20% of Latino students scored at or above proficient on the eighth grade math assessment, compared to 48% and 44% of their non-low-income and White peers, respectively. We also see smaller percentages of students who are Black, Latino, Indigenous, or from low-income backgrounds, and students with disabilities graduating from high school compared to their peers. While the overall graduation rate for the class of 2017-18 was 85.3%, it was lower for Black students (79%), Native American students (73.5%), students from low-income backgrounds (79.5%), and students with disabilities (67.1%).

As students of color transition into postsecondary education, they move into a public college system that doesn't reflect America's diversity: Not one state's public colleges enroll or graduate a representative share of Black and Latino students relative to state population.

In fact, since 2000, the percentage of Black students has decreased at nearly 60% of the 101 most selective public colleges and universities in the United States. Fewer than 1 in 10 of these colleges (9%) enrolls a percentage of Black students on campus that is proportional to the Black population of the state in which they reside. Since 2000, the growth of Latino enrollment at 65% of these institutions failed to keep pace with the growth in the state's Latino population. And only 1 in 7 of these colleges (14%) has a percentage of Latino students that is representative of their state's Latino population.

Once enrolled, the chance of completing college also differs for White and Black students, even within the same income group. At four-year institutions, White students are at least 11 percentage points more likely to complete a college degree than their Black counterparts, regardless of income group. The completion gaps are wide among low, lower middle, and upper middle income groups, but this discrepancy was the largest in the lower middle income group. White students were 17 percentage points more likely to graduate than their Black counterparts (67% vs. 50%), while among students from families with the highest incomes, the completion gap was considerable but somewhat smaller (11 percentage points).

And the racial disparities don't end there. Black students are vastly underrepresented in higher education, yet those that do attend college often bear a disproportionate student debt burden. Black students are more likely to borrow and default on their loans than their White peers. For federal loans, default occurs after a borrower is 270 days late and it is the most disastrous financial outcome of student debt. Defaulting not only ruins a person's credit, but makes future borrowing more expensive and can make it harder to get a job, rent an apartment, or buy a house or a car. Half of Black borrowers who entered college in the 2003-04 academic year defaulted on their student loans within 12 years, a staggeringly high number when compared to the nationwide default rate of 10%. Protective factors like degree completion or high family income, which would normally shield borrowers from adverse debt outcomes, don't necessarily protect Black borrowers. A Black bachelor's degree recipient is more likely to default than a White college dropout, and Black students from high-income families default at rates that are seven times higher than their White peers. Higher default rates among Black borrowers are not the result of over-borrowing or poor decisions, but are caused by structural racism that harms Black people financially and perpetuates the racial wealth gap.

These inequities are compounded by racial disparities in the labor market, where the Black unemployment rate is consistently double that of their White counterparts. Regardless of education level, the same racial disparities in employment persist: In May 2020, White bachelor's degree holders had lower unemployment rates than Black, Hispanic or Latino, and Asian American bachelor's degree holders. This structural disadvantage is a key contributor to the overall financial insecurity and inability to build intergenerational wealth among communities of color: Today's median Black family has a net wealth of $3,600, while the median Latino family has a net wealth of $6,600, compared to $147,000 for the median White family. The racial wealth gap is a product of slavery, Jim Crow, and racist federal housing policy. Combined with ongoing discrimination in employment and lending, these systemic barriers have effectively prevented many Black families from building wealth through homeownership, leaving them with a fraction of the wealth of White people.

The grim reality is that COVID-19 has made the inequities present in our education system, like those detailed above, even worse.

From its onset, the COVID-19 pandemic has underscored that not all adults have the privilege of working from home in accordance with states' social distancing or stay-at-home orders, and that those who are deemed "essential" and are required to place themselves at risk are disproportionately individuals of color or those from working-class, low-income backgrounds. Only about 1 in 5 Black workers and 1 in 6 Latino workers are able to work from home, compared with about 1 in 3 White workers. Research shows that predominantly Black counties account for over half of coronavirus cases in the United States, and nearly 60% of total deaths. It also shows that *social* determinants — including employment, access to health insurance and medical care, and poor air and water quality — are more predictive of infection and death from COVID-19 than are underlying health conditions. In Chicago, while Black residents are about 30% of the city's population, they account for nearly 70% of COVID-19 deaths. Stunningly, as of June 10, 1 in every 1,625 Black Americans has died from COVID-19, compared to 1 in 3,800 White Americans. Even more recent Centers for Disease Control data shows that a disproportionate number of Latinos are suffering from COVID-19 relative to their share of the U.S. population. In nearby Anne Arundel County, Maryland,

Latino residents account for 38% of all cases, despite only making up 8% of that county's population.

The economic toll on communities of color has been substantial. A new Associated Press poll finds that over 60% of Hispanic Americans say they have experienced some form of household income loss as a result of the pandemic, including job losses, unpaid leave, cuts in pay, and fewer scheduled hours compared with 46% of Americans overall. While 37% of Hispanic Americans and 27% of Black Americans say they've been unable to pay at least one type of bill as a result of the coronavirus outbreak, only 17% of White Americans say the same. A recent poll indicated that Latino and Black workers were more likely to be laid off due to the pandemic than their White peers, and that people of color who remain employed are more worried about losing their jobs.

The inequities impacting how Americans of different races, ethnicities, and incomes are experiencing the pandemic translate to educational inequities as well. Across the nation, schools are struggling to move to distance learning, as are teachers and administrators who may not have familiarity with learning management technology tools. Parents and educators alike are searching for promising practices and online learning resources, and many schools and districts lack large-scale experience with education technology. This spring, we also saw many high school students take at-home versions of Advanced Placement tests, which are often a factor in college admissions, despite not every student having the same access to an AP course or test. Additionally, not every student has a compatible device or access to high-speed internet to make online learning viable. As a result, a recent survey of teachers noted that student learning since schools closed has dropped to three hours a day, from six previously, and that lower-income students were down to two hours a day. Earlier in the pandemic, Los Angeles reported that about a third of its high school students were not logging in for classes. In states where schools remain closed for months or even longer, learning loss among students, particularly those who are already vulnerable, may carry far into the future, unless directly addressed through expanded learning opportunities.

Confronted with the uncertainty about the nature of COVID-19 and how long it may prevent the full resumption of in-person learning, parents and families are understandably concerned not only about their children's health and well-being, but also about their children's education at this unprecedented time. The Education Trust just conducted polls of parents in New York, Washington, Texas, and California. These polls show that nearly 90% of parents are worried that their children will fall behind academically because of school closings. Equity concerns about distance education seem particularly valid when we know that before the pandemic, 79% of White households had broadband access, while only 66% of Black families and 61% of Hispanic families had broadband service at home.

The Education Trust is grateful that many educators across the country have made one important shift during this crisis — showing their students even more clearly that they care by asking about students' well-being and connecting families with resources to provide some levity through fun virtual interactions with their students. This relationship-building between teachers and students was already happening in many places, but it was not happening nearly enough in places that serve a majority of students of color and students from low-income backgrounds. That connection is essential. In addition, Ed Trust's parent poll in New York revealed that 95% of parents want to have regular contact with or access to their child's teacher, but only 52% said their child's school has made that available. Our California poll revealed that Black parents were less likely than parents of all other racial groups to have been contacted by their child's teacher. We need to make sure this is something that is cherished in places where students face the most obstacles.

The pandemic also has had detrimental effects on college students forced to leave their campuses and return home to learn remotely, and especially on those who were working while enrolled and have lost income that's essential to continuing their education. The impact of the pandemic can also be seen in the disaggregated data showing which groups of students are worried about being able to graduate on time, and considering delaying or changing their education plans. Roughly three-quarters of undergraduate students have said they were worried about being able to stay on track and graduate, and those shares were higher among Black and Latino students. Another survey showed that 32% of Latino students, 24% of Black students, and 21% of Asian American students have canceled or delayed their education plans in light of the pandemic. College students are also impacted by the digital divide, as they return to homes that may not have reliable broadband access. Black and Latino students are also overrepresented within the population of students that were denied emergency financial aid by Secretary Betsy DeVos' interpretation of the CARES Act: undocumented students, incarcerated students, and students who have defaulted on their loans. All of these pressures take a toll on students' mental health: 80% said that the pandemic had negatively affected their mental health.

As noted in our Senate testimony earlier this month, our nation's students of color and their families find themselves enduring a pandemic that disproportionately impacts their health and safety, mired in an economic crisis that disproportionately affects their financial well-being, and living in a country that too often still struggles to recognize their humanity.

In response to these racial inequities, which have only grown in the wake of this pandemic, we urge Congress to take the following actions:

How Congress Can Act Boldly to Support and Strengthen P-12 Education in the Midst of COVID-19

Allocate Funds to Allow for Safe Reopening, Relief for Students, and Enable Learning to Continue

The first step toward making the system more equitable is to prevent the pandemic from making that task even harder. States and localities — which provide the vast majority of K-12 education funding — are bracing for major budget cuts as revenues continue to plummet. After the Great Recession of 2008, over 300,000 educators lost their jobs, and inflation adjusted state funding per pupil was still lower in 2017 than 2008. This time the cuts may be even larger. If we ignore the lessons of the last economic slowdown, students of color and students from low-income backgrounds will be hardest hit by these cuts. For example, while funding cuts to education were widespread following the Great Recession, an analysis of layoffs in Los Angeles found that Latino elementary students were 26% more likely than their White peers to have their teacher laid off; Black elementary students 72% more likely to have their teacher laid off.

The National Education Association projects that the United States could lose as many as 1.9 million education jobs if Congress doesn't extend financial relief to states and localities, and nearly half a million K-12 education jobs disappeared in April alone. The Learning Policy Institute estimates, based on projected state revenue losses for the end of this fiscal year and the next, that K-12 systems might need as much as $230 billion to stabilize their budgets. And those estimates are focused solely on making districts whole; they do not incorporate the additional costs that districts will face as a direct result of responding to COVID-19, including sanitizing schools, personal protective equipment, and providing devices and materials for distance/hybrid learning.

This is why over 70 education stakeholders have called on Congress to allocate at least $500 billion for state and local stabilization, and require that a proportional amount of these funds be directed toward K-12 spending. As

K-12 education makes up, on average, 35% of state general funds, Congress should allocate at least $175 billion for K-12 education. An investment of this size is essential to, at minimum, prevent the K-12 education system in America from becoming more inequitable in the wake of the pandemic.

These targeted federal stabilization funds, as well as the additional provisions outlined below, are necessary to ensure that schools are able to reopen safely and that states and districts are able to provide all schools — particularly underfunded, high-poverty schools that serve more students of color — with the resources they need to implement the Centers for Disease Control (CDC) considerations and each local health authority's guidance for keeping students and staff safe (e.g., adequate testing and contact tracing, use of PPE, protections for at-risk staff and students, social distancing, etc.). The funds will also be essential to maintain the nation's education workforce and implement equitable policies to the benefit of all students.

Ensure States and Districts Do Not Walk away from the Students Hit Hardest by This Crisis

While the federal government must provide financial assistance to address looming revenue shortfalls and budget cuts, states and school districts remain the primary actors in funding local education systems and deciding how equitably that funding is used. Federal stabilization money must be accompanied by strong requirements to ensure that states maintain their investments in education; to ensure that states and districts minimize cuts to their highest need districts and schools; and to prevent the U.S. Department of Education (ED) from steering funding away from low-income, public school students.

Specifically, the federal government must include *maintenance of effort* provisions that require state education spending levels to remain constant (i.e., at least at the same percentage of the state's total spending), even if the state's overall budget shrinks. Further, if spending cuts are necessary, the federal government must use a *maintenance of equity* provision to protect our highest-need schools by requiring *both* states and districts that receive additional federal funding to show that any necessary cuts are smaller per student in the highest-need districts and schools than the rest of the state or district.

Finally, we've already seen ED advise states and school districts to steer federal funding away from low-income, public school students into the hands of wealthier, Whiter private schools. Therefore, we urge Congress to prevent forthcoming regulations that would allow the Department of Education's recent misinterpretation of the Title I equitable services provision within the

CARES Act to be used to direct over $1.35 billion in CARES Act financial assistance away from public Title I schools primarily serving Black and Latino students to private schools that primarily serve White students, regardless of whether those schools are serving students from low-income backgrounds. Several states have already rejected this approach.

Ensure That Distance Learning is Possible for Every Student

Before the pandemic, 79% of White households had broadband access, while only 66% of Black families and 61% of Hispanic families had broadband service at home. More than one-third of all households with school-age children and incomes of less than $30,000 annually lack high-speed internet access. Additionally, Microsoft estimates that as many as 163 million people do not use the internet at broadband speeds, burdening students even further.

It is likely that distance learning will continue through the summer, into the beginning of next year, and intermittently if new cases of the virus emerge. The data we have from this spring is alarming. For example, data from California showed that 38% of low-income families and 29% of families of color are concerned about access to distance learning because they don't have reliable internet at home. Therefore, states and districts must have a plan in place to ensure that all students, including students from low-income backgrounds, have access to reliable, high-speed internet and devices and IT support to connect to virtual learning opportunities, and that educators have the support they need to effectively teach, assess, and connect with their students remotely. The lack of equitable access to broadband is not only a distance learning issue, but also an emergency preparedness issue in the event of further widespread closures.

Congress must allocate at least $4 billion through an Emergency Connectivity Fund via the Federal Communications Commission's federal E-Rate program to expand access to broadband services, Wi-Fi hotspots, and devices to ensure that all students have the ability to access online learning at home in the event of continued disruptions, and Congress should encourage districts to implement multilingual digital learning platforms to be fully inclusive. Congress should also encourage private companies to enable home broadband access for the students in the communities they serve at no cost during the pandemic.

Beyond the emergency response to ensure access during the pandemic, Congress should be looking at what it would take to ensure that the homework gap that affects at least 8 million K-12 students annually is closed for good. The same racial inequities in high-speed home Internet access exacerbated by the crisis will be present beyond it. America needs a national policy that recognizes that the Internet is an essential tool in continuing education outside of the classroom, both formally and informally, and that it is increasingly obvious that part of solving the racial inequities in education is solving the homework gap.

Address Learning Loss through Expanded Learning Opportunities

Students will likely return to classrooms with significant learning loss, which schools and teachers must be prepared to assess and address. Schools serving larger populations of students from low-income backgrounds are far less likely to be able to provide online learning opportunities for all students and, therefore, must find a way to make up for lost instructional time. In fact, an analysis done by McKinsey indicated that the average lost learning time for Black students due to the pandemic could be as much as 10 months; for Hispanic students, as much nine months; and for low-income students, over a year.

The stabilization funding described above — meant to make districts and schools whole — will not be sufficient to accelerate learning to make up for the billions of hours of instructional time that students lost this spring. That is why Congress should allocate dedicated funds to help schools facilitate expanded learning time, via summer school (online or in-person based on the most recent public health guidance available), extended day or year, intensive tutoring, or other evidence-based approaches to support students in completing unfinished learning and accelerating new learning.

This additional funding must be targeted to prioritize the equity gaps we know have been exacerbated by COVID-19 and to prioritize students, including students from low-income backgrounds, students with disabilities, English learners, and students experiencing homelessness or foster care, who have been most directly impacted by lost in-person instructional time. Additionally, educators will need sufficient time to prepare for the next school year and the substantially different work environment that they will be faced with, including altered or expanded school schedules, additional remote instruction, and curricular changes. This professional learning and planning time comes at a cost; Congress must allocate funding to cover it.

Address Students' and Educators' Social, Emotional, Mental, Nutritional, and Physical Needs

All students are experiencing stress, anxiety, and learning obstacles due to school closures and other COVID-19-related stressors. Many families are feeling the strain of ensuring students receive the care, attention, and educational resources they need to thrive. Parents and guardians are scrambling to maintain their own jobs, meet their families' basic needs, identify child care, and help engage their students in meaningful online learning. These challenges are even greater for some students and families, including students from low-income backgrounds and students of color, who already face steep economic and health inequities previously mentioned. Therefore, in addition to academic learning, schools must prioritize and center the social, emotional, mental, and physical health needs of these historically underserved students upon return to school.

At a minimum, Congress must ensure students' basic needs are met, including the more than 20 million students who depend on schools for their meals every day. In a national survey by Hunger Free America, 37% of parents reported cutting the size of meals or skipping meals for their children because they did not have enough money for food between mid-March and mid-April, when the survey was released.

Congress can directly address the food insecurity of students and their families through the Pandemic Electronic Benefits Transfer (P-EBT) program, which can ensure that students' nutritional needs are met throughout this summer and into the next school year. The program must also be expanded to cover children under 5 who are not currently included in this program due to the structure of the free-and-reduced-price lunch program.

Beyond basic needs, we know that over 75% of students receiving mental health care receive that care at school. Schools must also provide a positive and welcoming school climate, as well as quality dropout prevention and re-engagement programs — especially for the most vulnerable students. Therefore, it is critical that Congress allocate additional federal funding to support school counselors, mental health workers, psychologists, and social workers in the highest-need districts, and allocate resources to train teachers to understand and address the negative impacts of COVID-19 on students, especially those of color and from low-income backgrounds.

It is also critical to remember that we must ensure the safety and well-being of administrators, educators, and support personnel. Educators are experiencing greater stress and anxiety during COVID-19. When educators were asked in a recent survey conducted by the Yale Center for Emotional Intelligence about the most frequent emotion they felt each day of remote learning, their top five responses were: "anxious, fearful, worried, overwhelmed and sad," with anxiety being the most mentioned emotion. These emotions can often lead to teacher burnout. Therefore, we must support our educators by providing them with emotional support and mental health resources.

Congress Must Protect Students' Civil Rights

Finally, it is important to note that during this hectic and uncertain time, Congress must not abdicate its important role in protecting students' civil rights. Therefore, Congress must not provide blanket waivers of critical requirements under the Every Student Succeeds Act (ESSA) or the Individuals with Disabilities Education Act (IDEA) that protect all students' civil rights. ESSA and IDEA were designed to ensure all students have equitable access to a high-quality education. That goal has not changed even with the current crises this country faces. The existing waiver authority within ESSA provides sufficient authority for the U.S. Department of Education to meet states' needs. As ED has already acknowledged, the impact of COVID-19 will affect each state differently; therefore, case-by-case consideration of each state's needs remains the most appropriate path moving forward. Permitting blanket waivers to either law is dangerous and unnecessary.

The equity concerns exacerbated by COVID-19 must remain Congressional priorities beyond the pandemic. That means maintaining resources for expanding broadband access; extended, tailored learning time to accelerate learning; and keeping resources for students' and educators' nutritional, social, emotional, and mental health needs in place. This funding must be targeted towards the students that need it most. Additionally, the federal government must do more to promote diverse schools and classrooms, require data reported by schools, districts, and states to be disaggregated by race, and enforce students' civil rights during this uncertain time.

This is also the time to address the other structural inequities within our systems that have persisted for generations – long before COVID arrived. That means ensuring all students, but particularly students of color, have access to the critical resources they need to graduate ready for college and careers.

Congress must also support states and districts to advance equity in these areas:

Ensure Equitable Funding

As described above, districts serving large populations of students of color and students from low-income families receive far less funding than those serving White and more affluent students. Despite widespread attention to inequitable funding formulas — and courts that have declared them unlawful— too many states continue this unfair practice. Across the country, school districts with the most Black, Latino, and Native students receive roughly $1,800, or 13%, less per student in state and local funding than those serving mostly White students, and states and districts spend approximately $1,000 less per pupil on students educated in our nation's highest poverty districts than on those educated in the lowest poverty districts.

While money alone will not solve the deeply embedded systemic inequities our students face, it matters a great deal. Research shows that increased school spending leads to increases in graduation rates, higher wages, and a reduction in adult poverty, especially for students from low-income backgrounds.

To ensure equitable funding systems, Congress must support states to: (1) provide funding according to student need; (2) provide more funding to districts with low property wealth; (3) ensure that dollars are used well to improve student learning experiences and outcomes; and (4) be transparent about the funding system's design and monitor funding to districts. In addition, since ESSA requires that all states and districts report school-level per pupil expenditure data on state and local report cards, Congress has an especially important role to support states in sharing clear and transparent data on the amount of funding that schools actually receive. For many states, 2020 is the first year that they will be sharing this critical data with the public; Congress must ensure that the U.S. Department of Education is providing support to states to meet this requirement and enforcing the law when states do not provide this information in a timely manner.

Access to Strong and Diverse Educators

Research shows that teachers are the single greatest in-school factor for student success. Students with the strongest teachers receive what amounts to months' worth of additional learning each year. We also know that all students benefit from having at least one teacher of color, and students of color are more likely to attend school regularly, perform higher on end-of-year assessments, be referred to a gifted program, graduate high school, and consider college when they have had a teacher of the same race or ethnicity. Unfortunately, thousands of Black and Latino students attend a school where they have no same-race teachers. Even larger percentages of White students attend a school without a Black teacher and/or Latino teacher.

To ensure all students have access to strong and diverse educators, Congress must support states to: (1) set – then meet – clear goals at the state and district levels to increase access to strong and diverse educators; (2) target resources to the districts and schools that struggle the most to provide students from low-income backgrounds and students of color with access to strong teachers; (3) target resources to diversify the teaching workforce; (4) set high standards for how teachers are prepared and licensed to improve teaching quality for students in high-need schools and in historically underserved groups; and (5) make educator quality and diversity data more visible and actionable.

In addition, Congress must increase funding for Historically Black Colleges and Universities (HBCUs), Tribal Colleges and Universities (TCUs) and other Minority Serving Institutions (MSIs). These institutions prepare nearly 40% of Black teachers with bachelor's degrees in the United States. Congress should also fund the Augustus Hawkins Centers of Excellence Grant program for the first time since its creation in the bipartisan Higher Education Act of 2008. This program would provide critical funding to MSIs to provide increased and enhanced clinical experience and increased financial aid to prospective teachers of color, who, as detailed above, face higher burdens in college access and affordability than their White peers.

Access to and Success in Advanced Coursework

Research shows that when students are given access to advanced coursework opportunities, they work harder and engage more in school, and in turn have fewer absences and suspensions and higher graduation rates. And when these opportunities are provided to students of color, and their teachers receive training and supports, these students thrive alongside their peers. But, as shared earlier, too many Black, Latino, and low-income students, do not receive these opportunities.

To ensure all students have access to and success in advanced coursework, Congress must support states to: (1) use data to identify the barriers that prevent students of color and students from low-income families from enrolling in advanced courses and take action; (2) set clear and measurable goals for advancing access to and success in advanced coursework; (3) invest to expand advanced coursework opportunities — both courses and seats; (4) require and support districts to expand eligibility for advanced courses; and (5) support Black, Latino, and low-income students' success in advanced courses. Congress can act now to close opportunity gaps in access to advanced coursework by creating and funding grants to states and districts that can be used to implement open enrollment, establish universal enrollment or universal screening for advanced courses and programs, support districts in launching additional courses and innovative models that allow all students to benefit, purchase materials; cover the costs of advanced coursework exams for students from low-income backgrounds; and prepare and support educators to teach these courses.

Equitable State Accountability, School Improvement, and Reporting Systems

Not too long ago, students from low-income backgrounds, students of color, English learners, and students with disabilities — who had long gone underserved in our schools — were invisible, hidden behind averages. In 2015, ESSA, building on earlier federal legislation, challenged states to refine their accountability systems to provide the right combination of pressure and support for school improvement. The law leaves many key decisions up to states — decisions about what to measure, how to communicate how schools are doing on those measures, how to identify schools that need to take action to improve for any group of students, what to do to support school improvement efforts, and what to do if schools don't improve.

To ensure these systems are focused on supporting equity and achievement for all students, Congress must support states to: (1) only include indicators in state accountability systems that keep student learning front and center; (2) ensure that school ratings reflect how schools are doing for all groups of students; (3) establish criteria that honestly identify which schools need to take steps to improve overall or for one or more student groups; (4) provide meaningful support to schools that need to improve; and (5) report information that is understandable, easily accessible, and widely available. In particular, Congress must require states to administer statewide assessments during the 2020-21 school year. These assessments aligned to grade-level expectations are critical not only to helping families and educators understand how well students are learning, but also to supporting policymakers and leaders in identifying the places that are seeing promising results for all students so we can learn from those places.

Access to Equitable Learning Environments

Recognizing that school is where students spend the bulk of the time learning about themselves, their emotions and behaviors, and how to interact with others, over 90% of schools and districts report that they are working to support the social and emotional learning of students. Studies also show that social and emotional well-being is inextricably linked to the context in which students develop and the relationships they build over time. Too often, approaches to supporting social and emotional learning in schools ignore context, focusing solely on building specific skills (e.g., lessons on behavior).

Ignoring context carries significant risks, especially for those students who are already underserved by our education system: students from low-income families, students of color, LGBT youth, students with disabilities, and English learners. Failing to acknowledge the influence of the learning environment, or failing to address the processes and structures in schools that disadvantage some students, may do more harm than good. Congress must support states and districts to provide all students with equitable learning environments that foster belonging, challenge students, and provide the supports students need to thrive. This means, for example, funding and providing meaningful professional development and coaching on topics such as reducing bias and anti-racist mindsets; improving working environments and conditions to retain educators of color; and ensuring equitable access to and supports for success in rigorous and culturally sustaining coursework.

In addition, we must recognize that for Black children, attending school is an act of racial justice. In early 2019, when the current administration rescinded school discipline guidance that was put in place explicitly to ensure that Black children were not pushed out of school buildings, it sent a loud and clear message that it is okay for educators and school leaders to exclude these students from opportunities to learn. Congress must renounce that message and instead proactively support states and districts in identifying and addressing disparate school discipline policies and practices.

Congress Needs to Enact Equitable Reforms to Higher Education

Allocate Funds to Allow for Safe Reopening, Relief for Students, and Enable Learning to Continue

In response to COVID-19, Congress took important steps in the CARES Act that should be maintained into next year. Congress should look to build on its initial higher education stabilization in CARES by allocating an additional $50 billion in aid to help keep students from suffering economic hardship and assist nonprofit colleges and universities to remain financially stable while preparing for a safe reopening. Those funds should also be allowed to assist students who are incarcerated, undocumented, or otherwise barred from federal financial aid under other circumstances.

Congress should also take direct action to enable postsecondary learning to continue. The pandemic necessitates a doubling of the Pell Grant in light of the increasing financial uncertainty facing students who may be forced to halt their studies due to a lack of funding. Additionally, in light of the FAFSA renewal rate dropping below prior years, Congress should work with the Department of Education, as seen recently in a bipartisan letter from four U.S. Senators, to figure out how best to streamline the filing process to remove financial obstacles for students and their families, especially those directly impacted by the pandemic. To enable home learning, Congress should include the Supporting Connectivity for Higher Education Students in Need Act in its next response package, which would direct $1 billion to institutions that are primarily serving students of color and students from low-income backgrounds to ensure that students at those institutions can get the home Internet access they need to continue their postsecondary education. Finally, Congress should provide dedicated funds to support student success and completion. This funding stream should support students' academic and social needs that have been impacted by the crisis, such as mental health services and supplemental academic support. This could take the form of bridge programs, co-requisite instruction, and/or supplemental academic support for Pell-eligible students to make up for lost learning and increase the number of available advisers and counselors.

The student loan relief provisions in CARES gave relief to millions of borrowers facing tremendous economic pressure in the face of the recession, and those should be extended into next year. Congress should build on that relief by extending equitable, targeted debt forgiveness to millions of borrowers who were already struggling and are facing a near insurmountable repayment burden in the wake of the recession.

Protect, Increase, and Expand Pell Grants

The Pell Grant program is the cornerstone of federal financial aid. Created in 1972 as the Basic Educational Opportunity Grant, the program benefits over 7 million students annually and continues to serve as the primary federal effort to open the door to college for students from low-income backgrounds. Over one-third of White students, two-thirds of Black students, and half of Latino students rely on Pell Grants every year. Pell Grant dollars are well-targeted to those in need: 83% of Pell recipients come from families with annual incomes at or below $40,000, including 44% with annual family incomes at or below $15,000.

The Pell Grant program's impact is shrinking as the maximum award has failed to keep pace with the rapidly rising cost of college. The purchasing power of the Pell Grant has dropped dramatically since the program's inception. In 1980, the maximum Pell Grant award covered 77% of the cost of attendance at a public university. Today, it covers just over 28%, the lowest portion in over 40 years. If the maximum award continues to stagnate, the grant will cover just one-fifth of college costs in 10 years.

Doubling the Pell Grant is a rational response to the enrollment downturn due to the pandemic and the steady erosion of the purchasing power of the award. After prioritizing that step, Congress should also make the following structural reforms: re-index it to inflation, as it was before 2017, move the program to the mandatory side of the budget to avoid potential discretionary cuts to a program that functions like a mandatory program, and expand it and other federal financial aid to students who are incarcerated and students who are undocumented to maximize education opportunity and help close equity gaps.

Increasing Equity through Better Data and Funding Improvement Plans

Equity-focused accountability has the potential to refocus our higher education system on its most important purpose: successful outcomes for all groups of students. Congress must build upon current policy to create an accountability system that pushes institutions to serve students well, especially low-income students and students of color.

The first step in creating an equity-focused accountability system is maintaining and strengthening the protections we have in place currently. There is bipartisan support for closing the 90/10 loophole that sets up veterans as targets for predatory for-profits, and Congress should take that action, as well as moving the rule back to 85/15, per its original conception. Additionally, the recent gainful employment regulatory changes by the Department of Education removed the ability to hold accountable continuously poor-performing career education programs, and the recent borrower defense regulatory rewrite all but eliminated the right of defrauded or misled borrowers to get their federal loans discharged. Both of these changes should be reversed, and prior versions of the gainful employment rule and borrower defense rule restored.

In order to construct effective accountability and oversight systems, Congress must act to improve higher education data systems so they may provide reliable, consistent, and useable information. The bipartisan, bicameral College Transparency Act would overturn the ban on the creation of a student-level data system that would be immensely important in helping policymakers design systems that promote equity. Creating a student-level data system would make data on critical measures of student success like enrollment, persistence, retention, transfer, and completion, as well as post-enrollment outcomes such as earnings and employment, much easier to obtain and disaggregate by race, income, gender, ancestry, and other key criteria. The bill also contains privacy protections for sensitive student information essential to protecting the civil rights of all students.

In addition to maintaining and strengthening the accountability provisions currently in place, Congress must create pressure and provide support for the entire higher education system to improve, especially for the students from low-income backgrounds and students of color who are most likely to be underserved by today's system. Developing metrics that would establish minimum standards for institutions enrolling low-income students and students of color, and establish minimum standards for institutions regarding the performance, experiences, and outcomes for those low-income students and students of color are a prerequisite to holding institutions accountable for closing equity gaps in higher education.

However, any system that sets standards and walks away is one that is guaranteed to do damage to low-income students and students of color at institutions that need additional resources to respond to those standards. Investments in historically under-resourced institutions to support the implementation of evidence-based strategies that improve completion for students from low-income backgrounds and students of color are essential to making lasting, positive change for historically underserved students. In addition to investing more in Title III and Title V institutions, Congress should create a fund to support the development and scaling of interventions that improve completion.

Finally, take a rehabilitative approach to institutional improvement, not a punitive one. New standards that consider the reality that closing institutions can do tremendous damage to the students that are attending them should be implemented. This means consequences should be targeted at the programmatic level where possible, institutions should have time to adjust to new standards, continual growth and progress should allow for reduced consequences, and institutions that fail should be given support and the chance to submit improvement plans. However, when institutions are not meeting benchmarks, students, families, states and accreditors should be notified, and restrictions on enrollment and the elimination of Title IV eligibility must be on the table as eventual realities.

Investment in Student Success

Congress should invest in evidence-based policies to improve student success and close racial equity gaps. There is a growing body of evidence that wraparound support models like the City University New York's Accelerated Study in Associate Program (ASAP) are transformational for students. In New York City, ASAP nearly doubled three-year graduation rates for participants, up to 40% from 22%. While it required some upfront investment, due to the significant increase in graduation rates, CUNY ASAP drove down the cost per degree by 11%. These findings were replicated by three pilot programs in Ohio, which also nearly doubled three-year graduation rates and increased transfer rates to four-year colleges, and showed positive effects on enrollment, full-time enrollment, and credits earned. It also lowered the cost per degree. In order to scale these proven models, Congress should approve the Community College Student Success Act, which would provide grants to community colleges to scale ASAP-type programs. In addition to expanding ASAP, there are also promising practices around emergency student aid and microgrants that deserve further study, and Congress should support the development of these practices as well. Finally, students who are hungry cannot learn. Congress should make it easier for college students to enroll in the Supplemental Nutrition Assistance Program (SNAP) by eliminating the 20-hour work requirement that acts as a barrier for thousands of students.

Congress Must Protect Students' Civil Rights

The federal government has a vital historical role as the protector of civil rights and safety on college campuses. Colleges are venues for the exchange of ideas and the development and growth of students, not places where discrimination, hate crimes, or sexual assault are condoned. We support federal policies that encourage institutions to support a healthy campus racial climate, based on how accepted students feel on campus, how often they are able to engage across lines of difference, and how well the university supports diversity through events, clubs, and policies. Regular surveys of students and faculty on campus climate are essential practices to determine how to select and implement policies to ensure campus safety and equitable treatment. Federal, state, and institutional systems should include indicators that track and report incidents of bias or violence on campus. Federal requirements administered by the Equal Employment Opportunity Commission and Offices of Civil Rights can also provide some of this data to help inform Congress as they look to address these issues.

Conclusion

In closing, we cannot underestimate the impact that this crisis will have — and has already had — on all of our students, but particularly our children of color and children from low-income backgrounds. They and their families are already bearing the brunt of the crisis.

More than 118,000 people in the United States have died of the coronavirus, and more than 33 million Americans have filed for unemployment during the pandemic. Both in terms of deaths and lost jobs, people of color are disproportionately affected.

When students do eventually return to brick-and-mortar buildings, there will be students at the K-12 and postsecondary levels sitting next to each other with very different levels of learning. Young students whose parents had the resources and flexibility to help them learn via high speed internet while school was closed, and those whose parents had to work, possibly on the front lines, to make ends meet and who had less reliable internet access during the crisis have had substantially different remote learning experiences. We must ensure that the latter receive the support necessary to get the quality education they deserve. College students who went home to comfortable surroundings and families that didn't require them to provide financial and/or caregiving support have structural advantages that students who must also juggle financial or caregiving responsibilities at home while trying to focus on their studies or are plagued by worries about how to pay for college and stay in school amid the pandemic do not. If there is a post-pandemic return to the old "normal" — obscuring the inequities that we know exist — we will have learned nothing. The old normal is no longer an acceptable option — we must supply the resources and supports to ensure that equity gaps are closed for good.

If we fail to educate and protect students of color and students from low-income backgrounds, we have failed as a nation. We can choose to continue to shut out communities of color and low-income communities or we can make changes to allow for a more inclusive America — one that protects the most underserved and allows everyone to reach their full potential.

The challenges facing us right now are significant, but they are not insurmountable. The Education Trust stands ready to assist and support you in the work ahead.

Thank you for the opportunity to speak with you today. I look forward to taking your questions.

Chairman SCOTT. Thank you very much. Thank you very much.

And I thank all of our witnesses for their testimony. Under Committee Rule 8(a) we will now question the witnesses under the five-minute rule, and I will be recognizing committee Members in seniority order. Again, in order to ensure that the members' five-minute rule is adhered to, the staff will be keeping time, keeping track of time and use the chime to signal when one minute is left and when time is up entirely.

Again, they will sound a short chime when there is one minute left and a longer, more obnoxious chime when time is up. Please be attentive to the time and wrap up your time when your time is over and please remute your phone.

Again, if any member experiences technical difficulties during the hearing, you should stay connected on the platform, make sure you are muted with your mute button highlighted in red, and use your phone to immediately contact the committee's IT director whose name and number has been provided.

As chair, I will reserve my questions to the end and begin by recognizing the gentlewoman from California, Mrs. Davis, for five minutes.

Mrs. Davis.

Mrs. DAVIS. Thank you.

Thank you, Mr. Chairman.

And, Secretary King, it is very good to see you, sir. I certainly appreciate your public service.

One issue that goes underappreciated in higher education conversation today is that of campus climate. Today's colleges, as we all know, were built for the so-called traditional student population, largely made up of recent high school graduates from affluent families.

But we know that today's students are more diverse than ever. They are often older. They are the first in their family to go to college or from communities that have been poorly served by our Nation's colleges and universities, not to mention our early education and K-12 systems.

The protests for racial justice that have emerged across the country further underscore the need for our educational system to address systemic racism and ensure that students of color are well-served and supported.

Recently the President of Johns Hopkins University revealed that in 2014 they discontinued the practice of offering students preference in admissions for having family members who also attended the university, often called legacy admissions. And in the article he recognizes this was not an easy step to take. But this shift has allowed space for more Pell Grant-eligible students to enroll.

Secretary King, can you further explain some of the inequities associated with the practice of legacy admissions in higher education?

Mr. KING. Yes. The legacy admission policy has the impact of disproportionately advantaging students, White students—

Mrs. DAVIS. Mr. Secretary, I think we are having sound problems.

Chairman SCOTT. Ben, can you intervene?

VOICE. Mr. King, can you turn your volume on your mikes down? Leave your speaker. You are bouncing off your microphone and causing a bit of echo.

Mr. KING. All right. Is that better?

Voice. It is not, sir. It may be—let's see. The communication was good at the beginning of your testimony, sir. Let's see. Can you mute your microphone and then unmute it again just to try and see if that improves the quality?

Mr. KING. Sure.

VOICE. Mr. King, in the interest of time, I will jump offline with him and try to fix this. I think this may be something that we need to reset.

Chairman SCOTT. Ben, can you have him call in with audio over the phone?

VOICE. Yes.

Chairman SCOTT. Okay. Ben. Mr. King, let's see, if you could please use a phone and call your audio in.

Mr. KING. Okay.

Chairman SCOTT. Just mute your phone and call into—

VOICE. I will call—give you the number when you're ready, sir.

Mr. KING. Okay. Go ahead.

VOICE. It would be 415-527-5035, sir.

Mr. KING. 5025.

VOICE. 5035, sir.

Mr. KING. 35.

VOICE. Yes, sir. Let me know if you need the access code, Mr. King.

Mr. King, the access code is 996979932 and please follow any prompts in the affirmative. I think I can confirm you, Mr. King. Can you speak again, please?

I am sorry. I think you are on mute. And go ahead, Mr. King.

Mr. KING. All right. Can you hear me now?

VOICE. I can. So it will—now you will use your phone's mute capacity in order to mute your audio, sir, but this sounds very good. Thank you for your time and consideration, Mr. King.

Mr. KING. All right. Sorry about that. So in response to the question, good to see you, Congresswoman.

On the issue of legacy admissions, what we know is that the legacy advantage can translate into as much as a 45 percent increase in the likelihood of a student being admitted compared to a similarly situated who doesn't have the benefit of the legacy preference.

The consequence for our selective admission universities is that low-income students and students of color are at an enduring disadvantage and are dramatically underrepresented on those campuses and in those institutions.

So it makes sense, if universities are true to their commitments to a diverse student body, to eliminate legacy preferences. But to really ensure that students of color are fully represented in selective admission universities, more is needed.

Race needs to be taken into consideration in admissions policies. Financial aid needs to be provided to so that low-income students can have access to those institutions. More work needs to be done to recruit diverse fact to create a positive climate for students, and specific efforts need to be made to recruit students from high schools that serve large numbers of students of color.

But certainly eliminating the legacy admissions would be an important, strong step to improving diversity on our Nation's campuses.

Mrs. DAVIS. Thank you, Mr. Secretary. I appreciate that, because I think we all have to ask the question about the Federal role in that as well and it may be that encouraging and we also know that early admission plays a bit of a role as well.

Would you agree with that?

Mr. KING. Yeah. For many institutions the early admissions practice, again, advantages those students who have the most resources. If you think about access to school counselors, for example, we have some States where there are 500, 600 students per counsellor. And so counselors aren't able to support students. Students aren't able to take advantage of some of those early admission processes.

Mrs. DAVIS. Uh-huh, yeah. Well, thank you again.

How can our institutions of higher education lead the way in dismantling systemic racism and addressing the harm done to communities of color, even in a COVID world where students are going to be off-campus? What new approaches do we have to think about? I believe I have one minute left.

Mr. KING. Sure. Well, one immediate step is that campuses need to make sure that students can access higher education through distance learning. We know that low-income students and disproportionate students of color were at risk of not having the devices and Internet access they needed.

There is a congressional effort that Congresswoman Eschoo put forward to try to dedicate resources for higher ed to provide them that access. I think that is critical so we make sure that students can take advantage of higher ed this fall which will certainly be distant on some campuses, hybrid on others.

Mrs. DAVIS. Uh-huh, right. Thank you very much, sir. Good to have you with us.

Chairman SCOTT. Thank you.

Dr. Foxx, do you wish to be recognized at this point?

Ms. FOXX. Yes, sir, I do.

Chairman SCOTT. Dr. Foxx, you are recognized for five minutes.

Ms. FOXX. Thank you, Mr. Chairman.

Mr. Roy, prior to the COVID–19 pandemic, our country had record low unemployment across the board including for Black, Hispanic and Asian workers. What significant policies and economic conditions resulted in the historically low rates which existed before the pandemic?

And as Congress considers additional policy prescriptions for addressing the pandemic, how are the negative economic effects of the pandemic different from previous economic downturns such as the 2008 financial crisis?

Mr. ROY. Well, I will start, ma'am, with the second question, and then go back to the first. On the second question, we can hope that, if and when States and localities reopen their economies, there will be a relatively rapid rebound of businesses that did not run out of cash during the pandemic. The average small business has about 30 to 28 days of cash on hand if business shuts down. So, for those businesses, who knows how many of them will rebound.

But the ones that rebound, we should see unemployment recover relatively rapidly. And we saw that with SARS-CoV-1 in Asia. So that is my hope on that front, that, compared to the recession in 2008, where there was— there were underlying problems with the economy, particularly the inflation in housing prices, here we see something that hopefully can be relatively quickly solved if reopening can take place.

In terms of your first question—I am sorry. Now I have lost my— remind me what the first question, just briefly, was.

Ms. FOXX. Yeah. What are the—

Mr. ROY. Oh. The drivers of the low employment. Right.

Ms. FOXX. Fox right.

Mr. ROY. Right. So there were several things that, from a policy standpoint, led to record low unemployment prior to the pandemic. So that was something that was going on since the great recession from 2008, but the biggest drivers in the last several years have clearly been the Tax Cut and Jobs Act of 2017 and regulatory changes which have allowed manufacturing jobs and other industries to hire and expand in ways that have allowed employment to rise.

And, again, when employment rises, who benefits? Particularly, it is lower income workers, hourly wage workers that are disproportionately non-White.

Ms. FOXX. Right. I don't think there were any of those proposals in the HEROES Act.

Mr. Roy, as you have stated in your written testimony and in your research, a long-term shutdown is untenable, we have no choice but to reopen responsibly, even though a vaccine for COVID–19 has not been developed and research on treatment continues. Would you elaborate on the impact of the State and local shutdowns, whether it is possible to combat the pandemic and safely reopen at the same time and what effects this approach will have on communities around the country?

Mr. ROY. The most important thing to understand about COVID– 19 is the disproportionate impact it has not so much on race—so that is important, too—but on age. The fact is that 81 percent of all deaths due to COVID–19 are happening in people over the age of 65. And, as I mentioned in my testimony, 43 percent of all deaths are happening in the 0.6 percent of the population that lives in nursing homes.

On the flip side, COVID–19 from a mortality and severe illness standpoint is not really affecting younger people. Yes, there are isolated cases, but, in general, the probability of dying of influenza is much greater in young children than it is of COVID–19.

So that gives us an opportunity to reopen schools. Obviously, we have to take care to make sure that vulnerable teachers and other school staff are protected and that children who live with vulnerable grandparents, say, or other at-risk members of their household, that they are protected and they have the resources to learn outside of school, but we can reopen schools. Other countries are doing it, and that is an important thing for this committee to consider.

Ms. FOXX. Thank you.

You have already mentioned this. So I want to build on that point that you just made. Could you explain further the impact the actions of these Governors who forced nursing homes to accept COVID–19 patients who have been discharged from the hospital? Could you talk a little bit about the death rates and which States have experienced the highest rates of nursing home deaths?

And, Mr. Chairman, for your information, Mr. Thompson is back in the room.

Mr. ROY. So, in my written testimony, I have detailed Statebased data on both the share of overall COVID–19 deaths that are taking place in nursing home by State and also the percentage of nursing home and long-term care facility residents in that State that have died of COVID–19.

The worst State by far on that second metric is New Jersey. New Jersey is one of the States—11 percent of all residents of long-term care facilities in New Jersey have died of COVID–19—11 percent. And that is, in part, because New Jersey is one of the States, like New York, like Michigan, and several others, that forced nursing homes to accept people with active COVID–19 infections who were being discharged from hospitals, and that contributed significantly to the spread of COVID–19 in our long-term care facilities.

Ms. FOXX. And that is the same State where the State health director, I believe, took her own mother out of the long-term care facility before she enforced the rule to allow those people to come back in. That is one of the most shameful things that has happened in this country in my opinion.

Thank you, Dr. Roy.

Chairman SCOTT. Does the ranking member yield back?

Ms. FOXX. I yield back.

Chairman SCOTT. Thank you. The gentleman from Arizona, Mr. Grijalva.

Mr. GRIJALVA. Thank you, Mr. Chairman. I appreciate the hearing, and I appreciate the witnesses for being here.

Secretary King, good to see you again. We often talk about achievement gaps in education, often, and there has been a recent move to reframe those gaps as a result of—and, as a result, people are talking about opportunity gaps to highlight the systematic inequities in educational funding. These opportunity gaps are actually educational debt.

That debt has become even more apparent as a result of the COVID–19 pandemic and the debts that have long—that we have collectively failed to pay for a long, long time.

Mr. King, what will happen if Congress doesn't act with a level of urgency to pay back some of those debts for communities of color in the education arena, and as pressure to reopen schools—K-12, in particular—intensifies, the consequences of that cost that will be attendant to local communities as well as they prepare to respond to orders from States to open up those schools immediately?

Mr. KING. I am sorry. Good to see you, Congressman.

Mr. GRIJALVA. Good to see you.

Mr. KING. So, at this moment, what we know is that school districts are getting 90 percent or more of their funding from State and local dollars, and so those State and local budgets have taken a huge hit from the COVID–19 economic crisis, and that is going to translate into significant cuts to school district funding.

Some school districts are preparing around the country for 20, 25 percent cut in State aid. That will have a devastating impact. The NEA and others have estimated that could mean approaching 2 million jobs lost in the education sector, layoffs of teachers. It will also mean the elimination of programs, particularly programs that serve the most vulnerable students.

We also know that, if those cuts happen, districts will be much less able to do the kinds of practices that public health requires to have a safe reopen of schools. So we need Congress to step in with State stabilization dollars to prevent those cuts, and additional resources to address the consequences of COVID–19.

Mr. GRIJALVA. Thank you.

Mr. Roy, if I may, a question out of curiosity: In your verbal testimony, you mentioned the impact of small businesses, particularly the disproportionate negative impact on businesses owned by people of color and how that is so important to the recovery. You mentioned the unemployment in response to Dr. Foxx's question.

As we, as a Congress, struggle to make sure that the money that we are providing to local communities and to the administration for the implementation and the supplemental support of these small businesses that are disproportionately being affected now, do you think it is appropriate and necessary for, let's say, Secretary Mnuchin to release how the $650 billion that were provided for PPP and for other direct assistance to small businesses and businesses in general—that would give us a framework to see if—what impact that money is having. Do you think that all those figures should be released publicly?

Mr. ROY. I do, yes.

Mr. GRIJALVA. And, in doing so, I think it helps us guide how we need to structure making sure that the money goes to the greatest need. Is that correct?

Mr. ROY. One of my concerns about the way the PPP was designed by Congress is that it basically favored medium to large businesses over small businesses on a relative basis.

Mr. GRIJALVA. I agree.

Mr. ROY. Because, if you are a one- or two-person shop, you don't have the resources to be organized enough to draw that money down from PPP. The money ran out before [inaudible] people became more aware of what was going on. So the smallest businesses did not benefit from PPP nearly as much as they needed to.

Mr. GRIJALVA. Thank you.

I yield back, Mr. Chairman, and thank you for the hearing.

Chairman SCOTT. Thank you. Gentleman from Tennessee, Dr. Roe. Dr. Roe?

Mr. Thompson? Mr. Thompson?

Ms. FOXX. He is having trouble. Dr. Roe is one of our members at the funeral.

Chairman SCOTT. Okay.

Ms. FOXX. Mr. Thompson, I believe, is ready.

Chairman SCOTT. Mr. Thompson, recognized for 5 minutes.

Ms. FOXX. Well, sorry, Mr. Chairman. He is having a problem. Would you go to Mr. Walberg, and then come back to Mr. Thompson?

Chairman SCOTT. No problem.

The gentleman from Michigan, Mr. Walberg.

Mr. WALBERG. Thank you, Mr. Chairman. Can you hear me?

Chairman SCOTT. I can hear you.

Mr. WALBERG. That is great. I appreciate this.

And I notice that Representative Bonamici is in the room as it were right now, so certainly express our condolences to her at the loss of her mother.

Going back to a little of the statements that began about the HEROES Act, I think we need to understand that the HEROES Act is really just a messaging piece with no expectation that it would ever pass, and I—you know, I think it is cynical to even keep bringing it up as legitimate.

Also, there is a reason that major cities with terrible health and education outcomes are in long-held Democrat-controlled governments. That is a fact. Even in my boyhood home growing up in Chicago, challenges are there, but it has been the efforts of the longheld Democrat leadership that always complains about not having the outcomes we want, and, yet, the policies are still the same. And I think it is time to stop blaming the Republicans, who have been, especially in these last 3 years, very evidently been pushing real change that works and brought about economic growth in this country only impacted by COVID–19.

I think, also, until we stop opposing educational choice for minorities, like the D.C. Promise, the complaints ring hollow, and so I just want to point that out as well.

Mr. Roy, we know that COVID–19 is much more lethal for those over 65 years of age, like myself, with certain chronic conditions. Sadly, we now have a very sobering figure out there that shows nursing homes and assisted-living facilities have been some of the hardest hit victims of COVID–19. In my home State of Michigan, as of last Monday, almost 2,000 deaths have taken place among individuals who lived in nursing home facilities, which represents approximately one-third of the deaths Statewide.

Mr. Roy, your testimony mentions that over 40,000 seniors have tragically died under this care. What percentage of the U.S. population lives in long-term care facilities, and how does that compare with the share of COVID–19 deaths?

Mr. ROY. So, sir, as I mentioned in my oral and written testimony, 0.6 percent of Americans or U.S. residents live in nursing homes or assisted-living facilities, and, yet, they represent 43 percent Nationwide of all deaths from COVID–19.

Mr. WALBERG. Unbelievable. Unfortunately, Michigan was one of the handful of States, about five States, where the Governor issued an executive order forcing nursing homes to admit COVID–19-positive patients back into their facilities. Even more sadly, it is being reported that the State implemented this policy, contrary to recommendations it received from the State's leading nursing home association.

And so, Mr. Roy, how did this policy create such a dangerous situation for our Nation's seniors, and what should be done to address the challenges nursing homes face while caring for COVID–19 patients?

Mr. ROY. There is no doubt that Governor Whitmer's order to force nursing homes to accept patients with active COVID–19 infections worsened the state of nursing homes when it comes to COVID–19 fatalities. And we mentioned that one-third—you know, what the State is reporting as one-third of all deaths from COVID–19 in Michigan are coming from COVID–19 in nursing homes, first of all, the integrity of Michigan's data is not clear because Michigan has been one of the last States to actually report the data. They were the third to last State to report the data based on our work, and they also have had a big outbreak overall.

So, if you actually look at nursing homes with nursing home residents overall, 3 percent of all people who live in long-term facilities in Michigan have died from COVID–19, which is one of the highest rates in the country.

And so it is a real problem, and I think, in particular, what concerns me about Michigan is the fact that Michigan refused for many, many weeks to disclose their nursing home fatality data until basically CMS forced nursing homes to directly report their data to CMS and go around the State governments that were being cagey with their data.

Mr. WALBERG. Yeah, it was only about the last week or week and a half ago that Michigan began giving those—that data, but it was underreported as well. What can be done to address these data shortcomings moving forward to ensure we have the best information and make crucial policy decisions.

Mr. ROY. Well, what is good is that now CMS is requiring nursing homes to directly report their fatality data to the Federal Government. Now, the problem is that only starts on May 5th, that requirement. That only applies to nursing homes, not to assisted-living facilities, which are another form of long-term care facility less vulnerable seniors. So we are not going to get complete data from CMS, but at least that will help with the process.

The most important thing we have to do, obviously, is we have to protect the lives of the people who are living in these nursing homes. The way we have to do that is we have to have strict policies about patient visitation from relatives, but we also have to have strict policies about testing staff and making sure staff can't go from place to place, and much better oversight about infection control. A lot of these nursing homes were not designed to protect infections. That has been a huge problem, not just for this pandemic but in previous pandemics.

Mr. WALBERG. I yield back.

Chairman SCOTT. Thank you.

The gentleman from Connecticut, Mr. Courtney?

Mr. COURTNEY. Thank you, Chairman Scott, and thank you to all the witnesses for being here today.

I just want to begin by saying I am surprised to hear my good friend, Mr. Walberg, disparaging or dismissing the value of the HEROES Act provision for State and local assistance. Perhaps he missed it, but, just a couple of days ago, the U.S. Chamber of Commerce came out in favor of Congress acting to provide assistance to State and local government. They, again, are joining Jerome Powell, the chairman of the Federal Reserve Board, who has been, again, highlighting that in terms of fiscal stimulus that is still required, despite the best efforts by the Federal Reserve. And of course the National Governors Association, which is a bipartisan group, has strongly endorsed the provisions of the HEROES Act to bolster State and local support.

And, again, that is not because these individuals or groups have been hijacked in a partisan way. This is about math and the complete sort of erosion and collapse of State revenue that is happening across the country in red States and blue States. Again, it is just going to require that Congress take this measure up. And we actually are starting to see some signals out of the Senate that they are going to be moving towards bringing up some version of fiscal stimulus, which, again, is—basically listens to what the economic stewards of this country, particularly over at the Federal Reserve, have been calling for.

I would also like to bring up another measure of the HEROES Act, which, again, was alluded to in Ms. Williams' testimony, which, again, addresses another part of the fallout from this coronavirus recession, which is, again, the erosion of health insurance.

Ms. Wilson, in your testimony, again, you noted the fact that, at 13 percent unemployment, we are still about 30 percent higher than the peak of the 2009 recession and the impact that is having on employer-based coverage. I was wondering if you could sort of talk about that in a little more detail in terms of what that means to hourly workers, which, again, predominantly is or disproportionately consists more of workers and employees of color?

Ms. WILSON. Sure. So a couple of my colleagues at the Economic Policy Institute have estimated that, as of May 9th, about 16.2 million workers likely lost their employer-provided health insurance. What this means in terms of the racial disparities, we know that, going into the crisis, workers of color were less likely to have employer-provided health insurance to begin with.

The work—the hourly workers that you mentioned also are less likely to be insured through their employers so that providing coverage to these workers is important to their health, but it is also important in protecting communities and workplaces so that we can get everyone back to work safely.

Mr. COURTNEY. So—and the HEROES Act does two things. Number one, again, it requires that the States basically reopen their exchanges for special enrollment period. And, number two, it extends a 100 percent subsidy for COBRA so that, again, people who are losing their benefits along with their layoffs are—in fact, have some continuity of coverage. Is that right?

Ms. WILSON. Yes. That is my understanding, yes.

Mr. COURTNEY. So, now, Mr. Roy, in your testimony on page 10, you alluded to the fact that, you know, one of the impacts of the lockdown on public health is, in fact, the disruption of health insurance coverage. So do you support the COBRA subsidy provision, which, again, the U.S. Chamber of Commerce and the American Benefits Council has also come out and endorsed?

Mr. ROY. Well, I don't think that the COBRA subsidy program is the best way to improve—

Mr. COURTNEY.—yeah, we don't have a lot of time here—

Mr. ROY. If you would like, I would be happy to answer.

Mr. COURTNEY. Sure.

Mr. ROY. So the best way to do it is through improving the individual insurance market. So make the exchanges, the nongroup exchanges, better by funding reinsurance that allows the premiums to be lower in the ACA exchanges and, thereby, more accessible to people to people who need insurance between jobs.

At the end of the day, we need to move away from employer-based coverage, which is what the Chamber of Commerce wants; they want everyone to be tied to their job for health coverage. We should be moving to a system where individuals own their own health insurance.

Mr. COURTNEY. So, I mean, I agree with you about reinsurance, but I also think that, you know, in real time, we are watching people's healthcare coverage evaporate. And I will give you an example in Connecticut.

The Native American casino, Foxwoods, had 6,000 workers employed at the beginning of March. They have reopened. In fact, they went more aggressive than the Governor wanted. So it wasn't because, you know, they shut down because of a Governor-driven lockdown. But, anyway, they did reopen, but they only required 1,500 workers. So there is still 4,500 people who, again, starting on June 1st, lost their health coverage, and having that COBRA subsidy could at least extend that coverage and not disrupt their access to their doctors, their network of care.

Again, you know, fixing the exchange in terms of the long game, I couldn't agree with you more, but the fact of the matter is we are really trying to protect people in an emergency situation, and that is where, again, I think the COBRA subsidy, which is temporary— it is not a permanent fixture in the law—actually addresses a real need that is happening, and, again, which is disproportionately hitting hourly workers, which, in the case of Foxwoods, has, again, a high minority workforce.

Thank you. I yield back.

Chairman SCOTT. Thank you.

Is Mr. Thompson ready? The gentleman from Pennsylvania?

Mr. THOMPSON. Chairman, I am ready.

Chairman SCOTT. I am sorry. Who is that?

Mr. THOMPSON. This is G.T.

Chairman SCOTT. Okay. The gentleman from Pennsylvania, Mr. Thompson, is recognized for 5 minutes.

Mr. THOMPSON. Thank you. I am kind of making do here.

Mr. Roy, I want to thank you for making time today to join us here at the hearing. Obviously, due to COVID–19 and resulting State-mandated shutdowns, there has been a dramatic negative impact on the economy, workers, and families. Employment in the United States fell by more than 70,000 jobs in March and 20.5 million in April.

In my home State, Commonwealth of Pennsylvania, employment fell by more than 1 million nonfarm jobs in April, including declines in all 11 industry supersectors. However, due to the reopening of States, employment rose by 2.5 million. That is the largest number of jobs gained on record, and Pennsylvania total nonfarm jobs were up 198,300 over the month.

Mr. Roy, are you seeing signs that the economy is recovering and that jobs will continue to return? And what could prevent the— what is out there that may prevent the economy from rebounding quickly?

Mr. ROY. Well, Mr. Thompson, as I am sure you know, we are seeing some gradual improvement from the depths of the recent lockdowns on the recession. Particularly, as some States start to open, there is a clear correlation between the States that have reopened who never really locked down severely, like, for example, Florida and the economic performance of that State relative to others.

So that evidence at least gives us some hope that a rebound can happen relatively quickly as the economy is reopened, and I hope that we can get to that point as soon as possible. In fact, we should have gotten to that point for good sections of the workforce much earlier than we have up to this point.

Mr. THOMPSON. Well, thank you, and I—

Chairman SCOTT. Mr. Thompson, are you able to get your camera back on?

Mr. THOMPSON. Yes. Hold on a second.

Now it should be on, Chairman.

Chairman SCOTT. Okay. Well—

Mr. HAINES. Mr. Thompson is present on the video feed currently.

Mr. THOMPSON. It is a little confusing because I need the phone to speak, and just showing how handsome I am on the laptop. So kind of a dual role here.

Chairman SCOTT. Okay. Keep going.

Mr. THOMPSON. All right. Thanks, Chairman.

Chairman SCOTT. And if you would give him about 30 extra seconds for me interrupting him, I would appreciate it, Bernie.

Mr. THOMPSON. All right. Thanks, Chairman. I guess the message I would like to reinforce for all on this committee is, before we panic and look at creating all kinds of—that we ought to stay the course with what we have been doing prior to COVID–19 in terms of ladders of opportunity.

One of the things we have been able to work on in a bipartisan way has been career and technical education training, and I think—I know that there are issues now with people whose jobs have been lost because of the dictates of a Governor or impact of risk of coronavirus, but that—as a result, those jobs will be there, and I think the overarching need that we have is to focus on, again, getting people access to the types of job training, career and technical education training for those jobs.

Mr. Roy, to get America back to work, the White House and the CDC has issued guidelines for opening up America again, which include the three phases based on advice from public health officials. The guidelines are intended to help State and local officials make decisions about reopening the economy and getting people back to work while continuing to protect lives.

Mr. Roy, I know you have looked closely at the needs to reopen the economy safely. What additional points would you like to highlight for the committee on safely and responsibly reopening businesses and society?

Mr. ROY. Yeah. Our view at the Foundation for Research on Equal Opportunity and, as you may know from my written testimony, we have written extensively on how to reopen both the workplace and schools. Our view—

Mr. THOMPSON. Mr. Roy, I think you may be on mute.

Mr. ROY. Oh, I don't think I am on mute.

Mr. THOMPSON. Okay. I am not.

Mr. ROY. Okay. I will start again. I apologize.

As you may know from the white paper we put out at the Foundation for Research on Equal Opportunity on reopening workplaces and schools, our view is that the President's plan is actually too cautious, particularly when it comes to reopening schools, which can be done earlier, and reopening workplaces, particularly for younger members of the workforce who are at low risk for serious illness or death from COVID–19. And, in that context—

Mr. THOMPSON. I can't hear him. That is all right.

Mr. ROY. Yeah. I am sorry about that.

Well, to finish the answer for the record, maybe, I will just say that the most important things we need to do, one thing that a number of States have considered and more States should consider is starting the fall school year early to make up for some of the lost time from the spring.

And the other thing, you know, we would talk about is using—maximizing testing in particular targeted and at-risk populations that are asymptomatic, like, again, people with children who live with grandparents or other at-risk individuals and nursing home facilities because the more we can isolate and trace nursing home interactions, the more we can reduce the spread overall.

Mr. THOMPSON. Thank you, Chairman. I yield back.

Chairman SCOTT. All right. Thank you. Thank you, Mr. Thompson.

The gentlelady from Ohio, Ms. Fudge?

Ms. FUDGE. Thank you so much, Mr. Chairman.

Mr. Chairman, once again, my colleagues on the other side of the aisle live in an alternative universe with alternative facts. It ought to be interesting to me that Dr. Foxx and Mr. Walberg—I wonder if they are watching all the people marching in the streets today. These people are marching not because they just feel like marching. They are marching because of injustice.

You know, it would be nice if sometimes they would listen to what Black people actually think and not know what is best for us all of the time. That is if they know any Black people well enough to have that conversation with them.

Dr.—Secretary King, from your experience, what can we do at the Federal level to prevent students of color from falling further behind?

Mr. KING. Well, there is a long list, but I would start with a few priorities. One is we have got to save the childcare sector. Already, Black and Latino students are underrepresented in quality childcare, and, without $50 billion to stabilize the childcare sector, we are going to lose many of those providers.

In K-12, we know that schools are already highly segregated by race and class. You have the bill, the Strength and Diversity Act, which would help to address that and help us move towards more integrating schooling.

We also desperately need resources, resources to stabilize district budgets, but also resources to address learning loss. Students, particularly students of color, are less likely to have all of the things in place necessary to benefit from distance learning over the last few months. Many students will return to school many months— 9, 10 months behind in learning, will need additional support, afterschool time, extended school year, intensive tutoring to address those needs.

And they will also need socio-emotional and mental health support as well from many students who have been isolated from their relationship to school that matters so much for them.

Ms. FUDGE. Thank you.

Dr. Jones, how can we build trust between underserved communities and the local institutions, including hospitals and healthcare providers?

Dr. JONES. First of all, there has to be communication. So, I think that the hospitals need to be asking folks in the community, "What do you need?" There have to be perhaps community advisory boards and the like. There has to be an attention—is there something differential going on here by race in terms of our practice, in terms of sending people away from the emergency department?

So, the hospitals have to be unafraid to collect data by race and actually investigate possible differences in their practice by race, and there has to be investment in the community, in community health workers; in community, you know, health centers, even if they are not directly associated with the hospitals. There has to be some linkage.

It gets to the question of who is at the table and who is not? What is on the agenda is and what is not? As you said, so many people think that they can figure out what is good for those other people. We need to have the people who are impacted by decisions at the decision-making tables.

Ms. FUDGE. Thank you. And, to go further with you, Dr. Jones, can you talk just a bit, very quickly, about the impact of poverty on health outcomes for people of color?

Dr. JONES. Well, first of all, it doesn't just so happen that people of color in this country are overrepresented in poverty while White people in this country are overrepresented in wealth.

So, first of all, I mean, I have been writing so many notes, you know, talking about, well, you know, people, you know, frontline workers tend to be more people of color. That doesn't just so happen. So, we shouldn't take that as a baseline when we are trying to move people from there.

So, the first thing is it is because of historical injustices that are being perpetuated by present-day contemporary structural factors that we even see an association between social class and race so that even—and that goes—structural factors are part and parcel of structural or institutionalized racism.

So, even if we had the most successful antipoverty strategies in the world, if we do not also have the antiracism strategy, we would not take care of that, but the mechanisms are in housing. They are in our schools. They are in the investment in communities and in businesses. It is in green space. It is in sacrifice zones, the placement of communities of color around known polluting industries and the like.

So, poverty and race are correlated because of structural racism. We need to understand that, and we need to have both antipoverty and antiracism strategies.

Ms. FUDGE. Thank you so very much.

And, as I close, Mr. Chairman, I just want to note—I want you to know that I learned a long time ago: If you are not at the table, you are on the menu. Black people are sick of being on the menu.

I yield back.

Chairman SCOTT. Thank you. I thank the gentlelady from Ohio. The gentleman from Kentucky, Mr. Guthrie?

The gentleman from Alabama, Mr. Byrne? Mr. BYRNE. Thank you, Mr. Chairman.

I am very concerned about this topic. About a third of the people in my district are African American, but we know from the data about 50 percent of the people that have died from COVID–19 in my district are also African American. There is something going on there, and it bothers me greatly.

I have learned a lot from listening today. I have been doing a lot of research before today, but I think, as a Nation, we need to get to the bottom of this. Something is very wrong here, and we need to address it.

It is also true that a disproportionate number of people in my district who are African American have been affected economically. The worst thing we can do for them back in the spring of this year was to shut down the American economy, shut down our society, and shut down our schools.

There is no question that African Americans in my district were disproportionately affected when their jobs were wiped out. Small business people, African American small business people, lost their businesses as a result of it. And all children went home when they closed the schools, but some children had parents in households that could support them while they were trying to learn from home, and far too many African American children didn't.

So the best thing we can do here in Washington, besides trying to get to the bottom of what has happened here on the public health issue, is to get the American economy going again, because, without it, I am afraid we are only going to make inequality worse in this country.

You know, a lot of people, including a lot of people in my district, just can't do the jobs that they were trained to do on a Zoom meeting from their home. They just can't do that. When we take their jobs away from them, we take their opportunity away from them.

So, Mr. Roy, I would like you to discuss the pre-COVID–19 Trump economy's effect on disparities between White and minority unemployment rates in this country.

Mr. ROY. Thank you for the question.

So, as I mentioned in my oral and written testimony, before the pandemic, the disparities between the White and Black unemployment rates and the disparity between White and Hispanic unemployment rates had reached record lows, along with, as you know, the overall unemployment rate reaching record lows. And so that was something that I think we all could have taken the opportunity to celebrate at the time. Whether we did or not, I don't know. But those disparities have come back in tremendous force since the lockdowns have occurred, and you have all seen the charts from BLS that show this data very clearly.

And so that is—and what is interesting, too, by the way, is, if you look at Asian Americans, Asian Americans, for most of the 21st century, have had lower unemployment rates than Whites, but, as a result of the economic lockdowns, that completely changed. Now Asian unemployment is much, much higher than the White unemployment rates.

So that is a really useful, in a sense, illustrator of how the racial disparities that have been created by the pandemic as opposed to the structural racism legacy in slavery and segregation type issues that we have been discussing as well.

Mr. BYRNE. One of the things I have also noticed, Mr. Roy, is there has been an uptick in mental health issues as a result of lockdown. Do you have any information about how that uptick in mental health issues has affected minority communities?

Mr. ROY. Well, it is a huge problem in so many different dimensions, right? You have people who are already fragile from a mental health standpoint who are being pushed over the edge, and then you have ordinary people who are—who had what we might call median or normal mental health prior to the pandemic who are struggling now, and there is all sorts of ways this can happen, right?

You have the people who are in isolation, in their homes, not merely in terms of—in terms of their employment. You have people who may be in very crowded living facilities. This is particularly true, for example, in New York City, where people who live in intergenerational households with maybe three generations or more living in the same space are at greater risk of transmitting COVID–19, let alone having potentially mental health challenges.

So—and that is disproportionately a minority, particularly disproportionately immigrant phenomenon both in the United States and elsewhere.

So there are lots of things to be concerned about.

Mr. BYRNE. Last question is this: What is the effect of shutting down schools? What is the effect on minority kids?

Mr. ROY. Yeah. I mean, that is one of the most—the most difficult things to understand from a science standpoint, why we have been so aggressive at shutting down schools.

Shutting down schools can work with influenza because influenza does kill young people, but COVID–19 is not influenza. It is a very different disease that seems to largely spare younger children. And so, if you look at countries that have reopened their schools, in Europe and Western Europe in particular, they have done pretty well with school reopenings, and we should learn from their example.

Mr. BYRNE. That is great. Thank you very much.

And thank you, Mr. Chairman. I yield back.

Chairman SCOTT. Thank you.

The gentleman from the Northern Mariana Islands, Mr. Sablan?

Ms. Wilson? The gentlelady from Florida, Ms. Wilson?

The gentlelady from Oregon, Ms. Bonamici?

Ms. BONAMICI. Thank you, Mr. Chairman and Ranking Member Foxx and colleagues, thank you for the kind words of sympathy.

Thank you to our witnesses for being here for this important conversation.

I want to note I am a bit concerned about the suggestion that this is somehow a nursing home issue. Just a couple days ago, there was an article in Politico looking at a Harvard analysis of National Center for Health Statistics data, particularly focusing on the disparity in the Latinx community, and this is what it said: The danger is elevated, especially among younger minorities. Latinos age 35 to 44 have a coronavirus mortality rate nearly eight times higher than White people in that age group. And Black people in the same age range have a mortality rate nine times higher than White people. The inequity persists with Latinos age 25 to 34 and those 45 to 54, who have a coronavirus mortality rate at least five times higher than Caucasians.

So I am concerned that this is somehow an issue talking about what is happening in nursing homes, which of course is a concern.

I want to follow up on Secretary King's comments about childcare and early childhood education. We know the childcare sector already faced serious challenges, not just here in Oregon but across the country. There was a vast unmet need, high cost for families, and also insufficient compensation and benefits for early childhood educators.

Fixing the childcare system is important to children. It is important to families, and it is important to the economy, but it is also an issue of racial justice. As Secretary King recognized, the childcare workforce is overwhelmingly women and predominantly women of color. There are many barriers, especially with the children of color least likely to be put in supported childcare settings.

So we have some work to do. We need to make sure that resources are equitably distributed, and we need a dual focus. We need to stabilize the system, but we also need to vastly improve it. I recently released a report, Childcare in Crisis: Solutions to Support Working Families, Children, and Educators, in which I call for the passage of both the Childcare is Essential Act and the Childcare for Working Families Act, which together represent a critical Federal investment in the childcare sector that also advances equity.

Secretary King, how would you or how would providing equitable access to high-quality childcare and early childhood education benefit children and society as a whole, and what are the repercussions, particularly for low-income children and children of color if we continue the status quo?

Mr. KING. Thanks so much for that question. You know, the Nobel Prize-winning economist James Heckman has written about the return on investment on early childhood education that you can get a seven-to-one, eight-to-one return on investment because students who get high-quality early childhood education are more likely to rise from kindergarten prepared academically; they are more likely to graduate from high school; they are more likely to go on to college; and they are more likely to have long-term economic success; and, James Heckman has shown, long-term health benefits from having participated in quality early childhood education.

So the potential returns to an investment like the Childcare for Working Families Act is quite powerful and ought to be a rationale for bold action at this moment.

If we fail to invest in early childhood, what we know is you see the achievement gap already present in kindergarten—kids who are holding the book upside down because they are so unfamiliar with letters. We know there are a lot of folks who won't be able to go back to work if the childcare sector collapses, and that will disproportionately harm low-income communities and communities of color.

Ms. BONAMICI. I appreciate that.

And, Secretary King, I actually quote Professor Heckman in my report that I just released for that very reason, that this is a good investment that actually pays for itself over time, but also really gets our children, who are our future, off to a great start.

Dr. Wilson, Secretary King gave a compelling testimony about how harmful gaps in access to high-quality education affects longterm outcomes for children of color, and yet, as you note, educational attainment is not enough on its own to bridge the divide. So educational attainment is enormously important, but why is it insufficient in itself to close labor market gaps for workers of color?

Ms. WILSON. So educational attainment is important because it provides mobility. There is no question that a worker with a higher level of education is more likely to be employed and have higher wages than one with less education.

The problem that we see in the labor market is that, at the same level of education, we see disparities in employment as well as wages. And, in fact, over the last 40 years or so, the wage gaps— racial wage gaps have actually grown the most among the most educated workers in our economy.

So that raises another question of what is going on here, and I think it raise the issue of what we are here to discuss today, the role of racial discrimination and racism in creating unequal outcomes in our economy.

Ms. BONAMICI. So the Federal role in education is about [inaudible] as chair of the Civil Rights and Human Services Subcommittee, I intend to continue addressing it, and I yield back the balance of my time.

Thank you, Mr. Chairman.

Chairman SCOTT. Thank you.

The gentleman from Wisconsin, Mr. Grothman.

Mr. GROTHMAN. Thanks for having me.

It is a little bit difficult to be on here because it kind of appears in this committee we are supposed to always kind of look at people racially and just not look at people as people. So I have got to kind of switch my mind set for this committee.

First thing for Mr. Roy. Today—I don't know if you had a chance to look at it, but, yesterday, we had a total of 267 lives lost due to the COVID, which is, while not good news, is the lowest we have had since March 23rd. And I feel good about it because a lot of the so-called experts in the public health field were predicting disasters as States opened up their economy. But, instead, we have 267 lives. We have, I believe, now 10 days in a row of under a thousand lives lost. So it seems as though the so-called experts have rarely been so wrong.

Do you want to comment, Mr. Roy, on the fact that we only had 267 lives lost?

I am relying on the Worldometer website, which is what a lot of people tell me to look at because it has been cited nationwide. Do you want to comment on the relatively small number of deaths now that we have had so many States open up their economies compared to where we were a month ago?

Mr. ROY. Yes, Mr. Grothman. All of your points, I agree with. Both, there has been a precipitous decline in the daily death rate, and the predictions of what the death rate would look like today after States reopen their economies by certain experts were completely wrong—completely wrong.

And, by the way, we should emphasize that the impact of those experts' advice on low-income Americans, including minority Americans, has been disproportionately harmful.

Mr. GROTHMAN. Okay. You think we should be in the future a little more jaded about the public health establishment?

Mr. ROY. Well, here is the thing. You know, it is like CBO estimates. You can have a lot of expertise on the subject genuinely and still get predictions wrong. Predictions are not facts, and I think what happened here is you had a lot of people making educated guesses to the best of their ability, we might say, but they were just guesses, and yet we were expected to treat those guesses like they were certainty.

Mr. GROTHMAN. Thanks. My own personal weighing in, my little world that an individual Congressman gets, is there is a growing body of information that the way to avoid COVID is to have more vitamin D in your body, or at least there is a strong correlation between vitamin D and not getting the COVID. Are you familiar with that sort of thing, and would it be—perhaps be better off when we—rather than analyzing the chance of getting COVID by race, analyzing the chance of getting COVID by the amount of vitamin D in your body?

Mr. ROY. Well, as you know, correlation is not causation. The reason I mention that in this particular context is we don't know if the better response of people with high vitamin D is due to the presence of vitamin D or the fact that they are outdoors more. And what I mean by that is, if you are outdoors and you are exposed to sunlight and you are not in closed, confined areas with people who are COVID infected, that seems to be a major vector of transmission. Outdoor infection or transmission seems to be very, very low. But if you are in an enclosed space like a subway in New York City, for example, or a small apartment with the three generations of your family, that tends to be where the transmission occurs, or a nursing home, for example.

Mr. GROTHMAN. Okay. So you would say that a lot of this advice—at least in the State of Wisconsin, we were getting advice to stay indoors, lock yourself away. That was exactly the opposite of the advice that we should have been giving people?

Mr. ROY. In fact, it is quite possible that the lockdowns worsened transmission of COVID–19 by forcing people indoors and preventing them from being outdoors more and therefore being around other transmitters of the disease less.

Mr. GROTHMAN. I don't like to talk about race, like I said, but vitamin D, is there any difference by race that you are aware of?

Mr. ROY. Yeah, I don't know the data well enough to comment. So I will leave that one for now.

Mr. GROTHMAN. Some of my colleagues talked about difficulty getting into college racially and such. I know here, in the State of Wisconsin, very, very—maybe a smaller people of—percentage of color than normal, I am under the impression talking to people at our university systems, they already go out of the way through affirmative action to try to push more people of color into the universities. Is that typical around the country—

Mr. ROY. Well, you know—

Mr. GROTHMAN.—or is that just a Wisconsin thing?

Mr. ROY. It is difficult, but, you know, I will mention, as this came up earlier in this hearing, I am coming to you from Austin, Texas, and the University of Texas actually has a very interesting model in which they take the top—I think it is the top 10 percent of students from every high school in the State and guarantee them admission at the University of Texas.

And what that does is that allows you to find the high-achieving students in every high school, even if that high school is in a disadvantaged area. I feel like that model could be used more widely as an alternative to a form of race-based affirmative action.

Mr. GROTHMAN. Thank you for having this, Mr. Chairman.

Chairman SCOTT. Thank you.

Next, gentleman from California, Mr. Takano.

Mr. TAKANO. Thank you, Mr. Chairman. I thank you for this very important hearing on how COVID–19 has increased racial inequities in the country.

The shift to distance learning has exposed the educational inequities many students of color have been facing for decades as States start to open back up and grapple with the depleted budgets. It is the role of the Federal Government historically to ensure equity in every sector. And, recently, many competitive colleges, like the University of California's system, private schools such as Harvard University, have suspended the use of ACT and SAT scores in their admissions process to help level the playing field.

Mr. King, from your experience, how much of the college admissions process is reliant on these test scores?

Mr. KING. Yeah, well, there is no question that reliance on SAT and the ACT creates a disadvantage for students who have had less access to quality K through 12 preparation. There is also some evidence to suggest that those assessments, the more they are relied upon, the fewer Black and Latino students will be admitted.

But one worry I have, as folks move to test optional, is that just changing the use of test scores is unlikely to produce the kind of increase in Black and Latino representation that we ought to see, and so it is important that universities also take other steps. Financial aid is critical, making sure that resources are available to support students as they come to campus. It is critical that colleges and universities consider race as they are making admissions decisions. It is critical that they reach out to high schools that are in high-needs communities so students know about the opportunities. So the test optional piece can be a part of a package of efforts that would produce more diverse classes.

Mr. TAKANO. Well, Mr. King, do you believe that, you know, we have an opportunity here with SATs and ACTs now being very difficult to obtain because, of course, it is inadvisable to test large numbers of students in congregate settings—and I don't think it is—they found a way to do testing remotely for security purposes and integrity of the test. Is there an opportunity to reexamine college admissions generally?

Mr. KING. Yes. I mean, what I hope colleges and universities will do is look at their entire admissions process and ask what more could they do to make sure that they have a representative class— more low-income students, more students of color, more first-generation students. And they ought to consider not only the role of tests; they ought to also consider the role of extracurricular activity. They ought to credit the student who worked in their family's bodega each night the same way they credit playing on the lacrosse team, for example.

Mr. TAKANO. You know, unfortunately, you know, many of our— well, they—many schools will have IB programs, AP programs. Of course, these programs also rely on some form of testing. But I am worried about those schools that don't have, you know, a history of strong curriculum and that universities may be looking and favoring students who come from schools with a history of, you know, teachers who can teach these curriculum, which often aren't offered to low-income and minority students.

Mr. KING. That is exactly right. Black and Latino students are significantly underrepresented in access to AP and IB, and it is a problem both across schools and within schools. So students of color are less likely to be in schools that offer those courses, but, even when they are in schools that offer those courses, they are underrepresented relative to their percentage of the population.

We know that issues like implicit bias affect who gets referred to those courses. There are some States that are moving to an automatic default enrollment of students who qualify to try and reduce the role of implicit bias and perhaps teacher recommendations in the enrollment in those courses.

Mr. TAKANO. Of course, you know, I have long thought about how do we have an alternative to access to higher ed where the gateways are kind of characterized by testing, different kinds of admissions testing. I have long been interested in concurrent enrollment strategies, such as early college high schools. You know, what do you think about, you know, alternatives such as that?

Mr. KING. Yes. Dual enrollment, we know from large-scale studies can increase the likelihood that students graduate from high school and go on to college. So we ought to invest in dual enrollment. The challenge is the districts that need those dual enrollment programs the most are the ones with the least resources, and so we really need that infusion of additional dollars for K-12 and the higher-ed institutions that serve high-needs communities.

Mr. TAKANO. It does take resources to make sure that they have the teachers who are qualified to teach those courses, who know about the pedagogy. These school systems will need support in implementing the strategies of dual enrollment in early college high schools.

Mr. KING. That is exactly right. And we know that low-income students and students of color are disproportionately enrolled in the districts that are getting the least resources, and that is likely to get worse as States have to make huge cuts as a result of the COVID–19 economic crisis.

Mr. TAKANO. Well, you talk about maintenance of equity requirement. What do you mean by that? Well, we won't have time. I guess I will yield back, but wonderful to talk to you, Mr. King. Thank you so much.

Mr. KING. Good to see you.

Chairman SCOTT. Thank you.

Next, gentlelady from New York, Ms. Stefanik?

The gentleman from Georgia, Mr. Allen?

Ms. FOXX. Mr. Chairman, I just want to say Ms. Stefanik had to step out to another [inaudible] so thank you.

Chairman SCOTT. Thank you. I have been advised that she had to leave, but I wanted to call her name just in case she had gotten back in.

Mr. ALLEN. All right, sir. Can you hear me?

Chairman SCOTT. Mr. Allen from Georgia?

Mr. ALLEN. Yes, sir. Can you hear me?

Chairman SCOTT. I can hear you.

Mr. ALLEN. Great. Super.

Thank you for holding this hearing today, and one of the things that I brought up in the last hearing and I wanted to make sure that we, you know, had some feedback on this, is that, you know, in 2018, our Federal spending was about $4 trillion; discretionary, which is about 30 percent, is $1.2 trillion; mandatory was $3.8 trillion.

And then, in 2020, that has gone up substantially. We are at about $3 trillion in mandatory; $1.485 trillion in discretionary. And so it has gone up about $500 billion. And, you know, my question is simply this, and this is to Mr. Roy: We have spent about almost $4 trillion since COVID–19, and of course you have heard mention the HEROES Act here today, which is an additional $3 trillion, which would just about triple or more than triple discretionary spending. Mr. Roy, have you looked at the situation as far as discretionary—as far as this spending goes and its impact on the people of this country that are taking on—I have never liked debt. Obviously, I don't mind doing, you know, debt when you have collaeral and that sort of thing, but it looks like, to me, that we are on a downward spiral that is not going to be good for anybody in this country.

Can you comment on that, Mr. Roy?

Mr. ROY. Well, Mr. Allen, it is interesting because, tomorrow, I am actually testifying before the House Budget Committee on this very topic, how the combination of congressional spending and, of course, declining revenue from the lockdowns is going to lead to a massive explosion of the deficit this year.

And, by the way, all that does is move closer to us the ultimate fiscal reckoning, which will happen, when we have to crash Federal spending in order to deal with the fiscal crisis when nobody wants to buy Treasury bonds when the U.S. is insolvent.

And who will that harm? That will most harm the people who most depend on public assistance, public spending: Medicare, Medicaid, Social Security.

So, the more we destabilize our fiscal situation, the more we are putting at risk economically vulnerable populations.

Mr. ALLEN. You know we have had to deal with COVID–19 crisis and the next it looks like, if we don't do something about it, do you believe that fiscal crisis is coming upon us and coming upon us rapidly?

Mr. ROY. Yeah, I mean in both directions, right? Who knows? We can never predict when the fiscal crisis will come from the debt that we are piling on year after year, but we know it will come because of the laws of math, the laws of economics. We don't get an exception from those laws in the United States.

Mr. ALLEN. Exactly. And really the only way to overcome where we are is a strong economy. You know, as far as the workers that were affected or the workers that benefited from our strong economy which just three months ago was $22 trillion, going on $23 trillion, who benefitted the most from that strong economy?

Mr. ROY. Low-income Americans, minorities. As I mentioned in my written testimony, the disparity between the White and Black unemployment rates, the disparity between the White and Hispanic unemployment rates were at record lows prior to the pandemic and those disparities have now widened. The lockdown is driving those disparities.

Mr. ALLEN. As far as the biggest issue—and we have just got one minute to answer this question. The biggest issue I hear in my district is people who are on unemployment, including the $600 bonus, don't want to return to work. And there is a lot of animosity between the employers and the employees about returning to work. Have you looked at how this is affecting folks going back to work and rebuilding this economy?

Mr. ROY. There is no doubt that the $600 bonus is retarding the recovery, even in those States that have reopened, because people have a powerful economic incentive, and you can't blame them for it, a powerful economic incentive to stay on the sidelines.

So I would love for Congress to revisit that piece of legislation and reform the bonus so it is more targeted to the people who truly need the help.

Mr. ALLEN. Good. And, of course, the liability question is the other issue that we have got out there as far as employers worried about liability and bringing their employees back to work as far as lawsuits.

Mr. ROY. Yes.

Mr. ALLEN. What is your take on that?

Mr. ROY. It is absolutely a very important problem and if Congress sees fit to pass some sort of safe harbor to enable people to go back to work and for employers to reopen their doors, I think that would be very, incredibly important.

Mr. ALLEN. Right. Thank you, Mr. Roy.

And I yield back.

Chairman SCOTT. Thank you.

The gentlelady from North Carolina, Dr. Adams.

Ms. ADAMS. Thank you, Mr. Chairman. Thank you, Ranking Member, for convening this hearing today.

And to the witnesses, thank you for your testimony.

The HEROES Act requires OSHA to issue a temporary—emergency temporary standard that requires employers to develop and implement an infectious disease plan to protect workers from exposure to the coronavirus. This provision also makes it a violation of the OSHA Act to retaliate against workers for raising concerns to the employer or to the government about inadequate infectious disease protections.

Dr. Wilson, in your expert opinion is an enforceable safety standard a necessary step to economic recovery or would it, as opponents contend, impede economic recovery?

Ms. WILSON. I think it is a necessary step to economic recovery. As I mentioned, ensuring the health and safety of American workers and communities across the country are a critical step in building a solid recovery. We know from surveys that about 60 percent of those who work outside of their home express that they have concerns about contracting coronavirus. Among workers of color, Black and Latino workers in particular, that is closer to, like, 70 percent of those workers expressing concerns, in addition to the fact that they express greater concerns about retaliation as a result of speaking up against that.

So it is very important that the workers, as workers go back to work, have frontline workers who are already out there, that workers are empowered to advocate for touching on their own personal health and safety, as well as the health and safety of American workers.

Ms. ADAMS. Thank you very much.

According to research from the Brookings Institution, we can expect nearly 40 percent of borrowers to default on their loans by 2023. Now that doesn't even begin to recount for the impact of the COVID crisis, and to me this indicates a student loan default crisis.

And so as we know, certain students are at greater risk of default. The study finds that the rate of default for students at all-for-profit schools is almost four times that of students who attend community colleges.

Meanwhile, Black borrowers who completed a bachelor's degree default at five times the rate of White borrowers who complete their degrees and are even more likely to default than White borrowers who leave college without a degree. I am concerned that the student loan default crisis will worsen in the wake of COVID–19.

Secretary King, what can you tell us about those who struggle most to pay back their loans? And what do you see COVID–19, how do you see it impacting these struggling borrowers?

Mr. KING. Thank you, Congresswoman.

Certainly the racial wealth gap is driving the degree to which Black students are disproportionately likely to default on their loans at every income level. Even at the highest income level, Black students are some seven times as likely to default as White students.

The key is to provide targeted debt relief to try to address this and to ensure that college is more affordable. You look at the amount of the cost of attending a public college that was covered by Pell Grants in 1980. It was some 80 percent. Today that is down to 28 percent. We need to make sure that college is affordable for all students, and that investment in higher education will have long-term benefits for our economy.

Ms. ADAMS. Okay. Great. That was going to be my last followup question. What can Congress do? I believe you have answered that.

Again, thank you very much for your work. Thanks to each of our individuals who came and testified.

Mr. Chairman, I am going the yield back.

Chairman SCOTT. I thank you.

The gentleman from Pennsylvania, Mr. Smucker.

Mr. SMUCKER. Thank you, Mr. Chairman.

I appreciate this hearing on this important topic. I would like to thank, Mr. Roy, you for being here today. I really value your insight on these matters for not only the extensive research work that you have done, evaluating economic policies, but also your ability to speak to the healthcare impact, given your medical background.

So I want to go back to the discussion around the disproportionate deaths in nursing homes. My district is home to a high number of senior housing facilities, nursing homes, assisted living facilities, and other seniors, elderly residential communities. My State, Governor Wolf in Pennsylvania, was one of five governors who made the devastating decision to force nursing home to take COVID-positive patients.

Now think about this, and you mentioned this earlier. Many nursing homes were not in a good position to handle infection, to prevent the growth of infection. They were also at capacity. So I talked to nursing home workers and administrators who are extremely frustrated when they were at 98 percent capacity in one case, very difficult to isolate patients and so on. And we were moving patients. The governor was moving patients to the nursing homes when the hospitals were virtually empty and were best equipped to handle this.

The impact in Pennsylvania has been devastating. Nearly 70 percent of the deaths in Pennsylvania have occurred in nursing homes. To date, 6,400 deaths, 6,426 deaths in Pennsylvania, 4,389 of those were in nursing homes. To make that decision worse, at the same time the governor was not adequately prioritizing nursing homes for PPE. They were receiving PPE only after hospitals had what they needed. So, it was devastating.

Mr. Avery—or Mr. Roy, I should say. I am sorry. 4,389 deaths in nursing homes in Pennsylvania, how many of those can be attributed to that disastrous policy?

Mr. ROY. Well, Mr. Smucker, good to see you.

I don't know the answer to that because we have to look facility by facility and really do a retrospective analysis. I hope that those analyses are done by researchers as time goes on, we have more time to look at this particular problem. But as you say, it is a catastrophe.

Sixty-eight percent of all deaths in Pennsylvania are in nursing homes and yet—and by the way, the one thing that is really important to mention here is this was not some, oh, boy, you know, look at what happened here, you know, we shouldn't have done that.

At the time that Governor Wolf put this order into effect, at the time that Cuomo and Murphy and Whitmer and the other governors put these orders into effect, the nursing home community was up in arms, fighting these orders, arguing that they would devastate the facilities.

Mr. SMUCKER. You are exactly right. I talked to them. I was talking to them at the time. They were desperate for help, and it was in Pennsylvania and not New Jersey where the Secretary of Health quietly removed her own mother from a nursing home in the midst of this crisis. Think about that. Took her mother from a nursing home, despite moving patients to nursing homes and really simultaneously telling millions of Pennsylvanians that it was safe to keep your loved ones there. It is incredibly frustrating, and it makes me angry to understand what has happened here in Pennsylvania.

One of the things I haven't heard, and I am wondering if have you any information on this. Can you shed any light on disproportionate impact of nursing home residents who are minorities? Are there more minorities who have died in nursing homes as well as in the general population?

Mr. ROY. As I mentioned in my written testimony, we have tried to do that work. So we have done some basic correlations, a regression analyses of racial demographics at the State level and nursing home fatalities. At the State level we don't see a correlation. What we are hoping is that with the new CDC—excuse me—CMS data that is nursing home by nursing home and county by county, we can see if there are more correlations at the county level and at the facility level. But we don't know yet.

Mr. SMUCKER. One of the other—and I am running out of time quickly but we have continued to be in a lockdown and a shutdown in Pennsylvania for an extraordinarily long period of time. How do you think that would have changed, had we given adequate consideration to how many of the deaths were being—we were seeing them in nursing homes?

Mr. ROY. I mean, this is the two—the two points that I really want to drive home in this hearing. The first is that we didn't do enough to protect people in nursing homes who are disproportionately non-White.

The second thing is in a State like Pennsylvania where 70 percent or 68 percent of the deaths are happening in nursing homes, that means that the risk for the average Pennsylvanian who is not in a nursing home, the 99.4 percent of Pennsylvanians who don't live in nursing homes, their risk is cut by two-thirds which means you can do more to reopen the economy where you are opening schools safely for those individuals and we have unnecessarily harmed those vulnerable populations with lockdowns.

Mr. SMUCKER. Thank you.

Chairman SCOTT. Thank you.

The gentlemen from California, Mr. DeSaulnier.

The gentleman from New Jersey, Mr. Norcross.

John, you are muted.

Mr. NORCROSS. How is that?

Chairman SCOTT. You are good.

Mr. NORCROSS. Thank you.

First of all, Chairman, thank you for holding this. Ranking Member Foxx, good to have you on board.

I do want to follow up on a couple of items that we have talked about. I keep hearing about the fiscal health of our country. Obviously very important and for those who are discussing the debt, apparently that wasn't an issue when they gave away $1.3 trillion to top 1 percent which now shows it is not paying anywhere close and the unfunded war.

And that is what I was bringing up. If we were in a war, would we talk about the debt? No, we would do what we have to do as a country. And we are in a war except it is the virus.

Nursing homes, I keep hearing, are forced to accept people. So do hospitals. The difference is nursing homes were not prepared. Nursing homes, who take into consideration medical conditions, they didn't have the PPE. They didn't have the respiratory items in their atrium and HVAC systems. And the idea of saying they— the workers can only work in one nursing home. Pay them a living wage, and then they wouldn't have to go nursing home to nursing home.

So with that being said, I just want to talk about schools. When we look at what is going on—and I know my colleague just talked about the OSHA standards. Right now they are only guidelines.

Dr. Wilson, can you talk about the difference that schools, particularly in the areas with challenges to the budget, urban areas, that they are not getting direction now. If you have a standard, which we have talked about quite a bit here, we would know how to prepare for it.

We are in June, July, August, the construction period for schools. Yet we are not seeing schools follow any standards. Come the end of August, beginning of September, kids are coming back.

What is going to happen if they don't have their facilities set up for this COVID? Dr. Wilson?

Ms. WILSON. So I think that is a question that most of us don't look forward to seeing the answer to, for schools and facilities that are unprepared to welcome back students in large numbers, as well as teachers and faculty and staff.

So having the standards in place so that students are safe, so that teachers and staff are safe, is essential to reopening. That is a part of our recovery. Part of the recovery is about people having confidence that they can safely return to work, safely return to school, safely return to their way of living without putting their health at risk.

Mr. NORCROSS. Because right now, as I understand, most schools, they are 6 feet but they are not giving any guidelines. Many States have something call public OSHA which is determined by the State. Yet even those States aren't accepting these standards.

Do you see, come September, when the children go back, what confidence will parents have that the school is ready for it?

Ms. WILSON. Yeah I don't know that parents will feel very confident in sending their students back to school if we don't have consistent, enforceable standards that are in place, again, to protect the students, to protect the teachers, and protect other staff at the schools.

Mr. NORCROSS. So what we see is we heard about Safe Harbor and that discussion can happen. But, without any standards, everybody is doing their own thing. The lawyers are going to have a field day.

For those who are focused more on the economy than the people you represent, I just want to say one thing. There is an old saying. Those with the most toys or money when they die win. It doesn't matter how much money you have if you die.

I yield back.

Chairman SCOTT. Thank you.

The gentleman from Indiana, Mr. Banks. The gentleman from Indiana, Mr. Banks.

The gentleman from North Carolina are, Mr. Walker. The gentleman from North Carolina, Mr. Walker.

The gentleman from Kentucky, Mr. Comer.

The gentleman from Idaho, Mr. Fulcher.

The gentleman from Kansas, Mr. Watkins.

The gentleman from Kansas.

The gentleman from Texas, Mr. Wright.

The gentleman from Pennsylvania, Mr. Meuser.

Mr. MUESER. Thank you, Mr. Chairman. Thank you to all the witnesses for being here with us.

Mr. Roy, data suggests we had the strongest economy in 50 years prior to the COVID epidemic, pandemic. Does the data also support that this economy was very beneficial for low-income and minority Americans?

Mr. ROY. Yes, sir. The unemployment rate for African Americans, the unemployment rate for Hispanics, the unemployment rate for minorities overall was at record lows prior to the pandemic.

Mr. MUESER. Would you say during the course of the improvement in our economy that was the most significant improvement economically for Americans including low-income and minority workers?

Mr. ROY. Well, having the economic—having the unemployment rate at record lows is obviously an important achievement. It is not the only thing we have to do to ensure that all Americans prosper. Of course, we have to bring their incomes up, their wealth up, and things like that but certainly we were headed in the right direction.

Mr. MUESER. Right. Does the data projections suggest a safe opening will have dramatic improvements for low-income Americans and minorities?

Mr. ROY. Certainly I think the dispersion of policy responses we are seeing now, so, again, if you would compare Florida which never locked down very severely and then reopened early on relative to other States, the economic performance of all people and certainly of economically vulnerable populations is much greater there than elsewhere.

Mr. MUESER. Okay. So safe opening of schools, safe opening of small businesses very important for our overall economy but very important as well for low-income and minorities.

Mr. ROY. Especially so. And by the way, this is not just a 2020 thing. If you look historically at anytime in which we have had a severe recession, whether it was the early—recession of the early 1980s or the recession of 2008, minorities and low-income Americans were always the ones who were most harmed. Economic growth helps economically vulnerable people more than it helps the people who are already prosperous.

Mr. MUESER. Right.

So small businesses and particularly schools are very concerned about liability, once opening. Passing liability reform to hold harmless schools and businesses, I am told by schools, is critical. So a liability reform bill would be very important for low-income and minority students as well as workers.

Mr. ROY. It is essential. It is arguably the most important thing Congress can do. Obviously a lot of reopening policy is done at the State level but Congress is in a position to Act on this liability issue and it is arguably the single-most important policy we need to get the reopening, safe reopening to work.

Mr. MUESER. Right. You would also, I think, agree that a transportation infrastructure bill would be very important for all Americans including minority and low-income?

Mr. ROY. I think it depends on the details but, yes, you know, it would be useful particularly when it comes to, when you think about public transportation and the sanitary concerns of public transportation, that is something we need to address.

Mr. MUESER. You are a data-driven individual. I just want to ask about the nursing homes, your thoughts there. I am in Pennsylvania and, yes, we have—it is actually more than 70 percent. It is about 71, maybe 72 percent of our fatalities were in nursing homes. You stated 68 percent, but that might change on a daily basis.

When there was the Washington State and other areas in early March, we saw fatalities occurring, the corona just running through some of those nursing homes and seeing the fatalities, I mean, how can you—how can it be explained that two weeks after that on March 18th that some States, again, including Pennsylvania, ordered patients from the hospital with corona back to a nursing home and, as Congressman Smucker said earlier, meanwhile the nursing homes were at capacity, very limited space, and the hospitals were at 20 percent capacity maybe.

How can you explain that? How could somebody see the data and make that decision?

Mr. ROY. Well, it was clearly a reckless and catastrophic decision. I mean, what they would say, you know, in hindsight, I suppose, what Andrew Cuomo, for example, would say or Governor Wolf might say is, "Well, we were worried that the hospitals would get overwhelmed with COVID patients. That is why we wanted to force the nursing homes to accept the least severely ill of those actively infected COVID patients."

But that was a terrible—that was a completely wrong way to think about it because, if you were worsen the disease in nursing homes, you are going have more people come to the ICUs and more people come to the hospitals because the people who are most at risk of dying and being severely ill is the nursing home population. So they had their thinking backwards, but I think that was part of the thought process.

Mr. MUESER. Thank you.

Mr. Chairman, I yield.

Chairman SCOTT. I thank you.

The gentlelady from Washington, Ms. Jayapal.

Ms. JAYAPAL. Thank you, Mr. Chairman.

I have very surprised to hear some of the comments here around lockdown somehow harming our efforts and COVID, given that Washington State was the first State to have a case and we have managed it remarkably well through aggressive lockdown policies. I think the data has really shown that this was exactly the right approach.

Mr. Chairman, I wanted to focus my time today on people of color and healthcare. We know that people of color are disproportionately on the front lines as healthcare workers, janitors, postal service employees, and farm workers and that people of color are overrepresented among COVID–19 cases with Black Americans nearly four times more likely to die from COVID–19 than White Americans, and Latinx people comprising a greater share of COVID–19 cases than their share of the population in 42 States. They have allowed us, frankly, to stay safe while they have been risking their own lives and yet we continue to fail communities of color by not ensuring equitable healthcare for all.

We know that people of color disproportionately lack access to healthcare, representing over half of America's uninsured population.

Dr. Wilson, why do people of color disproportionately lack access to healthcare?

Ms. WILSON. I mean, a lot of the disproportionate lack of access to healthcare is related to the fact that, for so many of us, health insurance is connected to employment and we know that there are persistent disparities in the labor market, both in terms of employment outcomes but also in terms of the kinds of jobs and positions that people hold and the disparities that exist across those different kinds of occupations, whether you are a full-time employee or a part-time employee, et cetera.

So between those disparities in employment, on top of the occupational segregation that tends to put workers of color in occupation where they are less likely to have employer-provided health insurance, all of that contributes to these overall disparities in health insurance.

Ms. JAYAPAL. Thank you.

And, you know, I think that the crisis has made it clear that we have to address these inequities through untethering of healthcare from unemployment. What other steps, Dr. Wilson, should we be taking right now in the midst of this pandemic to address inequities and access to healthcare?

Ms. WILSON. I think it is important that we consider how in the current situation that we can make universal coverage available to everyone. That would include people not having to pay additional monies to be tested or to get treatment for COVID–19.

This is a unique situation that we find ourselves in. And it is important that people have the confidence to go and get the care, treatment, and testing that is so essential, not only for fighting the virus but also for building a solid recovery.

Ms. JAYAPAL. Thank you, Dr. Wilson.

I think that, you know, this pandemic has made it clear that when some members of our communities are excluded from equitable access to necessary resources and services, it hurts us all and I think the pandemic, obviously, you know, free testing, treatment, and any eventual vaccine for COVID–19 is critical.

But as more and more people lose their employment, lose their source of income, 44, almost 44 million Americans without—that have filed unemployment claims and 27 million minimum that have lost their healthcare, the reality is that they also have other healthcare needs that are going to need to be covered.

And that is why I have introduced the Medicare Crisis Program Act which would expand Medicaid eligibility to those who are uninsured and extend Medicare to recently unemployed individuals and their households during the COVID–19 crisis.

Dr. Wilson, should access to healthcare be tied to employment? How does this—who does this benefit and who does that leave out?

Ms. WILSON. Again, when we are talking about what needs to be done to make sure that we are living in a more equitable society, the fact that there are clear and persistent racial disparities and gender disparities in labor market outcomes suggest that necessarily tying health insurance to employment is not the best way of achieving a more equitable solution to the lack of health insurance unless we are also addressing those underlying disparities in the labor market.

Ms. JAYAPAL. Thank you so much for your testimony and for your work. I don't think anyone can make the case that the current healthcare system is working for us. I think COVID–19 has provided the clear case that when healthcare is provided by an employer and somehow tethered to your work, access to that healthcare is just as volatile as your employment status.

And so we are, you know, working very hard to rectify that and we must boldly call out the systemic inequities in our healthcare system and achieve health justice as a meaningful and necessary step towards racial injustice and in my view the best way to do that is to provide universal healthcare coverage for everybody from the Government, as so many other countries do.

Thank you, Mr. Chairman.

I yield back.

Chairman SCOTT. Thank you.

I notice the gentleman from Kansas has returned.

Mr. WATKINS. Yes, Mr. Chairman. Thank you.

Chairman SCOTT. Mr. Watkins, you are recognized for 5 minutes.

Mr. WATKINS. Thank you, Mr. Chairman. I appreciate it. And thanks to the panel for your insight, and it is so extremely important right now.

Mr. Roy, the CBO estimates that we may never return to the record low unemployment rates of recent years. I believe we can safely get people back to work faster than economic estimates. But what is your sense of how quickly jobs can return?

Mr. ROY. I think many jobs can return quickly. What I am more concerned with is not so much jobs returning quickly. I think a lot of jobs can return quickly as the economy reopens. I mean, I think there are certain sectors that are going to be more challenging, right? Hospitality is going to be more challenging. Bars are going to be more challenging. Airlines are going to be more challenging. But the bulk of the economy I do think can come back.

The one thing I worry about a lot is consolidation. We have had small businesses get absolutely crushed because they don't have the cash reserves and the leverage to stay afloat if we are going to lock down the economy for this long.

And I fear what we are going to see is a lot of big box, large, multinational corporations fill up the space that small businesses and entrepreneurs are not able to fill because they are more economically unstable.

Mr. WATKINS. Yeah. Thank you.

And Mr. Roy, we are beginning to understand the dramatic impact of COVID–19 and all the impact that these State-imposed lockdowns have had on the American work.

How damaging were State-imposed lockdowns, and can you comment on what the impacts were on small businesses versus large businesses?

Mr. ROY. So in the paper that I have mentioned that is in our— included in our written testimony on how to reopen the economy, we document a lot of the research that is out there on the fact that small businesses on average have about 28 days of cash in reserve if they don't have any revenue. And for certain types of businesses like restaurants, like retail shops, like repair shops, it is more like two weeks. So those businesses basically have gone belly-up. Over 100,000 small businesses have closed permanently as a result of the crisis. And the number, the true number, may be much, much higher.

So it is a serious problem and, you know, again, in terms of how we can get the economy back on track, the reopenings, the States that have reopened have shown a rebound, a pretty rapid rebound for the most part with the exception of some of the sectors I mentioned.

Mr. WATKINS. Okay. Thank you.

And obviously you mentioned that limiting companies' liability is such a critical component. Is there a precedence that I can look back to, to serve as maybe a baseline to understand effective policies?

Mr. ROY. You know, I am sure there is, Mr. Watkins. I would have to go back and look myself to see the one that really makes sense here. So I don't have a good answer for you on that right now.

Mr. WATKINS. Sure.

And, Mr. Roy, you mentioned earlier in response to Dr. Foxx that the Tax Cuts and Jobs Act, the deregulation, they were few of the main reason for such a strong economic—such a strong economy and that low unemployment before COVID–19. Can you expound upon that and touch on how we can continue to grow these policies and how could these policies help our economy bounce back in response to this downturn?

Mr. ROY. Well there is so many things to say about this. Of course, we don't have time to go through them all.

The regulatory initiative has played a big role. The Tax Cuts and Jobs Act, particularly reducing the corporate tax rates to a level that is more competitive with other countries meant that a lot of multinational countries that were moving jobs out of the United States to other countries like Ireland and Canada, are moving those jobs back to the United States.

Mr. WATKINS. Understood.

Thank you.

And, Mr. Chairman, I yield the balance of my time.

Chairman SCOTT. I thank you.

And I notice the—

Ms. FOXX. Mr. Chairman, I know you have favored the gentleman from Virginia before but today you are disfavoring him. You keep skipping over him and I have to speak up for him because he has been with us from the beginning and you have gone over him about four times.

So the next time you recognize a Republican, I would ask that you come back to Mr. Cline.

Chairman SCOTT. Thank you. I appreciate that. I apologize to my distinguished colleague from Virginia.

The—I notice the gentlelady from Florida has returned, Ms. Wilson.

Ms. Wilson, you are recognized for 5 minutes.

Ms. WILSON of Florida. Thank you so much, Chairman Scott, for your extraordinary leadership and Ranking Member Foxx for holding this hearing to investigate how the COVID–19 pandemic has widening racial inequities in education, health, and the workforce.

I want to thank all of the witnesses for their testimony today and this hearing, like others, challenges us to make more critically—to think more critically about the impact of systemic racism in our Nation. This is necessary if we are to move this country closer to the more perfect union spoken about in the preamble to our Constitution.

We must acknowledge the role that race plays in the distribution of wealth and benefits in this country if we are to ever address it. Part of that acknowledgment comes in the form of pointing out the disparity impact that catastrophic events have on Black and minority communities.

Many of us have heard the old saying that when America gets a cold, Black America gets pneumonia. Well, that happens to Black America when America has a pandemic and disproportionately negative health outcomes, disproportionately negative education outcomes, disproportionately negative employment outcomes.

So, I have a question. And my question is for Dr. Wilson. In the aftermath of the Great Recession, you and your fellow economists sounded alarm about elevated levels of long-term unemployment which disproportionately affected African American workers.

What is long-term unemployment, and do we need to be afraid that long-term unemployment will surge again among workers of color in this crisis?

Ms. WILSON. Thank you for that question.

Long-term unemployment is defined by people being unemployed for 26 weeks or longer. We saw extended—higher rates of longterm unemployment and extended durations of unemployment during the Great Recession because of the length of time it took for the economy to fully recover, thus reaching communities of color later in that recovery as opposed to sooner.

I think when we look at our current situation, it is reasonable to have concerns about whether we are going see that same kind of pattern. Looking at just one month out of data that we saw in May where the Black unemployment rate ticked up slightly where the overall unemployment rate actually declined suggests that recovery may not be as even as the initial impact that the pandemic had on the economy.

The long-term employment and the evenness of recovery are both issues that are important to keep our eyes on.

Ms. WILSON of Florida. What policy solutions can prevent longterm unemployment, particularly for workers of color, Black workers, Hispanic workers?

Ms. WILSON. So in order to prevent long-term unemployment, it is essential to get the economy reopened and people back to work as safely and quickly as possible. Prioritizing full employment, both in terms of monetary policy decisions as well as fiscal policy decisions, are things that can help with that.

Targeting efforts to create jobs in underserved communities where rates of unemployment are chronically and consistently much higher are ways to address both the public health issues, as well as the job issues.

Ms. WILSON of Florida. As you have pointed out, Black and Hispanic workers often continue to experience recession-level conditions long after the overall unemployment rate drops below 4 or 5 percent.

After the Great Recession, Black and Hispanic questions suffered for years after the economy appeared to be fully recovered for White workers. Thinking ahead to this economic recovery, I am curious whether you believe the Federal Reserve and policymakers need to shift how we define full employment. What effect could shifting this measure have on racial equity for workers?

Ms. WILSON. I think in order to more accurately evaluate slow employment, we have to consider the disparate rates of unemployment that exists across different communities. It goes beyond looking at one number, NAIRU, for example, that has consistently overestimated where unemployment should be in order to have a full and equally shared recovery.

So it requires that we pay attention to what is going on in different communities, and full employment cannot be declared until we see recovery happening in all communities, regardless of race, ethnicity.

Ms. WILSON of Florida. I yield back.

Chairman SCOTT. Thank you.

And now the distinguished gentleman, my distinguished colleague from Virginia, Mr. Cline.

And I apologize for skipping over you.

Mr. CLINE. Mr. Chairman, it is fine. I have been enjoying the conversation.

I just have a couple of questions for Mr. Roy.

You know, here in Virginia, our governor has placed quite a few restrictions on places of work and, you know, settings from state to state, workplace settings vary greatly with respect to how much risk of COVID–19 spread exists for workers and for customers.

Have these differences, the restrictions the different States, have they contributed to the impact of COVID–19 on minority communities and have the restrictions recognized these differences and should States continue to refine these restrictions based on the actual risk that is present?

Mr. ROY. Well, you know, one great example of this, Mr. Cline, is the towns that are on the border between Virginia and Tennessee. As you know, because Tennessee has pursued a policy of opening, they have also done a far better job of controlling the spread of COVID–19 in nursing homes but they have also had a much more open economy.

And So in Tennessee we are seeing much better performance for economically vulnerable population and also for medically vulnerable population, a much better performance than Virginia, all the way around. And yet Virginia is continuing to lock down, and I would say one of the most aggressive States in the country in terms of economic restrictions relative to their actual public health utility.

Mr. CLINE. Thank you. We are hoping that we can see some loosening of those restrictions and some improvements in economically vulnerable areas of the State. And I think that goes to your point.

Another question relating to higher education. Some students are really yearning to participate in the normal on-campus college experience. What should these students be aware of as they head to school in a couple of months, and what can they do to minimize the risk of contracting the coronavirus? And as a follow-up, how can students diminish the likelihood of passing the virus on to older family members that they have at home?

Mr. ROY. Another great question. This is something that is going to be part of the forthcoming report we are putting out at FREOPP on reopening schools and including postsecondary educational facilities.

So one thing that is important here is you want to obviously adjust campuses to have a little bit more physical distancing and that means maybe some students, particularly for most colleges, you don't have to have everyone in the dormitories. Most colleges, in fact, don't have enough housing space to house most of their students.

So allowing students and enabling students to come to classes from home is going to be very important, particularly those who are in more vulnerable populations.

On the flip side, maybe have you a student who needs to live in the dormitory because that is a way of avoiding or being around their grandparents or other at-risk individuals.

So it is important for the housing policies of universities and colleges and other postsecondary facilities to take that into account, to take the individual risks of students into account.

Obviously you want to be careful and you want to be safe, particularly around older faculty members, older members of the staff but in general people in the age bracket of colleges are at very, very low risk of severe illness and mortality from COVID.

And I would recommend to this committee, if members haven't already reviewed it, the testimony to the Senate Health Committee from Purdue President Mitch Daniels which was very compelling on all these points.

Mr. CLINE. I appreciate that. We have—not only does the Sixth District have more colleges and universities than any other congressional district, save one district up in Boston—I am not sure if it is Congresswoman Trahan's or a different one but we also have James Madison University in Harrisonburg which is a coronavirus hotspot.

It is going to be a scenario when they return to campus where there is going to have to be a lot of education and really a lot of work on the part of the whole community to ensure that the community stays safe and our efforts to bring the numbers down continues aggressively.

So thank you for your answers to those questions.

Whatever time I have remaining, I am happy to yield to the ranking member.

Ms. FOXX. I want to thank you.

Mr. Roy, as you mentioned in your written testimony, low-income students and students of color have experienced disproportionately negative impacts through closures. Given the body of research showing improved educational outcomes for participants of Choice Programs and their overwhelming bipartisan support among the public, do you think Congress should examine ways of examining school choice as we consider the possibility of future aid packages?

Mr. ROY. Yes. I mean, there is a lot of things to consider here. One is that school choice can be useful in allowing students to have in-person instruction in less hotspot areas. So if you live in an area where the pandemic has had an outbreak but you need get an education, school choice might allow you to get that education somewhere else.

Also one thing that is very important as a component of choice is not just choice of your school but choice in a particular class. For example, maybe there is a student who is really, really good at math but his own high school doesn't have the capacity to teach him, say, AP Calculus but he can through a virtual modular educational choice have the ability to get that instruction from a different school or a different teacher.

So there are a lot of different elements of disaggregating school choice into a broader concept of educational choice and our scholar at FREOPP, Dan Lips, has been one of the pioneers in that area.

Ms. FOXX. I would like to note that Tom Sowell has a wonderful editorial in the Wall Street Journal about the importance of school choice for minority and low-income students.

Thank you, Mr. Chairman.

Thank you, Mr. Cline.

Chairman SCOTT. Thank you.

The gentlemen from New York, Mr. Morelle.

Mr. MORELLE. Thank you so much, Mr. Chairman.

Mr. Chairman, I want to not only thank you for today but your leadership throughout the pandemic and for providing this committee with yet another opportunity to continue the critical work through these virtual hearings and briefings. So I very much appreciate all the work that you and your staff have done and just wanted to acknowledge that.

Since March, our Nation has faced insurmountable challenges and heart-wrenching losses. You know, the virus doesn't play by clear rules. So for months we have really largely relied on reacting to this unprecedented crisis to support our communities and our constituents.

But now, as we are regaining footing in many places, we have a very real opportunity, it seems to me, and a responsibility to take sort of intentional and preemptive action to safeguard the Nation, especially communities hardest hit by the pandemic against further fallout.

So, and there is no doubt, I mean, obviously we have talked about it at some length today, the racial and ethnic inequities that have existed for generations but the virus is now bringing that into stark relief and demonstrating how much our Nation—to our Nation how deep these inequities go.

I want to point out just a the bit of data from a group called Common Ground Health which is a not-for-profit in Rochester and the Monroe County Public Health Department. Here in Rochester we have four times the rate of infection, over five times the hospitalization rate, and two and a half times the mortality rate among our Black citizens and people of color in our communities. The statistics are unacceptable and they represent the deeply entrenched inequalities, inequities, and barriers to communities of color.

So as we have discussed in the hearing today and the hearing last week, the depths go deep. Last week we talked about education and the inequities in our educational system which are staggering, the digital divide, how difficult it is, how unprepared and underresourced many of our institutions serving low-income students are.

So with that in mind, you know, as we begin to rebuild our community, it is critical we look at recovery through the lens of addressing these underlying social determinants of health, education, and economic stability.

I had a couple of questions. Before I do that, I do want to acknowledge my good friend, Mr. King. He was, before Secretary of Education, was the Commissioner of Schools, the Commission of Education in the State of New York and he and I worked on many projects together. I wanted to acknowledge him and thank him for being here, as well as the other panelists. I do have a question for former Secretary King.

But before I do that, Dr. Jones, you had mentioned during your testimony that you essentially invited a questioner to ask about an allegory which helps talk about structural racism. I don't think anyone has done that. So if you don't mind, I would like to hear that, if you have a moment here to go through that.

Dr. JONES. Yes, I will do it very quickly, because I know you also wanted to ask a question of the Secretary.

So, this is an allegory, like most of them, that is based on something in my own real life that happened. The moral is that racism exists. Some—when I was a medical student, I was studying long and hard one Saturday with some friends. We got hungry. I had no food in the apartment. We decided to go into town and find something to eat. We find a restaurant. We walk in. We sit down. Menus are presented. Order – we place our order. Food is served. Not a remarkable story yet.

But as I sat there with my friends, eating, I looked across the room and I noticed a sign at the time. It was a startling revelation to me about racism. So, now I have intrigued you. What did the sign say? The sign said "Open." And if I hadn't thought anything more about it, I would have assumed that other hungry people could walk in, sit down, order their food, and eat.

But because I knew something about the two-sided nature of those signs, I recognized that now indeed because of the hour, the restaurant was closed, that other hungry people just a few feet away from me but on the other side of the sign would not be able to come in, sit down, order their food, and eat.

And that is when I understood how racism structures open/close signs in our society. It structures a dual reality. And for those who are sitting inside the restaurant at the table of opportunity, eating, and they look up and they see a sign that says "Open," they don't even recognize that there is a two-sided sign going on because it is difficult for any of us to recognize the system of inequity that privileges us.

It is difficult for men to recognize sexism, et cetera, et cetera. Yet those on the other side are very well aware there is a two-sided sign going on because it proclaims close to them they can look through the window and see people inside, eating.

So, for those inside the restaurant who asks, “Is there really a two-sided sign, does racism really exist,” I say I know it is hard for you to know when you only see ‘open’. In fact, that is part of your privilege not to have to know. But once you do know, you can choose to act. So, it is not a scary thing to name racism. It is an empowering thing.

It doesn’t even compel you to act but does equip you to act so that if you care about nose on the other side of the sign, which is an “if,” you can talk to the restaurant owner who is inside with you, say, “There are hungry people outside. Open the door. Let them come in. You will make more money or the conversations we can have.”

Maybe you will push food through the window or maybe you will try to tear down that sign and break through the door but at least you won’t be sitting back, “Huh, wonder why don’t those people just come on in and sit down and eat,” because you will understand something about that two-sided sign. I won’t go any more deeply into it. Thank you for asking.

Mr. MORELLE. Yeah. Thank you. I know my time has expired. So I will have to wait and get Mr. King and Dr. Wilson and I have other question for you, Dr. Jones, but I will yield the balance of my time. I appreciate very much all the panelists and the work they are doing.

Chairman SCOTT. Thank you.

The gentleman from South Dakota, Mr. Johnson.

Mr. JOHNSON. Thank you, Mr. Chairman. I appreciate it.

Mr. Roy, I was intrigued by the conversation that you and Mr. Cline were having about reopening in the fall and best practices. I think your answer focused—and Mr. Cline’s line of questioning focused largely on the collegiate system. Let’s talk a little bit the K-12 environment. If you were giving advice to school board members or administrators who wanted to make sure they reopened in an appropriate and safe way in the fall, what guidance would you provide to them?

Chairman SCOTT. Mr. Roy, you are muted.

Mr. ROY. Excuse me for that. I am sorry.

As I mentioned in my testimony, we have a paper forthcoming on this topic, which I am happy to share with you once it is out. It should be out in a few days.

The one thing I—let me start with one thing which is we are going to have to make some accommodations for people who can’t physically attend school. So if you are a child who lives with your grandparents or you have other at-risk individuals in your household, those are individuals that we are going to need to have stay at home.

There may be teachers who are elderly or otherwise at risk who similarly will need paid leave or other accommodations.

But leaving those two things aside, okay, so then what do you do for those particular individuals? One thing that we have been working on with some my co-authors with certain States is at those State-level, centralizing the virtual curriculum so that you don't leave the burden on an individual school district to create the virtual curriculum that runs in parallel to the in-person curriculum. Have that done at the State level so that if are you a student who does need to stay at home, there is—that process is scaled up more and leverages the resources of the State rather than at the district level.

And then for the people who do live—who are able to go to school, there is a lot—I think we can be more confident that the risk of transmission is low.

One thing I should mention by the way that I haven't mentioned yet is that we have a lot of research from outside the United States, in particular, that shows that transmission of COVID–19 in children is very, very low.

For example, in Iceland they did a study of the entire population of Iceland and found that there was not a single incident of a child transmitting COVID to his or her parents which is pretty remarkable if you think about it, given that live together and are around each other all the time.

So that gives us a lot of confidence that children are not vectors of transmission and that means a lot of precautions that schools are making regarding, well, we are going to only have classes of six people, say, or all the desks have to be, you know, 6 feet apart, we don't necessarily know if that is true. And I think there should be some flexibility in school districts to take that into account.

Mr. JOHNSON. Thank you very much, Mr. Roy.

And I would, Mr. Chairman, I would like to yield the rest of my time to the ranking member.

Ms. FOXX. Thank you, Mr. Johnson.

Mr. Roy, let's follow up on Mr. Johnson's questions. I think it was a good one.

As these restrictions are being raised, they are very blunt instruments. Everything shuts down. They are being lifted now. How should States and cities approach their decisions to lift restrictions and allow businesses and schools to reopen while keeping people safe? It is a very instructive example you gave us from Iceland.

Mr. ROY. Yeah. So we know that, for example, or at least there is a lot of evidence now that is accumulating that children are not vectors of transmission which should give us more confidence when it comes to reopening childcare centers and K through 12 schools and even, the you know, potentially postsecondary college instruction.

We have to do obviously do more research to confirm this, but we have very good reason to believe that would work.

And as I also mentioned, a lot of European countries—Germany, Switzerland, Austria—I could go on—have reopened schools without an impact on their caseload, their hospital load, et cetera, from COVID–19.

So all that seems to indicate that your vulnerability to COVID–19 is related to your—the nature—to the degree to which are you a vector of transmission. And so, again, for all those reasons, I think we have a reason to be hopeful and optimistic that younger populations can go back to work and also younger workers can go back to work.

So when it comes to reopening workplaces, I think one thing that States can do is think about industry, sectors, businesses in which the workplace is disproportionately younger because those are things you can bring back more quickly for States that are in the more hesitant cap.

Ms. FOXX. Thank, Mr. Johnson.

Thank you, Mr. Chairman.

I yield back.

Chairman SCOTT. I thank you.

The gentlelady from Pennsylvania, Ms. Wild.

Gentleman from California, mister—

Ms. WILD. I am here.

Chairman SCOTT. The gentlelady from Pennsylvania, Ms. Wild.

Ms. WILD. Thank you, Mr. Chairman. It took me a minute to unmute.

This questions is for Dr. Jones. Dr. Jones, only eight of the 60 retail drive-through COVID–19 sites that have opened as a part of the presidential administration's public-private partnership are located in Black communities. A company in my congressional district has received grant money for the development of rapid self-COVID tests and at-home tests.

How important is it that the Federal Government permit these tests to be purchased over the counter and without a prescription, and subsidize the cost of these tests and/or somehow make them free, and also require that insurance covers these tests with no cost sharing and that we protect and fund the U.S. Postal Service so that people can receive these rapid at-home tests without traveling to the store? That is a multipart question but kind of all part of the same piece.

Dr. JONES. Right. Well, it is very that important we increase testing in communities that have been the hardest hit. So, that is the first thing. I actually haven't researched the new at-home tests that you are talking about.

I would say that other additional ways to support testing and communities is to work with community organizations, to work with the why, to work with others who are placed in the community for even coming and because I don't know. So, I don't know about that particular test but I think there is something—

Ms. WILD. And just to clarify, the test is not yet available. The company is in the North Shore in my district and they are working on it and developing it but it is anticipated that it will be available later this year.

Dr. JONES. But I don't that think it should be, oh, if the test— center is not in your neighborhood, you are going to have to default to a home test. I think we need to make sure we have the same level of testing availability in all of our communities and perhaps more in the hardest hit communities.

So, nothing good or bad about that test. That doesn't answer the question of why do we not have more testing in our most heavily hit communities. And so, we need to have different partners, different strategies. We need to invest in, you know, minority-owned businesses in those communities to do the testing.

Because it could be that if you do your home tests, that—something about the connection about when the communication, when should you go based on what result, how should you pursue extra care might be lost. So, yes, good for that but not as a substitute.

Ms. WILD. Thank you very much. That is very helpful.

I would like to direct the next question to Dr. King and, Dr. King, if you could, I want to make this quick but we know that even before COVID struck, far too many students were leaving college before earning their certificate or degree and that this has been disproportionately likely to occur between low-income students and students of color.

I am deeply concerned that with the health pandemic that the small progress that we may have made on increasing the rate of college completion is going to be—is going to vanish.

Could you discuss the inequities in college graduation rates among different types of students and whether we have actually made progress in closing that completion gap among low-income students and students of color?

That is to Dr. King.

Chairman SCOTT. Dr. King, are you still on mute?

Ms. WILD. Did we lose Dr. King?

Mr. KING. Not on mute. Can you hear me?

Ms. WILD. Now we can.

Chairman SCOTT. Dr. King, are you still on mute?

Ms. WILD. Did we lose Dr. King?

Mr. KING. Not on mute. Can you hear me?

Ms. WILD. Now we can. Yes, thank you.

Mr. KING. Okay. That is good.

So we absolutely have significant disparities for low-income students and students of color in completion, and we know that some of that is driven by financial gaps. So those students are more likely to be negatively impacted by loss of employment, change in their family's financial situation. They are particularly vulnerable if their universities are struggling financially, which is the case for many of our public institutions, particularly as States look to make cuts as a result of the COVID–19 crisis.

So we need resources, but we also know that targeted investments like the CUNY ASAP program, which has doubled completion rates in community colleges through a mix of financial support and better advisement, those can make a huge difference and actually lower the per-graduate costs in the long run if we make those kinds of investments.

Ms. WILD. Thank you very much.

With that, I yield back, Mr. Chairman.

Chairman SCOTT. Thank you.

The gentleman from Pennsylvania, Mr. Keller?

Mr. KELLER. Thank you, Mr. Chairman, and thank you to the ranking member and our panelists today.

Mr. Roy, I just wanted to cover a couple things. I know a lot has been discussed about the nursing homes and what happened in my State of Pennsylvania as far as how it affected, while our population in nursing homes is relatively smaller, assisted livings, and the deaths are relatively high.

I take a look at them, and we have discussed on that side of it, but how did the other 45 Governors in the States that handled it better—were they looking at different information, or what do you think might have led them to make decisions that protected that population versus the Governors in like Pennsylvania and New Jersey, California, that had the problem with the deaths in these facilities?

Mr. ROY. Well, you know, I mean, I wouldn't want necessarily at this point in time rank Pennsylvania's Governor, you know, 45th or 47th or 40th. You know, I don't know that we can do that at this point, but I would say that, in terms of the States—let's put it this way. The States that have done the best—and I will use Florida as an example. What Florida did early on—their health secretary, Mary Mayhew, was very aggressive in resisting hospitals that were lobbying actively to have the permission to discharge COVID-infected patients—to offload them into nursing homes, and Mary Mayhew fought them on that very hard.

It was not an easy decision to fight the hospitals, which are very powerful lobbies in every State, and say, "No, you are not going to take those patients and get them out of your hospital and stick them in a nursing home as seeds because then you are only going to get more patients in your hospital with COVID later."

So she was aggressive about that, and she was also aggressive about limiting and restricting visitation rights, which of course is heartbreaking, right? If you had a loved one in a nursing home, you would want to go see them. You want to make sure they are okay. And that was a very difficult and painful decision that Florida did take early on that protected that population far better than other States did.

Mr. KELLER. Okay. Thank you. But one other thing I want to talk about—and it goes to my experience of having worked in a factory and later ran that larger manufacturing facility, and employers care about their employees, and they can actually keep them safe. We look through this whole pandemic and the shutdowns of larger operations, retailers, so on, being able to stay open, yet smaller businesses, which we know, in our small businesses, were more adversely impacted, which—whether it is minority businesses, but you know they were. So, you know, is there any reason to believe that the small businesses can't practice the same guidelines given the rules by CDC and so on that the larger retailers were able to do during the time that the economy was shut?

Mr. ROY. Well, you know, when it comes to—if you are referring to the fact that, in certain States, large retailers were allowed to open, but small retailers were not, absolutely that was an asymmetry and a terrible policy because those small businesses are the ones that make—help communities thrive, that help provide competition, that help provide lower cost to the consumer, for all different reasons, let alone the employment piece. It is really important to have those small businesses competing with the larger businesses.

So absolutely they have the capacity to, and we are seeing that in restaurants. For example, in Austin, again, where I live, Texas has allowed restaurants to open up to a certain point, and every restaurant cares about not just its workers but also its customers, to make sure that they have the confidence to patronize that restaurant knowing that it is going to be safe, that they are doing what they can from a cleanliness point of view. So businesses have the—have a powerful incentive to not only ensure that their employees are safe but that their customers are safe, and that is far more powerful than any government mandate.

Mr. KELLER. I agree with you on that, and I think that is part of the reason why we should look at some kind of liability protection for these businesses. That way, people can make the decision whether or not they feel safe patronizing a certain business, whether it be a restaurant or a retail operation.

The other thing I guess I would look at because we always talk about—you know, I have heard it talked about any kind of resurgence of cases when we start to open our economy, and we always talk about the positive cases and everybody is talking about how many more cases there are. But we are doing a lot more testing.

Is there another metric that we can look at to make sure that we are understanding the spread of this disease, maybe like the percentage of cases that are positive, you know, so that we sort of understand and make decisions based on good rational information?

Mr. ROY. Well, Mr. Keller, I am so glad you brought this up. This is such an important point.

We are seeing a rise in cases, and that is, in part, driven by the rise in testing, right? If 5 percent of people test positive and you double the number of tests, you might have double the cases, but we are not seeing a corresponding spike in deaths, and that is because a lot of the people who are testing positive at this point in the pandemic are less medically vulnerable. Either they are relatively younger people, or they just don't have as many preexisting conditions, like heart disease, high blood pressure, diabetes, et cetera.

So we don't yet know exactly because we don't have that granular level of detail, but we do know that the death rate from the cases we are seeing now appears to be significantly lower, and that is not surprising because, in pandemics of all kinds, what you see is that the most vulnerable people die first, and then the virus starts to affect less vulnerable people who don't die at the same level of frequency.

Mr. KELLER. Thank you, and I yield back.

Chairman SCOTT. Thank you.

The gentleman from California, Mr. Harder?

The gentlelady from Georgia, Ms. McBath?

Mrs. MCBATH. Thank you, Mr. Chairman, and thank you so much to our guests who are joining us here today. Thank you for joining us to talk about these very pressing issues.

And I just wanted to be completely clear. COVID–19 did not create these inequities that we are talking about today, but it simply has revealed, you know, long-borne suffering of the minority communities in America. Disparities in health, education, and the workforce are symptoms of years of racism, restrictive access to services, and high rates of poverty, and these symptoms are manifested in poor outcomes and are present in every part of American life.

As we learned from last week's hearing on the K through 12 funding, budget cuts due to COVID–19 will disproportionately impact students in lower income school districts where Black and Brown students make up a larger share of the student body. Students of every background absolutely, unequivocally deserve better.

A recent study showed that Black populations are at least 3.5 times more likely to die by COVID–19 than their White neighbors, and the Hispanic population is at least 2.5 times as likely to die.

It is incumbent on every member of our body, every member of this body, every citizen of the Nation to take seriously what we are witnessing before our very eyes, whether Democrat or Republican, whether you are Black, White, or Brown. It is time for all of us to take seriously the challenges that we are facing.

Dr. Wilson, my question is for you. There is a section that you entitled in your report that states—and I quote—the fallacy of race-neutral policy is further exposed by COVID–19. And why, in your observation, have race-neutral policies failed to offer genuine solutions to all the inequities, and what is an example of this failure in the COVID–19 area?

Ms. WILSON. So I think that the issue of race-neutral policymaking ignores many of the disparities that I highlighted in my testimony today that you just cited and ignores the fact that, even if a policy on its face is race neutral, meaning that it doesn't reference race in any way, it will not have race-neutral effects because the structures and systems in this society are not race neutral.

So any policy—every policy that is debated and passes day after day is going to have an effect on the way that [inaudible] income, wealth, and opportunity will flow. That is no different from our current crisis.

We have talked a lot about the efforts to slow the spread of the virus immediately by shutting down and the disparate effects that has had on workers of color who already faced higher rates of unemployment, who already had lower incomes, lower levels of wealth, and other kinds of financial resources that are critical for people to be able to weather this economic downturn.

So even when we implement a policy that is good for the Nation as a whole in terms of the public health and safety issues, because of these underlying disparities in health as well as wealth and other economic outcomes, we get these very different results in terms of how it impacts communities [inaudible].

Mrs. MCBATH. Thank you. Even within my own community—I represent Georgia's Sixth Congressional District—there is a North DeKalb portion of my district that—I see it as plain as day, the inequities within that portion of my district, the disparities of the largest cases of people that we have that have contracted COVID–19, and the largest numbers of individuals within my district that have been seriously affected and have even died have been in the part of my district that has the most number of diverse individuals and diverse people within the community. So thank you for that.

Thank you for your answer. These problems are enormous, and they continue to really raise the disparities that we see every single day, but no problem is greater than the American spirit, and I know that Americans have never shied away from a fight. I know that we will continue to work as hard as we possibly can, and we face no greater challenge at this point than creating a more equitable and free society.

And so this is my challenge to every one of my colleagues and all of my neighbors, to think very seriously about the type of society that you want to live in, the type of society that you want your constituents to live in. It is one where those with the least suffer the greatest in times of tragedy. Is that what we want? I don't think so.

So where whole parts of this great Nation are neglected and feel that they have no value, they deserve better, and so are we going to continue perfecting this union looking always toward the future and fight for a society that strives towards justice and equality. I would ask that of all my colleagues today.

Thank you, Mr. Chairman, and I yield back the balance of my time.

Chairman SCOTT. Thank you.

Dr.—gentleman from North Carolina, Dr. Murphy?

The gentleman from New Jersey, Dr. Van Drew?

The gentlelady from Washington, Dr. Schrier?

Ms. SCHRIER. Thank you, Mr. Chairman, and thank you to our witnesses.

I first wanted to make a quick comment, mostly to Mr. Roy about schools, simply because the vast majority of people commenting about schools say that we really don't know the role of children and transmission. We know they get it less often. We know they don't really have symptoms, but it is still kind of a big black box that we really won't know until schools open.

I also wanted to say that there is a general understanding that kids are better off in school. I don't think there is any question about that. They are barely affected, at least acutely. We don't know about long-term outcomes, but there is no question there.

The problem is that United States is not Iceland. The United States is fatter, less healthy. We have more type II diabetes. We have more kidney disease. We have more heart disease, all of the conditions that put you at much higher risk for this disease. Not just that, but kids who need most to be in school come from the families who we are talking about today that are at most risk of getting this disease and dying from it, and so I just wanted to clarify that point as a pediatrician.

I wanted to direct my question today to Dr. Wilson, because I— my district has a large Latino population, and we have seen them disproportionately hit by this disease, first because of working conditions that we have talked about, which are more crowded, fruit packing, agricultural jobs. But then, because 80 percent of transmission happens in the home and homes are more crowded, we have seen a greater amount of community spread.

Now, not just that. Since housing is part of how COVID is spread, we have always known that housing is tied to health outcomes, and in recent weeks, we have been talking about how housing is really fundamental to building wealth, building that nest egg, and achieving security. And I was wondering, Dr. Wilson, can you talk about housing, the changes we could make, perhaps even the difference between policies that help with rent versus the policies that help with ownership and the long-term outcomes of a change in policy there?

Ms. WILSON. Thank you for those questions.

Again, the structures and patterns that we observe in terms of housing access and housing affordability are directly related to a long history of policies that excluded certain populations—in particular, people of color—from building wealth through home ownership but also concentrated people and isolated people, economically and socially, in communities where the quality of housing was lower, the stock of housing was less available, was lower, thus driving up the cost of housing in many of these communities.

So I think that policies that address issues of affordability as well as housing quality are an important step in addressing the inequities that we see in terms of housing. They also spill over into unequal outcomes in health, as you indicated, as well as in employment and schooling.

Ms. SCHRIER. Thank you. I had another question about paid leave, sick leave, family leave, that we are finding that these same communities are really affected by not having the same access to leave, and then, also, if they are then in close proximity to people who are infected, they might need several series of quarantine time off, and I wonder if you could speak to we passed Families First to get 2 weeks of sick leave and to have up to 3 months of paid family leave, but what happens in these particular at-risk communities when you have to take time off, perhaps multiple times, when multiple close colleagues at work get this disease and you need to quarantine?

Ms. WILSON. So the connection between lack of paid leave and these other outcomes really puts workers in an impossible situation to make very difficult choices, in choosing between their health or their economic well-being. Without paid sick leave, workers forego earnings that are essential and critical to the economic well-being of their households because they are making decisions that are better for their health.

So by having paid sick leave more equitably and more broadly available to more workers, we really empower workers to make the kinds of decision that are best for optimizing both their health security as well as their [inaudible].

Ms. SCHRIER. Thank you very much, and I yield back.

Chairman SCOTT. Thank you.

The gentlelady from Illinois, Ms. Underwood?

Ms. UNDERWOOD. Thank you, Mr. Chairman.

The coronavirus pandemic has left no corner of our communities unscathed. Lives and livelihoods have been lost in my district in northern Illinois and in communities across the country, which is why I am also concerned with Mr. Roy's comments about the role of children as carriers for COVID–19.

There is a lot that we don't know, and the current guidance from the Centers for Disease Control and Prevention does point out that children are, in fact, at risk of infecting—I mean, at risk of contracting the disease, and could possibly be carriers. And so I think that, when we are addressing the United States Congress, we should continue to have fact-based findings to present to the committee, and then also make sure that we are encouraging the American people to consult with the national experts on this issue, which is the Centers for Disease Control and Prevention.

The damage from this crisis has not been inflicted evenly across our communities. The pandemic inside this pandemic is the disproportionate health and economic consequences of COVID–19 for communities of color, particularly Black Americans.

A recent Brookings analysis found that Black Americans between the ages of 65 and 74 are dying at five times the rate of their White counterparts, and the disparities are even larger for young adults. These racial graphs are glaring, but they are not surprising. They reflect a deeply entrenched racial inequity throughout our healthcare system, and one of the key drivers of these disparities is unequal access to care.

The uninsured rate for African Americans is more than 1.6 times higher than the rate for White Americans. To reduce disparities in health outcomes for both COVID–19 and other conditions, we must expand access to affordable healthcare, which is why I introduced the Healthcare Affordability Act, which would provide advance premium tax credits to more Americans and increase the size of those credits.

Dr. Jones, enhanced premium tax credits will bring affordable health insurance within reach for millions more Americans. How will expanded access to affordable healthcare reduce racial disparities in COVID–19 hospitalization and death rates?

Dr. JONES. So, it is very important. It is very important that we have access. And that is one of the ways that you value all of your people equally. So, if we really do care about those people, then we need to take away any kind of economic barriers.

I would also say that the healthcare system is the last-ditch salvation, so we need to make sure that last bit is there, that ambulance at the bottom of the cliff is there, but I would also say that does not absolve us from addressing—health is not created within the health sector, so we need to do that.

We need actually to strengthen—in all the ways that you said, to strengthen the ACA, to actually get to universal access, the high-quality healthcare, perhaps lower right now—

Ms. UNDERWOOD. Thank you.

Dr. JONES.—to make the age of Medicare eligibility and all of that.

Ms. UNDERWOOD. Thank you. Thank you. As the cofounder of the Black Maternal Health Caucus, I have been committed to reducing the alarming disparities in maternal health outcomes. In addition to introducing the Black Maternal Health Momnibus Act of 2020 with Congresswoman Alma Adams of this committee, I have also supported bipartisan efforts to extend Medicaid coverage from 60 days to 1 year postpartum.

Dr. Jones, recognizing that Medicaid covers more than 65 percent of African American births, can you describe the full importance of extending Medicaid coverage for a full year postpartum to close racial gaps in maternal health outcomes?

Dr. JONES. Well, because the maternal mortality rate difference between Black folks and White folks ranges from three to eight times, depending on what part of the country—

Ms. UNDERWOOD. That is right.

Dr. JONES. —the numbers of our mothers who are dying within the first year of childbirth is alarming. So, we do need to support them in all the ways that we can.

Ms. UNDERWOOD. Yes. It is about saving lives.

Dr. Jones, beyond extending postpartum Medicaid coverage, why do we need maternal health policies like the ones we included in the Momnibus, to improve data collection, [inaudible] social determinants of health, and provide targeted investments to improve Black maternal health outcomes?

Dr. JONES. We need to know what the problems are. So, we need to have our maternal mortality review committees with all of the data that they can have. We need to be able to list social determinants of health as risk factors—

Ms. UNDERWOOD. Yes.

Dr. JONES. —so, we can address them.

Ms. UNDERWOOD. Thank you. As we speak, scientists are working tirelessly to develop a safe and effective vaccine for COVID–19, yet the development of a vaccine is only the first step. We are going to need to rapidly deploy to every community across the country, and it needs to be done in an equitable way, and we know that African Americans currently have lower immunization rates than their White counterparts.

I am going to submit some questions for the record on that issue. I would like to thank the chairman for having this hearing and this opportunity to discuss these issues of critical importance.

As the committee knows, I am a public health nurse. We need to end these racial disparities in healthcare, whether it is COVID related or in our larger healthcare system, and make sure that, as we are communicating with the

American people during this pandemic, we are lifting up fact-based, evidence-based information to inform the American people.

And I yield back. Thank you.

Chairman SCOTT. Thank you.

Gentlelady from Connecticut, Ms. Hayes?

Mrs. HAYES. Thank you, Mr. Chair, and thank you to all the witnesses who are here.

Today, like I felt in so many other committees, I have just been listening and really just been overwhelmed, because I recognize that, once again, so many of my colleagues just don't get it. I, too, like the gentleman from Wisconsin, look forward to a time when people don't look at me racially and we don't have to deal with these issues in this way.

Last week, in this very same committee, we had a hearing about shutting down schools and what the budget cuts would look like after learning loss, but my response to that is so much bigger than just how our economy looks and how we are going to deal with these things economically. I can assure you, everyone on this committee, when my husband was diagnosed with COVID–19 and I stood over him waiting for his chest to rise to ensure that he was breathing, never once did I think about his job. Never once did I think about the economy reopening. I thought about my husband getting healthy, and I thought about us being safe.

So I—in that same vein, I am thinking, as we look forward to September and our schools open up, I was on a call last week with FEMA, and they indicated that they have no intention of supplying PPE for our schools. I live in a State that is already disproportionately impacted and has some very large equity gaps. In Fairfield County, 84 percent of our students graduate high school, and less than 5 miles down the road, in Bridgeport, about 74 percent of our students are high school graduates, and a parent was sentenced to 12 years in jail for what they called stealing education for sending her child to a school outside of their district. But that is how desperate people are to provide a good education for their children in this State.

Dr. King, it is so good to see you, and you opened up your comments with something that, as you know from prior conversations, is so near and dear to me, and that is the Brown v. Board of Education decision. And, like it, don't like it, whether it is uncomfortable or not, we have racial and equity disparities in our schools, in our public education system, and we as a committee have the ability to change those things.

As we look forward to September, Dr. King, can you talk a little bit about—I mean, we have heard about maximizing testing and opening earlier to make up for academic loss, but I am thinking about the trauma and what our teachers are going to be, and all the other things that are going to happen when children return to campuses.

Can you talk a little bit about what those inequities will look like after the COVID–19 pandemic and the State financial crisis if we do nothing to intervene?

Mr. KING. Sure. It is good to see you, Congresswoman.

Look, the impact of COVID–19 for kids, when I think about that, I think about the kid who relies on school, as many of your students did, for their positive relationships with adults and peers, and they have been without that. Some kids who are in homes where there is addiction, where there is abuse, where there is domestic violence, kids are in homes where there has been economic trauma, and so they have been without all of those supports.

And so when they come back to school in September, they are going to need more support, which means we need counselors, we need mental health services, we need an investment in the socio-emotional supports that students need, and that won't be there if school districts are forced to make huge cuts as a result of the lost State revenue.

Mrs. HAYES. Thank you. And I am happy that you used that word "investment" because thinking forward—and I will ask you, and I guess, Ms. Jones, I will ask you the same thing. Thinking forward, if we were to look at what types of investments we could make—I am sorry—to make public education more equitable, to address some of these underlying issues, I guess in the same way that we invested in small businesses and we invested in our larger economy, what would investments in our education system, in our children, look like moving forward?

Mr. KING. Well, we ought to close that $23 billion gap that the chairman talked about between students of color and White students in school spending. That is what a good investment would look like. A good investment would mean addressing the learning loss and the socio-emotional needs of students with supplemental dollars. Investment would mean doubling Pell grants and making it possible for low-income students to successfully pursue higher education.

Mrs. HAYES. Thank you. And I will switch over to Ms. Jones, and you hit on something because I know most of our education funding comes from municipal taxes, which already puts our kids at a disadvantage.

Ms. Jones?

Dr. JONES. Yes. So, we need to change that—local property taxes is the basis of funding schools—because if you have a poor neighborhood, poorly funded schools, another generation lost. We also need to invest very vigorously in early childhood education. We need to invest in teacher education. We need to have a model like Finland where you have a—you know, a mentorship position for teachers for 2 years after they graduate.

Thank you.

Mrs. HAYES. Thank you. I am not sure which bell that is, but, either way, I am done.

Thank you so much, Mr. Chair.

Chairman SCOTT. Thank you. Thank you.

Mrs. HAYES. Both are obnoxious.

Chairman SCOTT. Especially the second one.

The gentlelady from Florida, Dr. Shalala?

The gentleman from Michigan, Mr. Levin?

Mr. LEVIN. Thank you so much, Mr. Chairman, and happy Pride Month, everybody.

You know, President Trump and Secretary DeVos, just last week, claimed school choice is the civil rights cause of our time, and that is just honestly comical, but it is unsurprising because, in Michigan, we know that school choice causes segregation in our time.

We are seeing the impacts of these policies right now in Michigan's Ninth District. Mount Clemens School District in Macomb County has seen massive numbers of White students partaking in schools of choice to go to a nearby whiter school district. Michigan's school financing moves with the student, meaning that, when a student leaves to go to another school district, that funding goes with them.

As a result, Mount Clemens School District, with a majority Black student body, has faced major budget deficits for the past two decades and struggles to rebuild school infrastructure that hasn't been updated in more than 50 years. That is before the COVID crisis. These students are being intentionally left behind. There is no coincidence here.

Horrifically, Betsy DeVos is now trying to foist these harmful policies on the entire Nation as secretary of education. Just last week, the Department of Education finalized a rule that would funnel critical emergency money away from the school districts and students most impacted by COVID–19, as Congress intended—bipartisan, bicameral—and send it instead to private schools, even those serving the very wealthiest students.

Mr. King, I would like to ask you about this: Would you agree that school choice policies can, in place with funding models like Michigan has, disproportionately harm students of color by funneling money and, you know, other resources away from their schools?

Mr. KING. Yeah. There is no question that the vision of school choice that Secretary DeVos favors is one that is harmful to students, and the evidence is clear in Michigan, and it is both the problem of the funding structure; it is also the unregulated charter market, which has allowed for-profit charter operators who are not serving students well to proliferate without meaningful accountability. So this narrow vision of schools is part of the problem we have to solve.

Mr. LEVIN. Well, and I would just add that, here in Michigan, which Ms. DeVos—Secretary DeVos has had an impact on for many years, you—charters have almost no regulations, and it has been a very harmful thing.

What happens, then, to educational equity if we don't save our public schools? If we shift to the GOP idealized free market education system, which students will be hurt the most?

Mr. KING. There is no question it will hurt students of color and lower income students the most. Public education is the foundation of our economy.

In point of fact, the majority of kids of the Nation's public schools today are kids of color. We have no future as a society if we don't invest in their education. And, in the short run, one of the things we have to do is make sure that we correct the misinterpretation of the CARES Act that is literally taking dollars that were intended for public schools and sending them to private school.

Mr. LEVIN. Thank you.

And, you know, I feel like public education is really what built the middle class in this country, along with workers having the freedom to form unions.

Dr. Jones, how will policies like Secretary DeVos' proposed rule that we have been discussing further [inaudible] inequity and systemic racism in our education system? And you have got almost a minute to answer.

Dr. JONES. Almost a minute.

So, actually, these blinders that don't want to vigorously invest in the full excellent public education of all of our kids because people think there is no genius in the barrios or the ghettos or the reservations, we can get along very well, thank you, without them, those blinders are not just hurting those children; they are sapping the strength of the whole society because there is genius in all of our communities, and we could be doing so much better as a Nation or even as a world if we were to vigorously invest in public education.

So, what you are seeing is that there are whole communities that are being devalued for their genius, and, yes, vigorously investing in the full, excellent public education is what is going to save our Nation. That is one of the core—

Mr. LEVIN. All right. Thank you very much.

And, Mr. Chairman, before that horrible second bell, I yield back.

Chairman SCOTT. Tell me about it. Okay. Thank you.

The gentlelady from Minnesota, Ms. Omar?

The gentleman from Maryland, Mr. Trone?

Mr. TRONE. I am ready, Mr. Chairman, if it is—if I am up.

Chairman SCOTT. You are up, recognized for 5 minutes.

Mr. TRONE. Okay. Great. Thank you.

Dr. Wilson, your testimony highlights that Black-owned businesses have been hit hard by this crisis, in part, because they are disproportionately owned in industries that are vulnerable to shutdowns. You also note that Black families face vast wealth gaps compared to White families.

What effect do you believe this crisis will have on the wealth gap, but most importantly is, what should we be looking here in the Federal Government to try and address this wealth gap which is so profound and starts with homeowners—ownership, 40-some percent to 70-some percent? Then it goes over to owning businesses. How do we change this?

Ms. WILSON. So the wealth gap is one of the reasons that we are seeing such a disparate impact of COVID–19 in communities of color, at least in terms of the economic outcomes. As I mentioned before, having wealth, having savings puts you in a position to be able to weather the shutdowns and the things we have had to do in the interest of public safety. Without adequate savings, without adequate wealth, you have no cushion, or you are going to rapidly deteriorate any savings that you did have.

So I say that, if he we don't address the immediate crisis as well as think about addressing the wealth gap, we stand to see that wealth gap widening significantly, and that being both in terms of the impacts that we have seen on small business, as well as broader disparities in home ownership and other kinds of wealth-building techniques.

Mr. TRONE. Any ideas about how we can help minorities get into businesses? I mean, that is the big disparity. They are not starting the businesses; therefore, they aren't building up the equity. And then, of course, home ownership is the other piece where equity is, and, again, that lags too. So we need some ideas that we can drive that and stimulate it, prime the pump.

Ms. WILSON. Well, in terms of small business, it is important to recognize that Black business owners are less than 10 percent of all businesses owned in the United States. And, beyond that, if we think about the larger businesses that employ people, African American-owned businesses are only about 4 percent of those.

So the issues with Black owned business as a wealth-building tool, it is not so much starting the business, but in having opportunities to expand and grow those businesses so that they are able to build substantial wealth that is important in the communities in terms of making jobs available to folks, as well as building personal and community wealth.

So the things that need to be done to address that, we have to address, again, the racial disparities that exist throughout our system. Part of the reason why Black businesses don't have as many opportunities to expand and grow is because of the disparate predatory or lending practices that exclude Black business owners from getting the kind of capital that they need to expand their businesses, and normally we see these kinds of patterns with getting access to mortgage loans in order to purchase homes on top of the large income gaps and wage gaps that put people at lower levels of income with less to draw upon to make these kinds of investments.

Mr. TRONE. Let's jump over quickly to the racial inequities in the criminal justice system, Ms. Wilson. You know, if African Americans or Hispanics are incarcerated the same rate as Whites, we would have 40 percent less people in jail—40 percent. So that is the reality to this community—our communities of color disproportionately affected in an unjust justice system.

So what things do we need to do to help drive those unemployment numbers down for justice-impacted individuals so, when they come out, they can stay out and not have a circular system of recidivism?

Ms. WILSON. So there are a number of things that are being attempted in communities in cities across the country; specifically, ban the box provisions that prohibit an employer from asking people about their criminal background prior to—

Mr. TRONE. How big a difference do you think that ban the box makes? We have a bill that we just put in last week that I think does exactly that for the whole country. Talk about what a difference that makes.

Ms. WILSON. Well, I think that is an important first step, but there are other kinds of things that need to be put in place to support ban the box. That only gets your foot in the door. That just keeps you from being eliminated in that first round. So there are other kinds of policies and support that are important to help people reintegrate into society and into the workforce.

Mr. TRONE. Okay. Well, thank you very much, ma'am. I yield back before that bell rings.

Chairman SCOTT. Thank you. Thank you.

The gentlelady from Michigan, Ms. Stevens?

The gentleman from Nevada, Ms. Lee?

The gentlelady from Massachusetts, Ms. Trahan?

Mrs. TRAHAN. Thank you, Mr. Chairman, and thank you so much for the panel today. This was such a terrific hearing.

Communities of color have always experienced racial discrimination in healthcare settings. You know, dating back hundreds of years, race has been used as a weapon to undermine and dehumanize Black patients. As my colleague from Georgia mentioned, COVID–19 didn't create these disparities, but they have certainly— but it certainly has exacerbated them.

As Black and Brown patients struggle to access COVID–19 testing and treatment, Dr. Jones, according to the American Medical Association, only 5 percent of U.S. physicians are Black, 5.8 percent are Latinx, and only 0.4 percent are Native American. Black women account for only 2 percent of physicians in our country. How has the COVID–19 pandemic underscored the importance of increasing diversity in the field of medicine?

Dr. JONES. So, it has always been an important issue because more—if we train more physicians of color, then they tend to serve communities of color with a more respectful kind of way, and so, some of what we have seen with patients presenting at emergency departments and being sent back untested and the like and dying at home, that would be less likely to happen.

So, it is a chronic problem, and we need to address it. We need to address it not just in terms of medical school admissions, practices, but all the way back to early childhood education, that pipeline that starts very, very early on.

Mrs. TRAHAN. Great. And so, if you could just elaborate a bit on how increasing diversity in medicine and public health prevent discrimination and bias from affecting patient care.

Dr. JONES. So, we know that implicit bias exists among medical care providers. We have been knowing this for about 10, 15 years, even before we had the implicit association test, and so, physicians might look at a patient and think, oh, that patient couldn't afford, wouldn't comply, wouldn't understand, and not even give patients the full range of treatment options.

So, there are so many ways that these subtle biases against different groups, the assumptions that people draw, actually impair care, much less what happens when you have systems that also don't accept patients with Medicaid or don't whatever. So, it is a provider thing, and it is a system thing, and they go hand in hand because the more providers you have of color, then they are at the decision-making tables that can then change some of the system things that are going on.

Mrs. TRAHAN. I appreciate that.

What recommendations would you like to offer this committee as we think about how to address this issue? Are there incentives or programs that we could strengthen to address the lack of representation and diversity—

Dr. JONES. Yeah.

Mrs. TRAHAN. —across our healthcare continuum?

Dr. JONES. Something that has been in place for a decade is the National Health Service Corps, which got a little bit of a bump in the Affordable Care Act, but that enables students from low-income communities to actually go to medical school in the first place, and then they have a payback commitment in needed communities, medically underserved communities, where they are then more likely to stay. So, that is just one very specific thing. If that could become huge, then that would go a long way.

Mrs. TRAHAN. Thank you so much.

Thank you, Mr. Chairman. I yield back. Thank you, sir.

Chairman SCOTT. Thank you. Has anyone—Mr. Castro of Texas. Has anybody online or on air not been recognized?

If not, I recognize myself for a couple of questions, starting with Ms. Wilson.

Ms. Wilson, we have—Dr. Wilson, we have responded trying to stimulate the economy by using primarily unemployment compensation, food assistance, and other things. There have been other suggestions, like a payroll tax and capital gains tax holiday.

Which initiatives tend to stimulate the economy the most? Which give you the best bang for the buck?

Ms. WILSON. So, according to the recent analysis by economist Mark Zandi, we find that food assistance programs, SNAP program in particular, has the largest bang per buck. One dollar spend in food assistance will generate $1.67 in GDP a year from now. Unemployment insurance benefits are second with the bang for buck of $1.46.

Chairman SCOTT. And what about the payroll tax and the capital gain tax holiday? How do they score?

Ms. WILSON. So I don't recall off the top of my head the exact numbers there, but I will say that those typically have a bang for buck of under $1. So, whereas these direct payment assistance programs, such as unemployment insurance, SNAP, having a bang for buck well over a dollar, payroll tax and other kinds of tax incentives [inaudible] come in at under $1.

Chairman SCOTT. Thank you.

Dr. King, can you tell me a little bit about the importance after we—people have been out of school for so long, the importance of potential summer programs?

Mr. KING. Yeah. The summer creates an opportunity to try to make up for the ground lost. We ought to put in place summer programs in person where possible, given public health criteria and, if not possible, then through distance learning. But we know students are going to come back to school having lost as much as 70 percent of the ground of the school year in math, 30 percent or more in reading.

And the way that we address that is to provide additional instructional support, particularly critical for students with disabilities and English learners, who have been without services, in many cases, since March.

Chairman SCOTT. Thank you. And can you say something about how the funding public schools with the property tax affects equity?

Mr. KING. Yes. Well, the result of the property tax is huge disparities between districts. We know that districts with large numbers of students of color spend about $1,800 less per student than districts with large numbers of White students.

One of the things we can do to address this is to require, as a condition for new stimulus dollars, that States have to protect their highest-needs districts from cuts and that districts have to protect their highest-needs schools from cuts.

Chairman SCOTT. And so if you have property taxes, does that inherently create inequity?

Mr. KING. It does, and, in an environment where there is a financial crisis, what it means is that wealthy districts will be able to go back to their property tax owners, increase the property taxes a small amount, and generate significant revenue to absorb the cuts, whereas high-poverty districts don't have that wealth base, and the cuts will fall hardest on them.

Chairman SCOTT. And, Dr. Jones, can you say a word? We have talked about the COBRA subsidies. It is my understanding, if you lose your job, you lose your insurance, but, if you can get COBRA subsidy, you can continue your insurance. If you have to switch into the marketplace, you end up having to get a new insurance policy, get new providers, and even start your deductible all over. But then, when you get your job right back, you have got to go back, tell those providers, "It has been nice knowing you for a couple of months," and then start—get back your own providers, and then start your deductible all over.

Doesn't it make a lot of sense to try to do everything we can to maintain the continuity of your insurance?

Dr. JONES. It does. So, I think that extending COBRA, subsidizing COBRA coverage is a good idea.

Chairman SCOTT. Good. Thank you.

And, finally, Mr. Roy, I think we can all agree that it is a good idea to open schools as soon as possible if it can be done safely. If tests are not available, how do you reopen the schools safely?

Mr. ROY. Well, testing is one part of the equation. It is not the only one. So, for example, in Texas, where summer schools are able to reopen, a lot of schools are applying a hybrid approach where they are using temperature checks, which are not, of course—they are not nearly as definitive, but temperature checks plus symptomatic tests are questions to look at, whether children might have COVID infections.

But, again, it is more about risk management on the other side, like, before you get to the testing stage, really making sure that the kids are not transmitting the disease and that people who are at risk who work at those facilities, whether it is elderly teachers, staff, et cetera, and people who live in households where there are elderly grandparents, that they are removed from that setting. So it is more about, I think, preventing the risk of infection from happening in the first place than about testing, but testing can be part of the solution if we can scale it up, but you don't need testing to reopen the schools.

Chairman SCOTT. And, of course, if you don't know whether people are transmitting or not, if you wait until they are symptomatic because there is many will be transmitting before they are symptomatic, and one of the things that the HEROES Act includes is money for school construction. A lot of schools do not have proper ventilation, and that is one of the key safety requirements, to make sure you have good ventilation. So we are going to do everything we can, and everybody wants to open up as soon as possible. But, if you can't do it safely, I think we may have a problem.

So I want to thank all of our witnesses for their testimony.

Is there any other business? Anyone else have comments?

So I want to remind my colleagues that, pursuant to committee practice, materials for submission in the hearing record must be submitted to the Committee Clerk within 14 days following the last day of the hearing, so by 5 p.m. on July 5th, preferably in Microsoft Word format. Materials submitted must address the subject matter of the hearing.

Only a Member of the committee or invited witness may submit materials for inclusion. Documents are limited to 50 pages each. Documents longer than that can be incorporated by way of an internet link that may not be available in the future, so you want to be careful about that.

Without objection, I would like to enter the following into the record—following report: “Black Workers Face Two of the Most Lethal Preexisting Conditions for Coronavirus—Racism and Economic Inequality,” by Elise Gould and Valerie Wilson, published by the Economic Policy Institute.

Black Workers Face Two of the Most Lethal Preexisting Conditions for Coronavirus—Racism and Economic Inequality

Elise Gould and Valerie Wilson
June 1, 2020

“We’re all in this together” has become a rallying cry during the coronavirus pandemic. While it is true that COVID-19 has affected everyone in some way, the magnitude and nature of the impact has been anything but universal. Evidence to date suggests that black and Hispanic workers face much more economic and health insecurity from COVID-19 than white workers.

Although the current strain of the coronavirus is one that humans have never experienced before, the disparate racial impact of the virus is deeply rooted in historic and ongoing social and economic injustices. Persistent racial disparities in health status, access to health care, wealth, employment, wages, housing, income, and poverty all contribute to greater susceptibility to the virus—both economically and physically.

Though black and brown communities share many of the experiences that make them more susceptible, there are also important differences between these communities that need to be understood in order to effectively combat the adverse economic and health effects of the virus. This chapter, focused specifically on black workers, is the first in a series that will explore how racial and economic inequality leave workers of color with few good options for protecting both their health and economic well-being. A companion report highlights conditions for Hispanic workers.

Effects of the Pandemic on Black Workers

Economic Effects: Devastating Job Losses Are Hitting Black Workers and Their Families Especially Hard

There are three main groups of workers in the COVID-19 economy: those who have lost their jobs and face economic insecurity, those who are classified as essential workers and face health insecurity as a result, and those who are able to continue working from the safety of their homes. Unfortunately, black workers are less likely to be found in the last group. They have suffered record numbers of job losses over the last two months (March 2020–May 2020), along with the ensuing related economic devastation. They also are disproportionately found among the essential workers in the economy today—continuing to go to their workplaces, risking their health and that of their families because they are unable to sustain adequate social distance from their co-workers and customers.

Spiking Unemployment Rates

The labor market has continued to deteriorate, as evidenced by massive numbers of unemployment insurance claims through the middle of May (Shierholz 2020). As of May 16, nearly one in four workers have applied for unemployment insurance benefits, either in the regular program or through the new Pandemic Unemployment Assistance program, since stay-at-home orders first went into effect. Furthermore, in the first month of job losses, for every 100 workers who were able to file for UI, 37 additional workers tried to apply but could not get through the system to make a claim (Zipperer and Gould 2020). While many of those who initially couldn't get through have likely been able to in subsequent weeks, it is also likely that would-be applicants face ongoing challenges and that the reported number of applicants understates the magnitude of the problem.

The latest national data available to assess the impact of job losses for black and white workers separately is the Current Population Survey for April 2020. The labor market started deteriorating in March but fell off a cliff in April. While the losses have certainly continued, the April data gives us a first look at how black and white workers are faring.

Figure A shows the unemployment rates for white and black workers in February, March, and April of this year. February provides a benchmark for the pre-pandemic economy. As will be described in greater detail later, the black unemployment rate has, even in the tightest of labor markets, been persistently and significantly higher than the white unemployment rate. Both began rising in March and then skyrocketed in April. As of the latest data, the black unemployment rate is 16.7%, compared with a white unemployment rate of 14.2%.

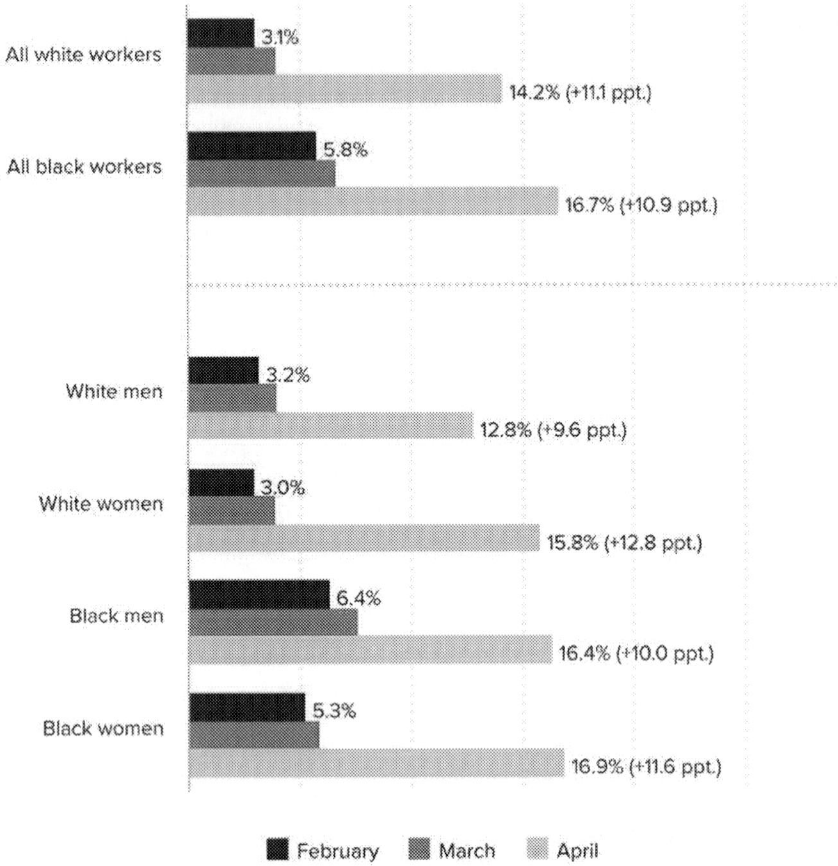

Note: White refers to non-Hispanic whites, Black refers to Blacks alone.
Source: EPI analysis of Bureau of Labor Statistics Current Population Survey public data.

Figure A. While unemployment skyrocketed for Black and white workers in the COVID-19 labor market, the unemployment rate is higher for Black workers. Unemployment rates by race, and by race and gender, February–April 2020.

And while these differences are notable, they mask even greater disparities that are apparent when we look at unemployment rates by race and gender. White men experienced a large, but relatively smaller, rise in unemployment. Still, the white male unemployment rate is now higher than the highest point the overall unemployment rate reached in the depths of the Great Recession (10.0%, in October 2009; see EPI 2020). White women experienced the largest increase in unemployment, while black women now have the highest unemployment rate of the four groups analyzed. (It should be noted that across race, gender, and ethnicity, Hispanic women actually have the highest unemployment rate as of April 2020—about one in five Latina workers are unemployed. Further data on Hispanic workers will be provided in a forthcoming report).

Falling Employment-to-Population Ratios

The unemployment rate is a commonly used measure of labor market slack. One limitation, however, is that it relies on would-be workers to either be on temporary layoff or have looked for work in the last four weeks to be counted as unemployed. In this economy, with the health requirements to stay home and with sectors being completely decimated, it is likely that many would-be workers are not actively looking for work and therefore would not be counted in the official unemployment rate. For this reason, policymakers should look to other measures to determine when to turn on and off policy triggers to support workers and the economy (Gould 2020b). One such measure is the employment-to-population ratio (EPOP), or the share of the population with a job. Figure B displays the EPOP for the same groups shown in Figure A.

Employment losses were stark across racial lines between February and April. Black workers saw slightly greater losses in employment than white workers (10.6 vs. 9.5 percentage-point losses). This translates into an employment loss of 17.8% among black workers and 15.5% among white workers. More than one in six black workers lost their jobs between February and April. As of April, less than half of the adult black population was employed. While the economic devastation is widespread, as we show in this chapter, black workers are less able to weather such a storm because they have fewer earners in their families, lower incomes, and lower liquid wealth than white workers.

As with the unemployment rates, women suffered greater job losses than men. Black women experienced a drop in their EPOP of 11.0 percentage points. Put another way, 18.8% of black women workers lost their jobs between February and April. At 45.5%, white women haven't seen such a low share of the population with a job since the late 1970s, when white women were still increasing their participation in the labor market in general.

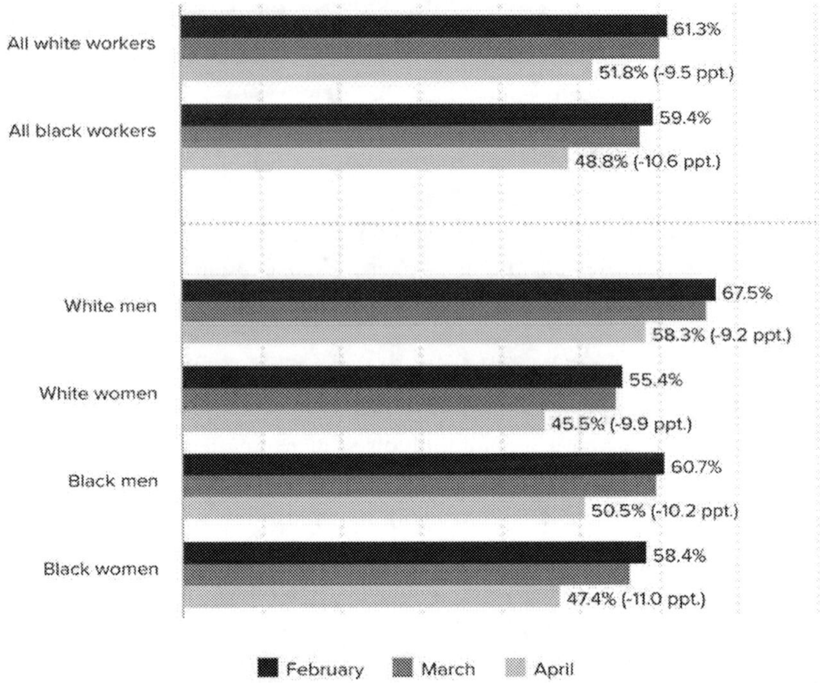

Note: White refers to non-Hispanic whites, Black refers to Blacks alone. The employment-to-population ratio is the share of the population who are working.

Source: EPI analysis of Bureau of Labor Statistics Current Population Survey public data.

Figure B. Employment has dropped sharply in the COVID-19 labor market—Black women face the largest losses.
Employment-to-population ratio by race and gender, February–April 2020.

Health Effects: Black Workers and Their Families Are Facing Greater Health Risks

Black Workers Are More Likely to Be in Front-Line Jobs That Are Categorized as 'Essential'—Forcing Them to Risk Their Own and Their Families' Health to Earn a Living

Not only are black workers losing their jobs at an incredible pace, those who aren't losing their jobs are more likely to be found on the front lines of the economy in essential jobs. Rho, Brown, and Fremstad (2020) conducted an important and useful study of six sectors of the economy that are considered essential and in which most workers are on the front lines of the COVID-19 labor market. Their results, displayed in Figure C, show that black workers make up a disproportionate share of these essential workers who are forced to put themselves and their family members at additional risk of contracting and spreading COVID-19 in order to put food on the table.

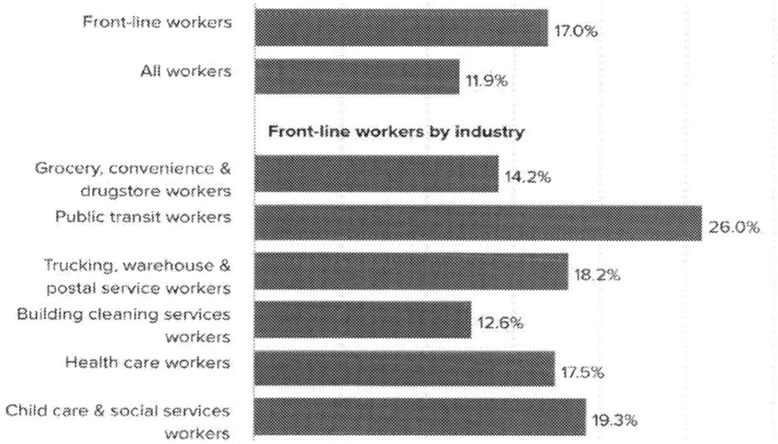

Notes: The front-line industry categories used here are the categories used in the CEPR report (see Source below for more information). Sample is a 2014–2018 five-year estimate.

Source: EPI analysis of data from the Center for Economic Policy Research (CEPR) report A Basic Demographic Profile of Workers in Frontline Industries (April 2020).

Figure C. Black workers are more likely than other workers to be in front-line jobs. Black workers as a share of all workers in a given industry.

Black workers make up about one in nine workers overall; they represent 11.9% of the workforce. However, black workers make up about one in six of all front-line-industry workers. They are disproportionately represented in employment in grocery, convenience, and drug stores (14.2%); public transit (26.0%); trucking, warehouse, and postal service (18.2%); health care (17.5%); and child care and social services (19.3%). While, in the near term, this protects them from job loss, it exposes them to greater likelihood of contracting COVID-19 while performing their jobs.

African Americans Have Disproportionately High COVID-19 Death Rates and Are More Likely to Live in Areas Experiencing Outbreaks

Given the disproportionate representation of black workers in front-line occupations where they face greater risk of exposure to COVID-19, it is not surprising that illness and deaths are disproportionately found among black workers and their families. As shown in Figure D, African Americans' share of those who have died from COVID-19 nationally is nearly double (1.8 times higher than) their share of the U.S. population. The ratios are even higher in some states: in Wisconsin and Kansas, the rate of African American deaths is more than four times as high as their share of the population in those states (Meepagala and Romer 2020). By comparison, whites account for a smaller share of deaths than their share of the population.

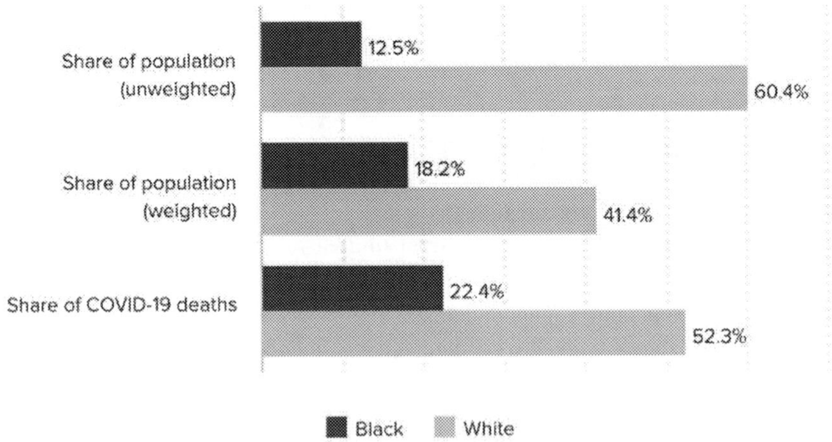

Notes: White refers to non-Hispanic whites, black refers to blacks alone. All shares are as of May 13, 2020. Shares of COVID-19 deaths are based on provisional death counts. Weighted population shares reflect the racial distribution of the geographic locations where COVID-19 outbreaks are occurring, and help to ascertain whether disproportionate deaths are occurring within certain racial groups.

Source: Centers for Disease Control and Prevention (CDC), Provisional Death Counts for Coronavirus Disease (COVID-19): Weekly State-Specific Data Updates.

Figure D. Black Americans make up 12.5% of the U.S. population but account for 22.4% of COVID-19 deaths.
Shares of population vs. shares of COVID-19 deaths, by race.

The Centers for Disease Control (CDC) also reports weighted population distributions in an effort to reflect racial/ethnic distributions of the geographic locations where COVID outbreaks are occurring. These weighted population distributions indicate that African Americans represent a larger share of the population in areas where outbreaks are occurring than their representation in the population overall (18.2% compared with 12.5%). Therefore, one of the reasons for disproportionately higher rates of COVID deaths among African Americans is the fact that they are more likely to live in areas that have experienced COVID outbreaks. Even accounting for this fact, African Americans still have higher death rates than their weighted population shares would indicate.

Underlying Factors

The devastating effects of COVID-19 on the economic and physical well-being of black Americans were entirely predictable given persistent economic and health disparities. In this section, we describe some of the underlying economic and health factors behind the unequal outcomes observed thus far. These same factors will ultimately prolong the effects of the pandemic on black workers and their families long after the immediate threat has passed.

Underlying Economic Factors Exacerbate the Effect of the COVID-19 Recession on Black Workers and Their Families

Black workers and their families were economically insecure before the pandemic tore through the United States. The pandemic and related job losses have been especially devastating for black households because they have historically suffered from higher unemployment rates, lower wages, lower incomes, and much less savings to fall back on, as well as significantly higher poverty rates than their white counterparts. This prior insecurity has magnified the current economic damage to these workers and their families. The next seven figures illustrate the differences in socioeconomic status between white and black workers, households, and families.

Higher Unemployment Rates

Let's start with the labor market. Historically, black workers have faced unemployment rates twice as high as those of their white counterparts. When the overall unemployment rate averaged 3.7% in 2019, the white non-Hispanic unemployment rate was 3.0% and the black unemployment rate was twice as high, coming in at an average of 6.1% over the year. This difference cannot be explained away by differences in educational attainment. Figure E shows that at every level of education, the black unemployment rate is significantly higher than the white unemployment rate, even for those workers with college or advanced degrees.

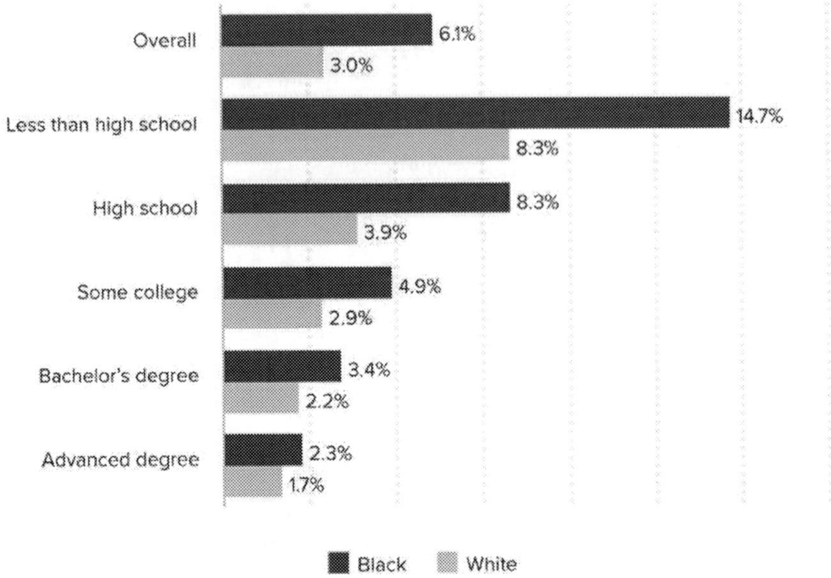

Notes: White refers to non-Hispanic whites, Black refers to Blacks alone. Educational categories are mutually exclusive and represent the highest education level attained for all individuals ages 16 and older.

Source: Economic Policy Institute, State of Working America Data Library, [Unemployment by race and education], 2019.

Figure E. Black workers are far more likely to be unemployed than white workers at every level of education.
Unemployment rates by race and education, 2019.

Significant Wage Gaps

Among the employed, black workers face significant pay penalties. No matter how you cut the data, black workers face significant pay gaps in the labor market, and research has shown that these pay gaps have grown since 2000 and in the decades before (Gould 2020a; Wilson and Rodgers 2016). On average, black workers are paid 73 cents on the white dollar. We know from a host of economic research that a person's wages are not a simple function of individual ability. Instead, workers' ability to claim higher wages rests on a host of social, political, and institutional factors outside their control (Manning 2003; Card, Devicienti, and Maida 2011). Because of historic and current

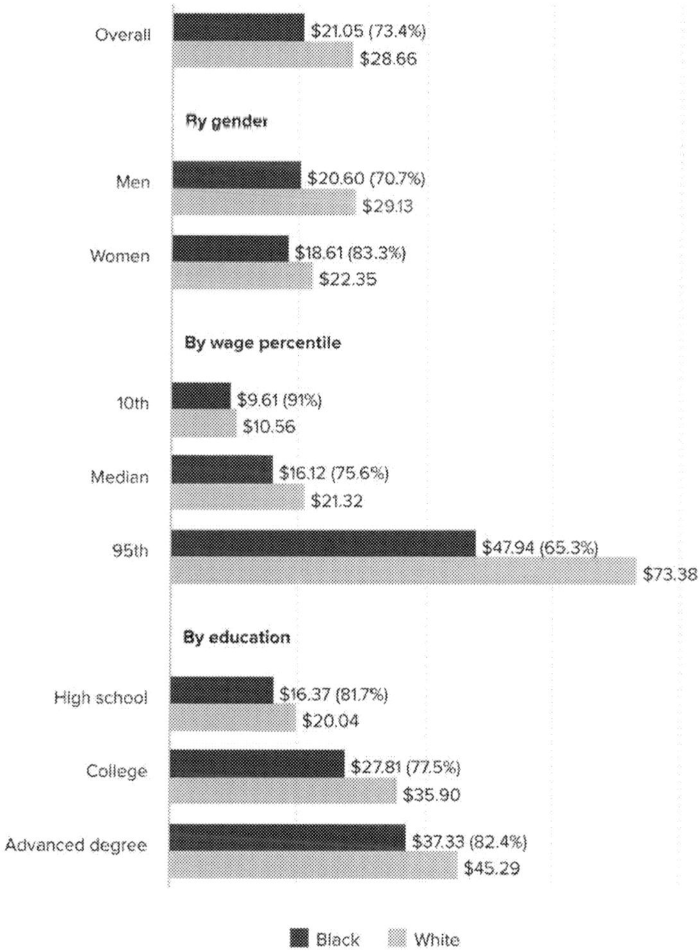

Note: White refers to non-Hispanic whites, black refers to blacks alone.

Source: Authors' analysis of Economic Policy Institute, State of Working America Data Library, [Median/average hourly wages], 2019, and of EPI Current Population Survey Extracts, Version 1.0 (2020), https://microdata.epi.org, adapted from State of Working America Wages 2019.

Figure F. Black--white wage gaps are wide no matter how you slice the data. Average wages of black and white workers, by gender, wage percentile, and education, 2019.

privilege in the labor market (National Advisory Commission on Civil Disorders 2016), white men enjoy exceptionally high wages. Therefore, the gap between white men and black men is particularly stark. Black men are paid only 71 cents on the white male dollar. Black women, who face both gender and race discrimination, are paid even less—64 cents on the white male dollar.

As Figure F shows, black–white wage gaps persist across the wage distribution as well as at different levels of education in the pre-pandemic economy. The black–white wage gap is smallest at the bottom of the wage distribution, where a wage floor—otherwise known as the minimum wage—keeps the lowest-wage black workers from being paid even lower wages. The largest black–white wage gaps are found at the top of the wage distribution and are explained in part by occupational segregation—the underrepresentation of black workers in the highest-wage professions and overrepresentation in lower-wage professions—and the pulling away of the top more generally.

Similarly, across various levels of education, a significant black–white wage gap remains. Black workers can't simply educate their way out of the gap. Even black workers with an advanced degree experience a significant wage gap compared with their white counterparts.

Benefits Gaps

Not only is black worker pay significantly less than that of their white counterparts, but their benefits are as well. Along with health insurance, discussed in more detail below, two benefits are acutely important at this particular time: paid sick days and the ability to work from home. These two workplace benefits help shield workers from economic losses by allowing them to take paid time off to care for themselves or family members and allowing them to stay out of harm's way and still earn a paycheck by working from home. Figure G illustrates how black workers are less likely than white workers to enjoy these benefits.

The Family First Coronavirus Response Act was an important first step in providing vital paid sick days, but somewhere between 6.8 million and 19.6 million private-sector workers were left without paid sick days as a result of the firm-size exemptions in the law (Gould and Shierholz 2020). Obviously, those loopholes need to be closed, and workers—regardless of race or ethnicity—also need a permanent fix to this basic labor standard.

Given what we know about job losses and essential workers, it's not surprising that significantly fewer black workers can telework than white workers. Fewer than one in five black workers in the pre-pandemic economy were able to work from home. This inability to keep their jobs and stay safe makes it even harder for black workers to maintain economic and health security during this difficult time.

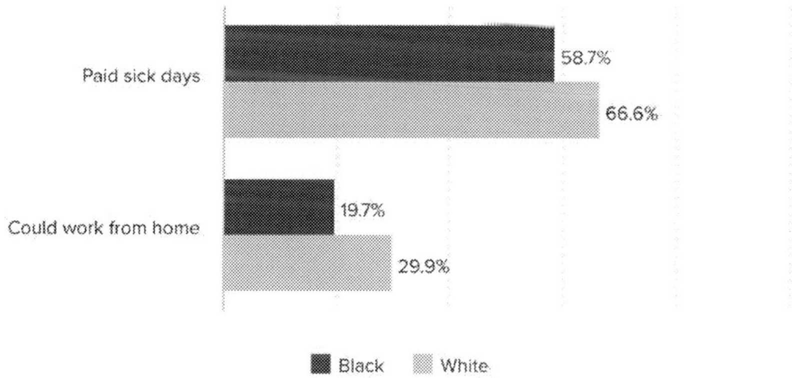

Sources: U.S. Bureau of Labor Statistics, Job Flexibilities and Work Schedules, 2017 and 2018; U.S. Bureau of Labor Statistics, American Time Use Survey microdata.

Figure G. Black workers are less likely to have paid sick days and less likely to be able to work from home than white workers.
Shares of workers with paid sick days and the ability to work from home, by race.

Lower Household Incomes and Higher Poverty Rates

Significant gaps in both employment opportunities and wage levels translate into lower incomes and higher poverty rates in the pre-pandemic economy, as shown in Figure H.

In 2018, median household income for white households was 70% higher than for black households ($70,642 vs. $41,692). On top of decades of preferential wealth accumulation for white families versus black families (Rothstein 2017; Darity et al. 2018), lower incomes are one of the reasons that black families haven't been able to build up savings to weather storms such as the one our country finds itself in today.

At the bottom of the income distribution, the black poverty rate is two-and-a-half times the white poverty rate. One in five black people in this country live below the poverty line—that's below about $26,000 annual income for a family of four. Job loss for those living at such low incomes is absolutely shattering.

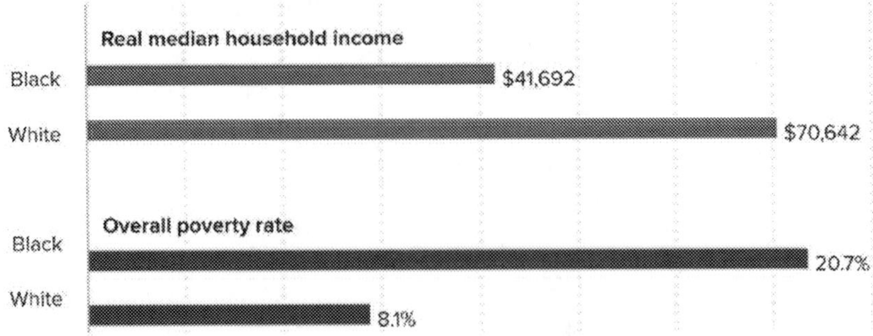

Notes: White refers to non-Hispanic whites, black refers to blacks alone. Black households are households in which the head of household is black. White households are households in which the head of household is white. The poverty rate is the share of people whose family income is below the official family-size-adjusted poverty threshold.

Source: EPI analysis of Current Population Survey Annual Social and Economic Supplement Historical Poverty Tables (Tables 3, H-5, and H-9). Adapted from Racial and Ethnic Income Gaps Persist Amid Uneven Growth in Household Incomes (EPI 2019).

Figure H. Black households have lower incomes and higher rates of poverty than white households.
Real median household income and overall poverty rate, by race, 2018.

Lower Shares of Households with Multiple Earners

In the pre-pandemic economy, black workers were less likely to have multiple earners in their household (shown in Figure I). Half of all black households had only one earner, while nearly half of all white households had at least two earners. This racial disparity in the number of household earners is not just a function of how many working-age adults live in the household, or family structure, but is another measurable consequence of the persistent 2-to-1 ratio between the black and white unemployment rates. The inequities black workers experience in the labor market have larger consequences for the economic vulnerability of black households because it is far more likely that when one household member loses their job, it translates into a complete loss of income for that household. Black households are less likely to have a second earner to fall back on to make ends meet.

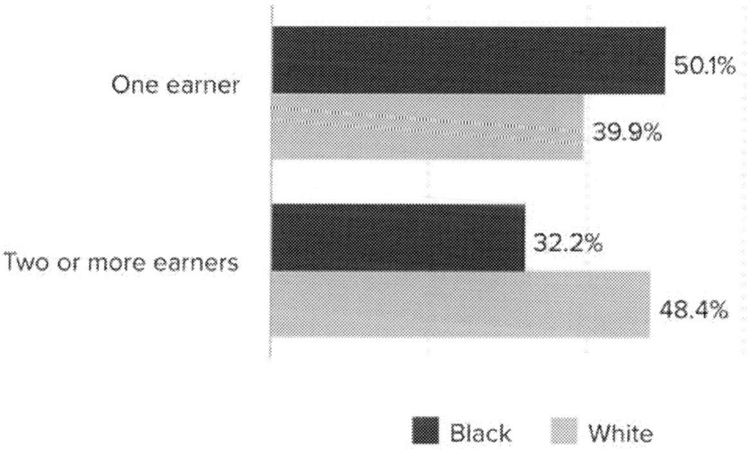

Notes: White refers to non-Hispanic whites, black refers to blacks alone. Black households are households in which the head of household is black. White households are households in which the head of household is white. Nonelderly households are those in which the heads of household are ages 18–64.
Source: Authors' analysis of Current Population Survey Annual Social and Economic Supplement microdata, 2018.

Figure I. Black households are less likely to include multiple earners than white households.
Shares of nonelderly households with one earner vs. two or more earners, by race, 2018.

Higher Shares of Households Headed by Single Parents

Single working parents, a subset of one-earner households, face the added burden of needing to balance the competing demands of work, online distance learning, and child care responsibilities. Black women, in particular, as shown in Figure J, find themselves at the nexus of these overlapping responsibilities since they are 3.6 times as likely as white women to be single heads of households with children under age 18 (14.4% of black households compared with 4.0% of white households).

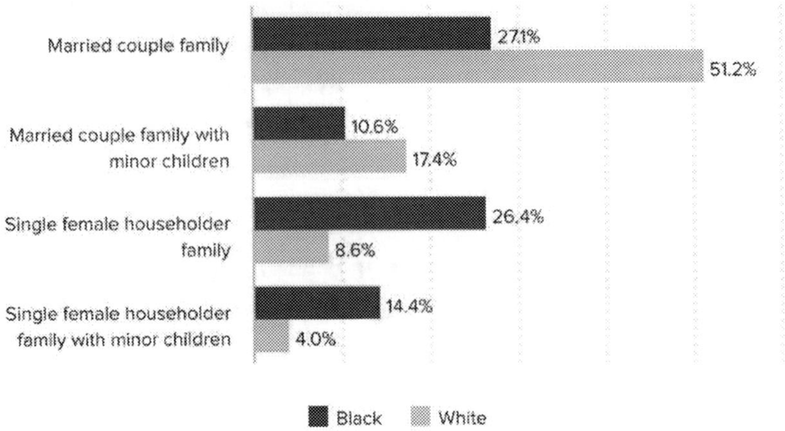

Note: White refers to non-Hispanic whites, Black refers to Blacks alone. Black households are households in which the head of household is Black. White households are households in which the head of household is white.

Source: U.S. Census Bureau, 2018 American Community Survey 1-Year Estimates, Table S0201.

Figure J. Black women are more likely to be single heads of households and single parents than white women.
Shares of Black and white households by selected family type, 2018.

Less Cash Reserves

On top of lower wages and incomes and higher poverty rates, black families have significantly less access to liquid assets than white families. It's been long established that black families face a large and persistent wealth gap. Darity and others have shown that no matter how it's measured, the racial wealth gap is large and persistent (Darity et al. 2018). To weather a financial loss, families often must dip into their liquid assets to pay for their living expenses. If they lose their job or experience a serious health shock, their only hope of making ends meet and continuing to pay their rent or mortgage and put food on the table is to rely on their savings. Wealth is often tied up in housing assets, particularly for black families, and therefore is inaccessible when dealing with sudden and large losses in income.

Figure K displays one component of wealth, the total value of all transaction accounts for black and white families. Transaction accounts include checking or savings accounts, cash, prepaid cards, and directly held stocks, bonds, and mutual funds. These are assets that can quickly be used to purchase goods and services, unlike less liquid sources of wealth like homeownership or assets in 401(k)s. Overall, white families hold, on average, more than five times as much liquid assets as black families do, $49,529 versus $8,762. This makes white families far more capable of weathering the storm of COVID-19, whether it be job loss or another financial hit.

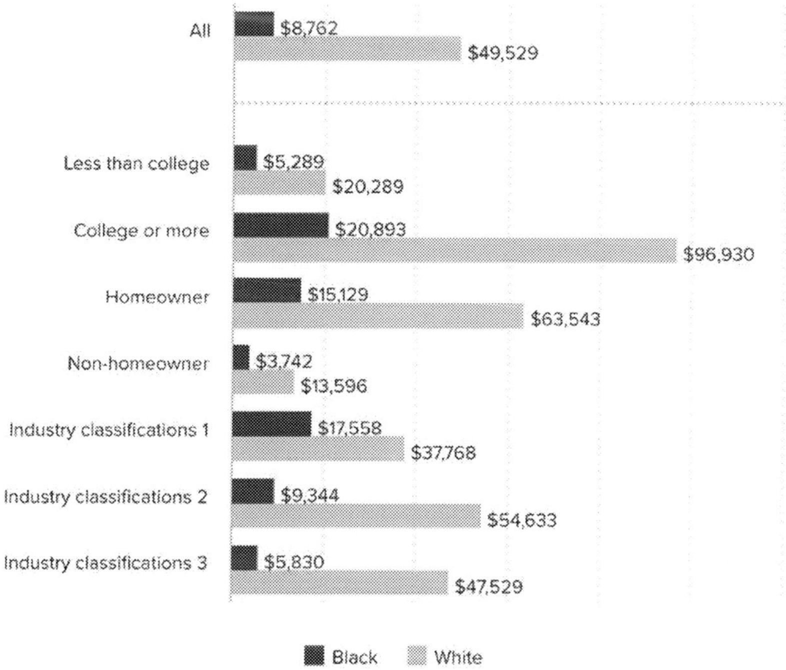

Notes: White refers to non-Hispanic whites, black refers to blacks alone. Transaction accounts include checking or savings accounts, cash, prepaid cards, and directly held stocks, bonds, and mutual funds. Industry classifications 1 include mining, construction, and manufacturing. Industry classifications 2 include transportation, communications, utilities and sanitary services, wholesale trade, finance, insurance, and real estate. Industry classifications 3 include agriculture, retail trade, services, and public administration. Race is the race of the survey respondent; industry classifications are for head of household. Education is the education level of the head of household.

Source: EPI analysis of Federal Reserve 2016 Survey of Consumer Finances combined extract data accessed from the UC Berkeley Survey Documentation and Analysis website. The 2016 survey is the most recent survey available.

Figure K. Black families have significantly less cash reserves to draw upon than white families.
Total value of all transaction accounts, for black and white families, by education, homeownership, and employment sector (mean values, 2016 dollars).

The attainment of higher education does not bridge this divide. This gap remains large when we compare white and black families whose heads of household have the same level of education. In fact, the absolute gap in liquid assets between black and white families is far larger among those *with* a college degree or more versus those with less than a college degree. White families headed by a college-degree holder have nearly five times the access to money in transaction accounts as similarly degreed black families. The gap persists whether the black family owns a home or not. The gaps in liquid assets differ by what sector the family head works in, but no matter how the data are cut, white families have far more access to liquid wealth.

It is not surprising then that research by Ganong et al. (2020) finds that income volatility has a much greater impact on the spending of black households than white households. They report that these differences in ability to smooth consumption leads to a 50% reduction in black families' ability to spend on essential goods and services as compared with white families when they are faced with similar income losses.

Underlying Health Factors Put Black Workers and Their Families at Greater Risk for Contracting COVID-19

Black workers also face greater underlying pre-pandemic health insecurities that make them more susceptible to the coronavirus. According to one demographic assessment of vulnerability, an estimated 30% of the country's overall population live in the counties at greatest risk of health and economic disruption from COVID-19, while a much higher share—43%—of black Americans (17.6 million) live in those same counties (Fitzhugh et al. 2020). Below we explore some of the factors contributing to the greater risk of adverse health outcomes related to COVID, including preexisting health conditions, lack of health insurance, housing conditions, and population density.

Preexisting Health Conditions Compound the Risks Faced by Black Workers

Preexisting health conditions—such as diabetes, hypertension, asthma, and diabetes—are associated with greater risk of death from the coronavirus. As shown in Figure L, African Americans experience all of these illnesses at higher rates than whites. The greatest racial disparities exist in the prevalence of diabetes (1.7 times as likely among African Americans as among whites) and hypertension (1.4 times as likely).

Air pollution has long been known to increase risk of heart and respiratory disease, heart attacks, asthma attacks, bronchitis, and lung cancer (Sass 2013). Therefore, environmental racism—the disproportionate impact of environmental hazards on health outcomes among people of color—is a contributing factor to these racial health disparities. According to a 2018 report by a group of scientists at the EPA National Center for Environmental Assessment, published in the *American Journal of Public Health*, people of color are disproportionately affected by air pollution due to their proximity to particulate-matter-emitting facilities (Mikati et al. 2018). African Americans suffer the most, with exposure 54% above average.

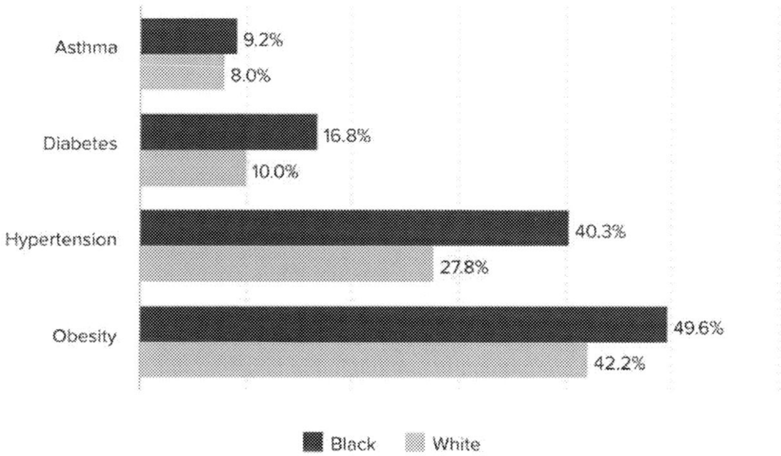

Notes: White refers to non-Hispanic whites, black refers to blacks alone. Age-adjusted prevalence of asthma, diabetes, and hypertension among adults ages 18 and over. Age-adjusted prevalence of obesity among adults ages 20 and over.

Sources: National Center for Health Statistics, National Health Interview Survey 2018; National Center for Health Statistics, National Health and Nutrition Examination Survey, 2013–2016, 2015–2016, and 2017–2018.

Figure L. African Americans have higher rates of chronic illnesses associated with greater vulnerability to COVID-19.
Age-adjusted prevalence of asthma, diabetes, hypertension, and obesity among black and white adults.

Lack of Health Insurance Also Negatively Affects Health Outcomes among Black Families

Early diagnosis and treatment are essential to minimizing the severity of chronic illnesses, and regular health care is important for promoting better overall health. The lack of health insurance often results in a choice to delay receiving health care until one's condition is critical. Figure M shows that black workers are 60% more likely to be uninsured than white workers. This is likely an additional contributing factor to the disparity in chronic illnesses described above, but it also might result in uninsured workers waiting longer to seek care for suspected coronavirus symptoms.

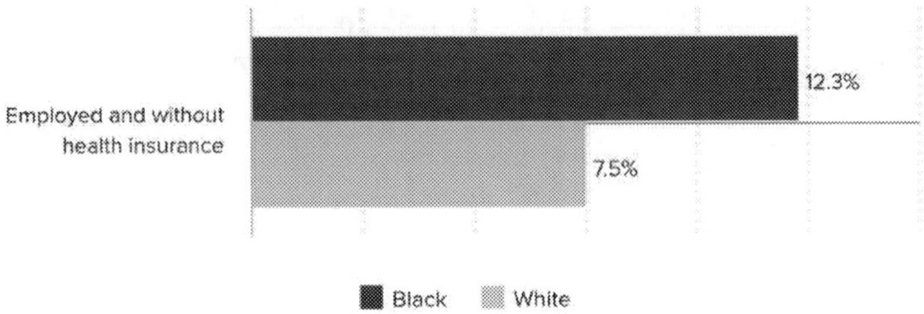

Note: White refers to non-Hispanic whites, black refers to blacks alone.
Source: Authors' analysis of 2018 American Community Survey microdata.

Figure M. Black workers are 60% more likely to be uninsured than white workers. Shares of workers without health insurance, by race, 2018.

Black Workers and Their Families Face Greater Risk of Exposure to the Coronavirus Because They Are More Likely to Live in Densely Populated Housing

The health and economic risks associated with COVID-19 are not limited to individual workers, but also affect their families and communities. The high rate of contagion associated with the coronavirus has made social distancing critical to slowing the spread of infection. However, in smaller or more densely populated home environments, it can be more difficult to effectively isolate vulnerable family members from those who have been infected or who face greater risk of exposure to the virus because of their work conditions. For example, those who live in multi-unit dwellings, such as apartment or condo buildings, tend to reside in more densely populated areas where more people share highly trafficked common spaces than those who live in single-unit detached dwellings. As shown in Figure N, 54.5% of African American households live in single-unit structures, compared with 74.2% of white households. On the other hand, 29.2% of African American households live in structures that include five or more units—more than double the rate of white households.

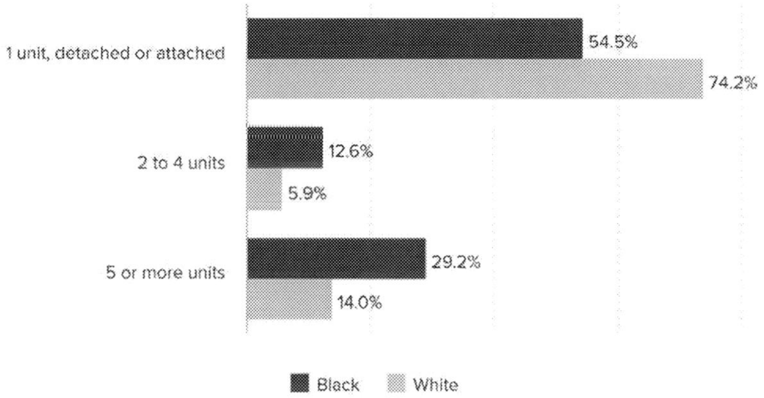

Note: White refers to non-Hispanic whites, black refers to blacks alone. Black households are households in which the head of household is black. White households are households in which the head of household is white. Totals may not sum to 100%. Structures categorized as mobile home, boat, RV, van, etc. are omitted.

Source: U.S. Census Bureau, 2018 American Community Survey 1-Year Estimates, Table S0201.

Figure N. Black households are more than twice as likely to live in densely populated housing structures as white households.
Shares of black and white households by type of housing structure.

Black Workers Are More Likely to Live in Multigenerational Households with Older Family Members Who Are at High Risk of Contracting the Virus

African Americans are also more likely to live in multigenerational households where there may be older family members who are considered high risk. As shown in Figure O, black workers are twice as likely as white workers to live in households with three or more generations, such as a grandparent living with children and grandchildren. While older people have been encouraged to isolate themselves as a preventative measure, this presents a challenge in homes where other members of the household must work outside of the home.

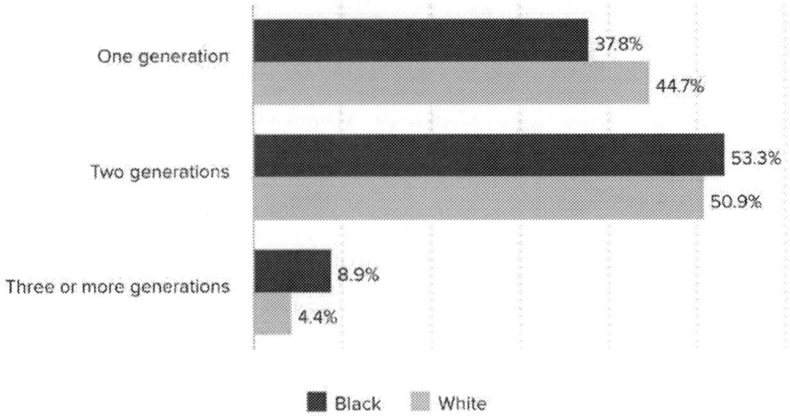

Note: White refers to non-Hispanic whites, black refers to blacks alone.
Source: Authors' analysis of American Community Survey 2018 microdata.

Figure O. Black workers are twice as likely to live in households with three or more generations than white workers.
Shares of workers by number of generations in their household, 2018.

Policy Divides: The Fallacy of Race-Neutral Policy Is Further Exposed by COVID-19

The once-in-a-generation challenges presented by the coronavirus have required leaders in government and private industry to respond quickly in order to minimize the threat to public health as well as the economic harm. Consistent with the scale of the crisis, many of the actions taken have been widespread in terms of the number of people helped, and the magnitude of the interventions has been unprecedented. Still, even such a broad-reaching response can yield uneven results because of differential access to the resources needed to equitably implement the response.

The Digital Divide Creates Disadvantages for Working and Learning Remotely

Decisions to close schools and most businesses have meant that work and learning are taking place at home and online, requiring access to computers and digital connectivity. While the majority of households in the United States have a computer and internet access, racial disparities exist. Figure P reveals that 5% fewer black households than white households have a computer in the home and 10% fewer have a broadband internet subscription. This racial disparity in computer and internet access is often referred to as the digital divide.

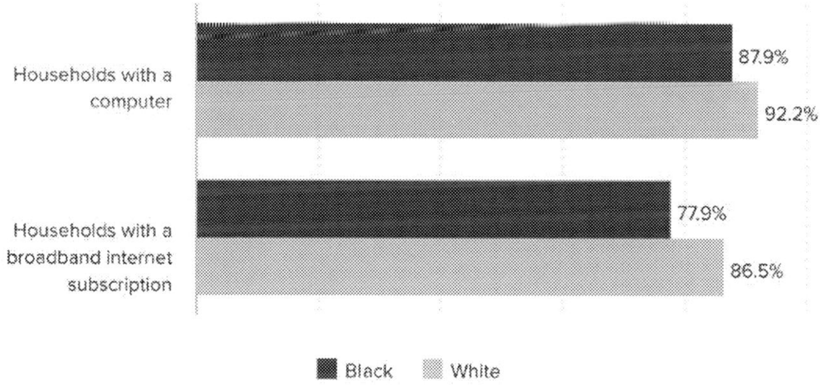

Note: White refers to non-Hispanic whites, black refers to blacks alone. Black households are households in which the head of household is black. White households are households in which the head of household is white.
Source: U.S. Census Bureau, 2018 American Community Survey 1-Year Estimates, Table S0201.

Figure P. Black households are substantially less likely to have a computer or internet access at home than white households.
Shares of black and white households with a computer and broadband internet access, 2018.

The Unbanked Face Delays in Receiving CARES Act Cash Assistance

One of the first critical interventions undertaken by Congress in the wake of the pandemic was the passage of the Coronavirus Aid, Relief, and Economic Security (CARES) Act. One of the provisions of this act includes a one-time payment of $1,200 to individuals with adjusted gross income below $75,000, and $2,400 to married couples filing taxes jointly who earn under $150,000. Families with children are also eligible to receive an additional $500 per qualifying child. Considering that the median black household income is well below those thresholds (Figure H), they are more likely to qualify; however, racial differences in access to bank accounts have presented challenges for disbursing the money to unbanked households quickly via direct deposit. According to a 2018 report from the FDIC, 16.9% of black households were unbanked in 2017, meaning no one in the household had a checking or savings account, compared with just 3.0% of white households (Apaam et al. 2018).

Black-Owned Businesses Are More Concentrated in Vulnerable Industries, but Face Challenges in Applying for Paycheck Protection Program Loans

Providing support to small businesses has been a top priority of legislation designed to lessen the harmful economic effects of the pandemic. While less than 10% (9.4%) of all U.S. business owners are African American, black-owned businesses are more likely to be in vulnerable industries. According to one estimate, 40% of the revenues of black-owned businesses are earned in the five most vulnerable sectors—including leisure, hospitality, and retail—compared with 25% of the revenues of all U.S. businesses (Fitzhugh et al. 2020).

In this analysis, we use the April 2020 decline in payroll employment by industry as a measure of which businesses have been most affected by reduced demand and are therefore more vulnerable to business failure due to the pandemic. According to the Bureau of Labor Statistics, the industries with the largest total job losses in April were in accommodation and food services, retail, and health care and social assistance. As shown in Figure Q, 27.6% of black-owned businesses are in those three sectors, compared with 19.7% of white-owned businesses. The large number of job losses in these industries is due in part to the fact that they employ many more people than other industries. Another way of measuring the impact of losses is to consider job losses as a share of March (the previous month's) payroll employment. Based on this measure, the largest percentage losses in payroll employment were in arts, entertainment and recreation; accommodation and food services; and other services. These three industries account for almost a third of black-owned businesses (32.3%), but just 18.8% of white-owned businesses.

The CARES Act also established the Paycheck Protection Program (PPP), which offers loans to small businesses to use for payroll costs, mortgage interest, rent, and utilities—loans that are forgivable on the condition that the businesses retain or rehire employees at their pre-pandemic levels of pay (SBA 2020a). At least 75% of the forgiven amount must have been used for payroll costs. While a very small share of black-owned businesses are employers—only 4.2% have employees, compared with 19.6% of all businesses and 20.6% of white-owned businesses (U.S. Census Bureau 2016a)—sole proprietorships, independent contractors, and self-employed individuals are also eligible to apply (SBA 2020b). Loans for this group of businesses can also be forgiven if 75% of the loan is used to replace 1099-MISC income or net self-employment income.

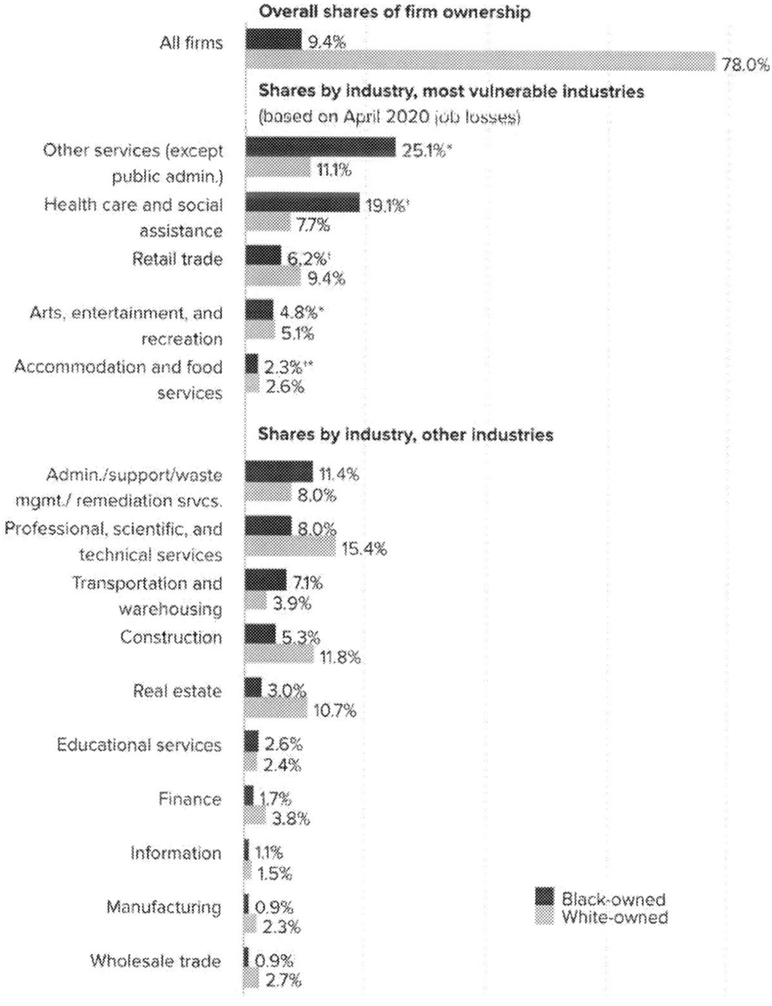

Notes: †Indicates the three industries that saw the largest declines in payroll employment in April 2020. *Indicates the three industries that saw the largest percent change declines in payroll employment in April 2020. Totals may not sum to 100%. Industries making up less than 1% of total share (agriculture, mining, utilities, management of companies and enterprises) are omitted.
Source: Authors' analysis of U.S. Census Bureau, Survey of Business Owners (2012).

Figure Q. Black-owned businesses are a small share of overall business, but are most likely to be in industries impacted by COVID-19 shutdowns.
Shares of firm ownership by industry.

Despite such broad eligibility criteria for the PPP, there have been a number of anecdotal accounts of black business owners who have faced barriers to applying for loans in the first place, even as large publicly traded companies, including popular restaurant chains, were among the first to get loans—quickly depleting the $350 billion that was originally allocated (Flitter 2020). One of the main barriers cited by small black-owned businesses has been a lack of preexisting banking relationships with the larger lenders that were first to get the program up and running in their systems. The biggest shortcoming of the PPP was that its total funding level was capped, which made it a zero-sum dash to be the first to apply.

Although a second round of $310 billion in funding was approved in late April 2020 to cover unmet demand, if the program had initially been uncapped and everybody who qualified was guaranteed to get it, there may have been less harm in a business having to wait longer to get an application processed. The defining features of parallel plans in the United Kingdom and Denmark is that they are open-ended and hence not zero-sum among businesses (White 2020; Thompson 2020).

Conclusion

The global impact of COVID-19, both in lives lost and economic devastation, is likely to leave a lasting mark for years to come. The best path forward includes making sure that we use the painful lessons learned during this crisis to better prepare ourselves for the next one. The disparate racial impact of COVID-19 illustrated in this chapter should come as no surprise given the ongoing legacy of racism that continues to produce unequal outcomes affecting nearly every aspect of life in the United States. If we are to protect African Americans from suffering under the same needlessly heavy burden during the next economic or public health crisis that they are suffering under now, we must work diligently to address long-standing underlying racial disparities in economic and health outcomes.

Acknowledgment

We are grateful for the valuable research assistance of Daniel Perez.

References

Apaam, Gerald, Susan Burhouse, Karyen Chu, Keith Ernst, Kathryn Fritzdixon, Ryan Goodstein, Alicia Lloro, Charles Opoku, Yazmin Osaki, Dhruv Sharma, and Jeffrey Weinstein. 2018. *2017 FDIC National Survey of Unbanked and Underbanked Households*. Federal Deposit Insurance Corporation, October 2018.

Card, David, Francesco Devicienti, and Agata Maida. 2011. *Rent-Sharing, Hold-Up, and Wages: Evidence from Matched Panel Data*. IZA (Institute for the Study of Labor) Discussion Paper no. 6086, October 2011.

Darity Jr., William, Darrick Hamilton, Mark Paul, Alan Aja, Anne Price, Antonio Moore, and Caterina Chiopris. 2018. *What We Get Wrong About Closing the Racial Wealth Gap*. Samuel DuBois Cook Center on Social Equity and Insight Center for Community Economic Development, April 2018.

Economic Policy Institute (EPI). 2020. *Economic Indicators: Jobs and Unemployment*. Last updated May 8, 2020.

Fitzhugh, Earl, Aria Florant, J.P. Julien, Nick Noel, Duwain Pinder, Shelley Stewart III, Jason Wright, and Samuel Yamoah. 2020. *COVID-19: Investing in Black Lives and Livelihoods*. McKinsey & Company, April 2020.

Flitter, Emily. 2020. "Few Minority-Owned Businesses Got Relief Loans They Asked For." *New York Times*, May 18, 2020.

Ganong, Peter, Damon Jones, Pascal Noel, Diana Farrell, Fiona Greig, and Chris Wheat. 2020. "*Wealth, Race, and Consumption Smoothing of Typical Income Shock*." University of Chicago, Becker Friedman Institute for Economics Working Paper no. 2020–49. http://dx.doi.org/10.2139/ssrn.3583707.

Gould, Elise. 2020a. *State of Working America Wages 2019: A Story of Slow, Uneven, and Unequal Wage Growth Over the Last 40 Years*. Economic Policy Institute, February 2020.

Gould, Elise. 2020b. "The Unemployment Rate Is Not the Right Measure to Make Economic Policy Decisions Around the Coronavirus-Driven Recession: Policymakers Should Use the Employment Rate to Continue or Stop Economic Assistance." *Working Economics Blog* (Economic Policy Institute), March 20, 2020.

Gould, Elise, and Heidi Shierholz. 2020. "Senate Coronavirus Bill Is Crucial—But It's a Fraction of What's Needed." *Working Economics Blog* (Economic Policy Institute), March 18, 2020.

Manning, Alan. 2003. *Monopsony in Motion: Imperfect Competition in Labor Markets*. Princeton, N.J.: Princeton Univ. Press.

Meepagala, Shawn, and Carl Romer. 2020. "*Mapping Racial and Ethnic Differences with COVID-19*" (interactive data tool). Center for Global Data. Accessed May 29, 2020.

Mikati, Ihab, Adam F. Benson, Thomas J. Luben, Jason D. Sacks, and Jennifer Richmond-Bryant. 2018. "Disparities in Distribution of Particulate Matter Emission Sources by Race and Poverty Status," *American Journal of Public Health* 108, no. 4: 480–485. https://doi.org/10.2105/AJPH.2017.304297.

National Advisory Commission on Civil Disorders. 2016. *The Kerner Report*. Princeton, N.J.: Princeton Univ. Press.

Rho, Hye Jin, Haley Brown, and Shawn Fremstad. 2020. *A Basic Demographic Profile of Workers in Frontline Industries.* Center for Economic and Policy Research, April 2020.

Rothstein, Richard. 2017. *The Color of Law: A Forgotten History of How Our Government Segregated America.* New York: Liveright.

Sass, Jennifer. 2013. "Air Pollution Linked to Deadly Lung Cancer." *Expert Blog* (Natural Resources Defense Council), October 17, 2013.

Shierholz, Heidi. 2020. "Nearly One in Four Workers Has Applied for Unemployment Benefits." *Working Economics Blog* (Economic Policy Institute), May 21, 2020.

Small Business Administration (SBA). 2020a. "*Paycheck Protection Program*" (web page). Accessed May 2020.

Small Business Administration (SBA). 2020b. "*PPP Loans for 1099 Independent Contractors*" (web page). Accessed May 2020.

Thompson, Derek. 2020. "Denmark's Idea Could Help the World Avoid a Great Depression." *Atlantic*, March 21, 2020.

U.S. Census Bureau. 2016a. "Statistics for All U.S. Firms by Industry, Gender, Ethnicity, and Race for the U.S., States, Metro Areas, Counties, and Places: 2012" [Table]. Data from the *Survey of Business Owners (2012)*, published September 25, 2016. Accessed May 2020.

U.S. Census Bureau. 2016b. *Survey of Business Owners (2012)*. September 2016.

U.S. Census Bureau. 2018. "*Table S0201: 2018 American Community Survey 1-Year Estimates, Selected Population Profiles*." Accessed May 2020.

White, Andreas. 2020. *Transatlantic Trends from the UK's Coronavirus Job Retention Scheme and the Paycheck Protection Program in the US.* Kinsley Napley, May 7, 2020.

Wilson, Valerie, and William M. Rodgers III. 2016. *Black–White Wage Gaps Expand with Rising Wage Inequality*. Economic Policy Institute, September 2016.

Zipperer, Ben, and Elise Gould. 2020. "Unemployment Filing Failures: New Survey Confirms That Millions of Jobless Were Unable to File an Unemployment Insurance Claim." *Working Economics Blog* (Economic Policy Institute), April 28, 2020.

Chairman SCOTT. I want to, again, thank our witnesses for their participation today.

Members of the committee may have additional questions that they will submit. It would be hoped that you would answer them as soon as possible. The hearing record will be open 14 days in order to receive the responses.

And I would remind our colleagues that, pursuant to the committee practice, witnesses—witness questions for the hearing must be submitted by the Majority Committee Staff or Committee Clerk within 7 days. Questions submitted must address the subject matter of the hearing.

I now recognize the Ranking Member for her closing statement.

Ms. FOXX. Thank you, Mr. Chairman.

I want to thank our witnesses for participating in this hearing today but, again, say we should return congressional precedent and hold our hearings in person. Running the country through virtual proceedings and proxy votes is unacceptable.

As we consider how to mitigate the impact of COVID–19 on families and communities, we must highlight the benefits that come to children and families in two-parent households. The likelihood of poverty in a two-parent family drops to 9 percent from as high as 39 percent in single-parent families.

This is crucial to remember as the percentage of two-parent households have dropped from 88 percent to 69 percent since 1960. While America's single parents make tremendous efforts on their families' behalf and may not have other options, we can encourage and remove barriers to raising children in two-parent homes.

Before COVID–19, unemployment was at record lows, including minority unemployment, and the flourishing economy ushered in under the Republican-led Congress and the Trump administration benefited workers, employers, and families alike.

The coronavirus and related State-imposed shutdowns have caused devastating job losses. The positive news: there is a path forward. We have seen from the May jobs report last month, with 2.5 million jobs added to the economy, that reopening our economy safely is helping Americans get back on their feet.

Mr. Chairman, I also would like to ask unanimous consent that the June 21 editorial from The Wall Street Journal, "Failure in the Virtual Classroom," be included in today's hearing record.

THE WALL STREET JOURNAL.

Failure in the Virtual Classroom

A study finds that many schools barely cared if kids did any work.

By The Editorial Board
June 21, 2020 5:49 pm ET

The remote-learning experiment isn't going well. This month the University of Washington's Center on Reinventing Public Education published a report looking at how 477 school districts nationwide have responded to the Covid-19 crisis. Its findings reveal widespread neglect of students.

The report found only 27% of districts required teachers to record whether students participate in remote classes, while remote attendance has been abysmal. During the first two weeks of the shutdown, some 15,000 Los Angeles students failed to show up for classes or do any schoolwork.

The Philadelphia Inquirer reported that, 10 weeks in, "the Philadelphia School District registers just 61% of students attending school on an average day." The same week the Boston Globe reported that only "half of students are logging into online class or submitting assignments online on a typical day."

Students have an incentive to ditch digital class, since their work counts for little or nothing. Only 57.9% of school districts do any progress monitoring, the report found. The rest haven't even set the minimal expectation that teachers review or keep track of the work their students turn in. Homework counts toward students' final grades in 42% of districts. And some schools that do grade offer students a pass/incomplete.

Teachers unions never want teachers' performance judged by student achievement, so they've lobbied to ensure a lack of accountability and assessment during the shutdowns. They dressed up this demand in the language of social justice: Because the pandemic has not visited the same hardships on all families, the only equitable solution is to deprive *all* students of for-credit instruction, they claim.

Chicago Teachers Union President Jesse Sharkey said that "customary forms of grading are inappropriate in a global health crisis" and asked "how can such an uneven playing field produce fairness and justice for minority students?" United Teachers Los Angeles lobbied for no student to receive a failing grade, or a worse grade than they had before the shutdowns. The union declared that "we are pressing [the school district] to not mandate summer school for students who earned a D grade," which they said was "simply an issue of fairness."

The current and past presidents of the District Teachers Association for the Mountain View-Los Altos High School District in California jointly wrote in April that "in effect, assigning letter grades to our students is equal to assessing their access to technology and Wi-Fi, their housing security and ableism."

In reality, this "equitable" treatment dooms poor and minority students to a lasting educational disadvantage. In April, the National Assessment of Educational Progress reported only 24% of eighth graders scored proficient or above in civics, while 15% showed proficiency in U.S. history. And that was before school districts decided to write off the spring semester as a loss.

Rich parents can afford tutoring or can transfer their kids to costly private schools where learning continues and homework still counts. The least privileged kids will be stuck. With no grades or tests to identify those who have fallen behind, children will be pushed into the next grade regardless of whether they're ready. Many will never catch up. Where's the outrage over this injustice?

Ms. FOXX. And I want to give some quotes from it to explain some of the problems that we are having right now that nobody has discussed.

The title Failure in the Virtual Classroom, the remote learning experiment isn't going well. This month, the University of Washington Center on Reinventing Public Education published a report looking at how 477 school districts nationwide have responded to the COVID–19 crisis. Its findings reveal widespread neglect of students. This should concern all of us, Mr. Chairman.

The report found only 27 percent of districts required teachers to record whether students participate in remote classes while remote attendance has been abysmal. During the first 2 weeks of the shutdown, some 15,000 Los Angeles students failed to show up for any classes or do any schoolwork.

The Philadelphia Inquirer reported that, 10 weeks in, the Philadelphia school district registered just 61 percent of students attending schools on an average day.

The same week, the Boston Globe reported that only half of students are logging into online classes or submitting assignments online.

Students have an incentive to ditch digital classes since their work counts for little or nothing. Only 57.9 percent of school districts do any progress monitoring. The rest haven't even set the minimal expectations that teachers review or keep track of the work their students turn in.

We are failing our students, and it is because primarily, as this article points out, of teacher unions, and they go on to quote the people in the teacher unions.

It really—we need to get the schools open and do anything we possibly can.

I also want to point out that, to tie it back into the economic situation, yesterday, The Wall Street Journal editorial board pointed out that, quote, States that are reopening faster are recovering faster and easing more economic suffering. Specifically, the editorial board writes: Nine of the 10 States with the highest jobless rate are run by Democrats, who have tended to demand that the economy should stay locked down and, in some cases, are still resisting opening. One exception is Colorado, where our former colleague, Democratic Governor Jared Polis, was one of the first to reopen. His decision is paying off as Colorado's jobless rate in May fell to 10.2 percent from 12.2 percent in April. To lead our country back to a thriving economy, we can and we must reopen America.

There is also one other thing that I noticed in one set of comments that were made near the end of this hearing, and that was the comment that it is better to basically give welfare than it is to help people get a job, and, Mr. Chairman, that goes against everything we have ever known in this country, which is you get a better bang for your buck from welfare than by people going to work, and I just don't think that is true.

I think everything that we can do to help people go to work, it diminishes poverty. It gives people options. And I hope that we will take some more focus on that in the future and talk about those statistics, too.

With that, Mr. Chairman, I yield back.

Chairman SCOTT. Thank you. I thank you for your comments on the impact—economic impact of certain initiatives. That is actually arithmetic. Some investments in the economy do better than others, and that is just a fact. The [inaudible] tax and capital gains tax holiday do virtually nothing to stimulate the economy whereas some of the other supports do much better.

But there is a lot that we can do to help our Nation get through this pandemic. In end the—and also reduce the racial disparities as we do it. We want to thank our witnesses for their guidance and pointing out that the HEROES Act is a major step in the right direction to get us through this pandemic.

If there is nothing more to come before the committee, the committee now stands adjourned, and I thank our witnesses again.

Thank you.

Congressional Research Service
Informing the legislative debate since 1914

MEMORANDUM June 19, 2020

To: House Committee on Education and Labor

From: Bernadette Fernandez, Specialist in Health Care Financing, bfernandez@crs.loc.gov, 7-0322
Ryan J. Rosso, Analyst in Health Care Financing, rrosso@crs.loc.gov, 7-9995
Evelyne P. Baumrucker, Specialist in Health Care Financing, ebaumrucker@crs.loc.gov, 7-8913
Adrienne L. Fernandes-Alcantara, Specialist in Social Policy, afernandes@crs.loc.gov, 7-9005
Victoria L. Elliott, Analyst in Health Policy, velliott@crs.loc.gov, 7-2640
Jameson A. Carter, Research Assistant, jacarter@crs.loc.gov, 7-9963

Subject: **Information Requested about Racial Disparities in Private Health Insurance and Medicaid and COVID-19 Related Issues**

This memorandum is in response to your request for information regarding racial disparities and health coverage, specifically in the context of the Coronavirus Disease 2019 (COVID-19) pandemic. You provided questions to the Congressional Research Service (CRS) as a starting point for this project; the final set of issues addressed in this memorandum is the result of discussions between you and CRS. Per such discussions, the memorandum specifically explores disparities with respect to private health insurance (including employer-sponsored health benefits), Medicaid, and the State Children's Health Insurance Program (CHIP) only and does not address other forms of coverage. Relevant background information applicable to these sources of coverage is incorporated into the answers as necessary.

Given that the pandemic is a recent event, information about the effects of the pandemic on existing racial disparities in health coverage is limited. Furthermore, given the time constraints associated with this request, CRS's ability to perform original analysis was also limited. As such, CRS relied heavily on existing research to respond to your questions as submitted, which are in bold below. We synthesized historical and current information (when possible) concerning racial disparities in health coverage. We also include discussion of recent research and government efforts that are directly relevant to the issues raised in your questions related to the current pandemic. Due to the afore-mentioned time constraints, we were not able to provide a thorough analysis of all issues raised in your questions, but attempted to broadly identify policy and implementation issues, provide examples for illustrative purposes, and cite relevant sources of information.

This memorandum is written in a Questions and Answers format to align with the memorandum request. Your four questions are pasted below verbatim, in the order submitted to CRS. Given that disparities in health coverage may be of general interest to Congress, information included in this memorandum may be provided to other congressional requesters or incorporated into other CRS products for general distribution. Your identity as a requester would not be disclosed in either case.

Responses to Submitted Questions on Racial Disparities in Health Coverage and COVID-19 Related Issues

Question 1. What percentage of unemployed workers of color work in industries/occupations that provide employer-sponsored health care coverage?

In discussing this question with CRS, you indicated a preference for an explanation of any data limitations associated with your stated question and a response from CRS to related questions that could be answered using available resources. The rest of this response provides that information.

CRS is not aware of any survey data sources that provide population estimates of the industry/occupation of individuals that became unemployed since the start of the COVID-19 pandemic in the U.S. and/or corresponding recession.

CRS is aware of two existing surveys that could *separately* provide statistics on the following measures prior to the beginning of the pandemic: (1) the percentage of unemployed workers by race and Hispanic origin and by industry/occupation[1] and (2) the percentage of employees at surveyed firms who are offered employer-sponsored insurance by industry/occupation.[2] However, the survey parameters do not allow the two data sources to be merged to answer your question as submitted. Some of the methodological issues are subsequently outlined below.

First, the two data sources are surveying different populations. One source is a survey of individuals that would identify the percentage of unemployed workers by race and Hispanic origin and by previously worked industry/occupation. The second source is a survey of employers that identify the percentage of employees who are offered employer-sponsored insurance at such firms. These two surveys are not linked and have different sampling units. Given these differences, it could not be assumed that an unemployed individual who previously worked in a particular industry/occupation would be offered health insurance at the same rate in which the industry/occupation offered employer-sponsored health insurance.

Second, the two surveys provide point in time estimates of two different populations at the time that each survey was administered. Some individuals who were unemployed at the time they were surveyed returned to work *after* the timeframe surveyed. The offer rate of employer-sponsored insurance may have changed for a variety of factors (e.g., business' economic concerns) in between when the survey was administered and the individual returned to work. Furthermore, an individual would be returning to a job that is hiring at that time the individual is seeking a job. The rate of which *hiring* firms offer employer-sponsored insurance within an industry/occupation may be different than the rate in which *all* firms within an industry or occupation offer employer-sponsored insurance.

Third, it could not be assumed that an individual would return to work in the same industry/occupation that they previously worked.

As such and per CRS' conversation with you, the following question has been answered:

What percentage of workers in each industry/occupation were offered employer-sponsored health insurance, by race and Hispanic origin, and did workers of any race or Hispanic origin have offer rates that were statistically different than the percentage of White workers that were offered employer-sponsored health insurance in the same industry/occupation?

[1] U.S. Census Bureau, *Current Population Survey Data Tables*, https://www.census.gov/programs-surveys/cps/data/tables.html.

[2] U.S. Bureau of Labor Statistics, *Employee Benefit Survey*, https://www.bls.gov/ncs/ebs/benefits/2019/benefits_health.htm.

CRS typically relies on survey data when trying to respond to questions about different groupings of Americans. One such source is the Census Bureau's Annual Social and Economic Supplement to the Current Population Survey (CPS ASEC), which provides annual estimates on income, poverty, and health insurance coverage in the United States.[3] The most recent release of CPS ASEC data predates the COVID-19 pandemic and provides estimates for 2019.

CRS analyzed CPS ASEC data to estimate the number of working Americans who reported being offered health insurance by their employer in 2019.[4] This information is presented by industry and occupation in **Table 1** and **Table 2**, respectively. The industries and occupations included in the CPS ASEC survey are determined by the Census Bureau and are self-reported by the respondents.

As evident in the industry-centered table (**Table 1**), there is a wide range of employer-sponsored health insurance offer rates across industries, which range from 43.5% to 88.3% across 13 industries. Workers in the public administration, mining, and manufacturing industries reported being offered employer-sponsored insurance at the highest rates (88.3%, 85.2% and 84.1%, respectively) in 2019. On the other end of the spectrum, workers in the agriculture/forestry/fishing/hunting, leisure/hospitality, and other services industries reported being offered employer-sponsored insurance at the lowest rates (43.5%, 46.7%, and 52.0%, respectively).

Table 1. Percentage of Workers by Industry Who Were Offered Employer-Sponsored Insurance, 2019

Industry	Offered Employer-Sponsored Insurance	Lower Limit of Offer Rate	Upper Limit of Offer Rate	Standard Error
Agriculture/forestry/fishing/hunting	43.5%	38.2%	48.9%	3.3%
Mining	85.2%	80.5%	89.9%	2.9%
Construction	61.4%	59.1%	63.6%	1.4%
Manufacturing	84.1%	83.0%	85.2%	0.7%
Wholesale and retail trade	65.8%	64.2%	67.3%	0.9%
Transportation/utilities	77.2%	75.5%	78.9%	1.0%
Information	81.0%	78.0%	84.0%	1.8%
Financial activities	81.2%	79.5%	82.8%	1.0%
Professional/business services	75.6%	74.3%	77.0%	0.8%
Educational/health services	76.7%	75.9%	77.6%	0.5%
Leisure/hospitality	46.7%	45.2%	48.3%	0.9%
Other services	52.0%	49.5%	54.5%	1.5%
Public administration	88.3%	87.0%	89.7%	0.8%

Source: CRS analysis of CPS March Supplement, 2019. Additionally, the 2019 ASEC research file for offer and take-up of employer-sponsored health insurance. The March Supplement is used primarily for occupation classes, industry classes, work status, and race, while the research file is used for offer rates.

[3] U.S. Census Bureau, *Current Population Survey Data Tables*, https://www.census.gov/programs-surveys/cps/data/tables.html.

[4] Jameson A. Carter, Research Assistant, performed the statistical analysis.

Notes: Workers are defined as those who were employed in the prior week, and who are not self-employed. The survey is conducted from February to April so these weeks vary. Therefore, these 2019 estimates only contain information from the spring. A worker was defined as receiving an offer if they were the policyholder of employer-sponsored insurance in the reference week or, if they were not a policyholder, if their job offered employer-sponsored insurance that they were eligible for.

All of these estimates are derived from a sample, which is an incomplete measurement of the U.S. population. CRS used standard errors to characterize just how incomplete these estimates could be. Standard errors are a measure of the extent to which an estimate can be expected to deviate from a true value for the full population. That is, how much these specific offer rate calculations might differ from the reality faced by Americans. Furthermore, researchers often turn to confidence intervals in order to characterize standard errors, as these intervals use statistical maxims to gauge statistical precision. Note that the lower and upper limits reported in this table represent the bounds of a 90% confidence interval. For example, for persons employed in the agricultural industry you would interpret the 90% confidence interval as such, "The 90% confidence interval for offer rates of Agricultural workers ranged from 38.2% to 48.9%. If the 2019 ASEC were repeated 100 times, the true offer rate would fall within an interval constructed in this way 90 times. That is, if the true offer rate does not fall within the interval reported in this table, it is due to an issue in the sample that occurs 10% of the time." See,
https://www.census.gov/content/dam/Census/library/publications/2018/acs/acs_general_handbook_2018_ch07.pdf and https://www.ncbi.nlm.nih.gov/pmc/articles/PMC4742505/.

As evident in the occupation-centered table (**Table 2**), there is a wide range of employer-sponsored health insurance offer rates across occupations, which range from 39.0% to 85.1% across 10 occupations. Workers with a management/business/financial occupation and professional/related occupation reported being offered employer-sponsored insurance at the highest rates (85.1% and 81.6%, respectively) in 2019. On the other end of the spectrum, workers with a farmer/fishing/forestry occupation and service occupation reported being offered employer-sponsored insurance at the lowest rate (39.0% and 53.2%, respectively).

Table 2. Percentage of Workers by Occupation Who Were Offered Employer-Sponsored Insurance, 2019

Occupation	Offered Employer-Sponsored Insurance	Lower Limit of Offer Rate	Upper Limit of Offer Rate	Standard Error
Management/business/financial jobs	85.1%	84.1%	86.1%	0.6%
Professional/related jobs	81.6%	80.8%	82.4%	0.5%
Service jobs	53.2%	51.9%	54.5%	0.8%
Sales/related jobs	63.0%	61.3%	64.6%	1.0%
Office/administrative support jobs	74.1%	72.9%	75.3%	0.7%
Farming/fishing/forestry jobs	39.0%	33.2%	44.8%	3.5%
Construction/extraction jobs	58.4%	55.8%	61.0%	1.6%
Installation/maintenance/repair jobs	77.4%	75.2%	79.7%	1.4%
Production jobs	78.5%	76.9%	80.1%	1.0%
Transportation/material moving jobs	66.9%	64.9%	68.8%	1.2%

Source: CRS analysis of CPS March Supplement, 2019. Additionally, the 2019 ASEC research file for offer and take-up of employer-sponsored health insurance. The March Supplement is used primarily for occupation classes, industry classes, work status, and race, while the research file is used for offer rates.

Notes: Workers are defined as those who were employed in the prior week, and who are not self-employed. The survey is conducted from February to April so these weeks vary. Therefore, these 2019 estimates only contain information from the spring. A worker was defined as receiving an offer if they were the policyholder of employer-sponsored insurance in the reference week or, if they were not a policyholder, if their job offered employer-sponsored insurance that they were eligible for.

All of these estimates are derived from a sample, which is an incomplete measurement of the U.S. population. CRS used standard errors to characterize just how incomplete these estimates could be. Standard errors are a measure of the extent to which an estimate can be expected to deviate from a true value for the full population. That is, how much these specific offer rate calculations might differ from the reality faced by Americans. Furthermore, researchers often turn to confidence intervals in order to characterize standard errors, as these intervals use statistical maxims to gauge statistical precision. Note that the lower and upper limits reported in this table represent the bounds of a 90% confidence interval. For example, for persons employed in the agricultural industry you would interpret the 90% confidence interval as such, "The 90% confidence interval for offer rates of Agricultural workers ranged from 38.2% to 48.9%. If the 2019 ASEC were repeated 100 times, the true offer rate would fall within an interval constructed in this way 90 times. That is, if the true offer rate does not fall within the interval reported in this table, it is due to an issue in the sample that occurs 10% of the time." See,
https://www.census.gov/content/dam/Census/library/publications/2018/acs/acs_general_handbook_2018_ch07.pdf and https://www.ncbi.nlm.nih.gov/pmc/articles/PMC4742505/.

CRS then estimated the percentage of workers in each industry and occupation who were offered employer-sponsored insurance, by race and Hispanic origin. These estimates incorporate the respondent's self-reported responses to the survey questions on race/ethnicity and reflect the CPS ASEC survey response categories related to race and Hispanic origin.[5] The category of "Multiracial, non-Hispanic" is the combination of all categories where multiple races were indicated. The race and ethnicity categories are mutually exclusive. Statistical significance testing (at the 90% level) was subsequently performed to determine whether each estimate was significantly different from the estimate for the "White alone, non-Hispanic" grouping within a given industry or occupation category. In some instances, there was not a large enough sample size to make such analysis and corresponding cells were labeled with a "—".

As evident in the industry-centered table (**Table 3**), there were no statistically significant differences in the employer-sponsored insurance offer rates between Black workers and White workers in any industry category in 2019. However, there were numerous industries in which Hispanic workers were offered employer-sponsored insurance at statistically significant lower rates than White workers in the same industry. This was most pronounced in the construction and professional/business services industries. The rate in which Asian workers were offered employer-sponsored insurance in particular industries occasionally did not have any statistically significant difference from the offer rates for White workers in the same industry. In two of five industries that indicated a statistically significant difference (information and professional/business services), Asian workers were offered employer-sponsored insurance at higher rates than White workers in the same industry.

Table 3. Percentage of Workers within Each Industry Who Were Offered Employer-Sponsored Insurance, by Race and Hispanic Origin, 2019

Industry	White alone, non-Hispanic	Black alone, non-Hispanic	Hispanic, any race	Asian alone, non-Hispanic	Multiracial, non-Hispanic	AIAN alone, non-Hispanic
Agriculture/ forestry/fishing /hunting	47.2%	—	38.6%	—	—	—
Mining	86.3%	—	78.7%	—	—	—
Construction	70.6%	65.2%	45.6%*	62.9%	—	—
Manufacturing	87.1%	83.5%	72.6%*	84.5%	81.1%	81.0%

[5] U.S. Census Bureau, *ASEC 2019 Public Use Data Dictionary*, https://thedataweb.rm.census.gov/pub/cps/march/06_ASEC_2019-Data_Dictionary_Full.pdf.

Industry	White alone, non-Hispanic	Black alone, non-Hispanic	Hispanic, any race	Asian alone, non-Hispanic	Multiracial, non-Hispanic	AIAN alone, non-Hispanic
Wholesale and retail trade	67.8%	65.7%	60.8%*	61.0%*	58.8%	71.0%
Transportation /utilities	79.7%	79.8%	68.6%*	71.6%	75.8%	—
Information	82.1%	76.6%	78.8%	90.7%*	—	—
Financial activities	81.4%	84.7%	76.1%	84.6%	81.7%	—
Professional/ business services	78.4%	75.0%	59.1%*	86.6%*	75.3%	—
Educational/ health services	78.1%	76.2%	70.5%*	79.1%	72.7%	66.3%*
Leisure/ hospitality	46.8%	51.5%	44.3%	45.8%	42.9%	53.3%
Other services	55.7%	59.6%	43.7%*	36.4%*	—	—
Public administration	89.6%	89.0%	85.7%	77.7%*	86.1%	80.6%

Source: CRS analysis of CPS March Supplement, 2019. Additionally, the 2019 ASEC research file for offer and take-up of employer-sponsored health insurance. The March Supplement is used primarily for occupation classes, industry classes, work status, and race, while the research file is used for offer rates.

Notes: The estimates comprise the respondent's self-reported responses to the survey questions on race/ethnicity and reflect the CPS ASEC survey response categories related to race and Hispanic origin. The category of "Multiracial, non-Hispanic" is the combination of all categories where multiple races were indicated. The groupings listed in this table are mutually exclusive. AIAN = American Indian and Alaskan Native.

These are point estimates and in order to compare between groups, statistical significance testing was conducted. All point estimates noted with a * have been tested for being significantly different (at the 90% level) from the "White alone, non-Hispanic" grouping *within each occupation*. Therefore, comparing offer rates between occupations is not advisable. Further, comparing offer rates between any two race and/or Hispanic origin groupings is not advisable, other than comparing any one race or Hispanic origin category with White workers. Significance is in part due to the error around an estimate. While a point estimate may be reliable enough to be reported on its own, differences between races and Hispanic origin may not be significant because of the error around the estimate. Cells with "—" denote that the category's estimates were derived from fewer than 75,000 weighted observations and/or that the standard errors were high enough that the estimates were not considered reliable.

As evident in the occupation-centered table (**Table 4**), offer rates for employer-sponsored insurance for Black workers were not statistically different than the offer rates for White workers in any occupation in 2019. However, in almost all occupations, Hispanic workers were offered employer-sponsored insurance at statistically significant lower rates than White workers in the same occupation. This was most pronounced in the construction/extraction occupation.

The lack of statistically significant differences between certain races/ethnicity and White workers in certain industries and occupations (**Table 3** and **Table 4**) may in part reflect federal requirements on employers regarding how employer-sponsored health insurance must be offered. Specifically, employers offering employer-sponsored health insurance to certain employees must make that coverage available to all *similarly situated* individuals.[6] Similarly, all restrictions on such benefits must apply to all *similarly situated* individuals. In this context, a group of *similarly situated* individuals is identified by a "distinction

[6] 29 C.F.R. § 2590.702(b)(2).

between or among the groups of participants [that] is based on a bona fide employment-based classification consistent with the employer's usual business practice."[7] Depending on the employer, a bona fide employment-based classification could be full-time versus part-time, different geographic locations, membership in collective bargaining units, different occupations, etc.

Table 4. Percentage of Workers within Each Occupation Who Were Offered Employer-Sponsored Insurance, by Race and Hispanic Origin, 2019

Occupation	White alone, non-Hispanic	Black alone, non-Hispanic	Hispanic, any race	Asian alone, non-Hispanic	Multiracial, non-Hispanic	AIAN alone, non-Hispanic
Management/business/financial jobs	85.3%	89.6%*	79.6%*	86.3%	84.6%	77.8%
Professional/related jobs	81.8%	82.5%	76.2%*	86.1%*	73.7%*	78.8%
Service jobs	54.3%	62.1%*	47.1%*	44.6%*	50.5%	48.9%
Sales/related jobs	65.8%	60.5%	57.5%*	53.7%*	55.0%	—
Office/administrative support jobs	75.0%	76.7%	70.0%*	70.6%	72.3%	79.8%
Farming/fishing/forestry jobs	41.2%	—	35.8%	—	—	—
Construction/extraction jobs	68.2%	69.0%	44.1%*	—	—	—
Installation/maintenance/repair jobs	79.8%	78.9%	68.8%*	76.0%	—	—
Production jobs	82.1%	82.7%	68.2%*	74.0%*	78.7%	—
Transportation/material moving jobs	69.2%	70.1%	60.8%*	58.6%*	58.5%	—

Source: CRS analysis of CPS March Supplement, 2019. Additionally, the 2019 ASEC research file for offer and take-up of employer-sponsored health insurance. The March Supplement is used primarily for occupation classes, industry classes, work status, and race, while the research file is used for offer rates.

Notes: The estimates comprise the respondent's self-reported responses to the survey questions on race/ethnicity and reflect the CPS ASEC survey response categories related to race and Hispanic origin. The category of "Multiracial, non-Hispanic" is the combination of all categories where multiple races were indicated. The groupings listed in this table are mutually exclusive. AIAN = American Indian and Alaskan Native.

These are point estimates and in order to compare between groups, statistical significance testing was conducted. All point estimates noted with a * have been tested for being significantly different (at the 90% level) from the "White alone, non-Hispanic" grouping *within each occupation*. Therefore, comparing offer rates between occupations is not advisable. Further, comparing offer rates between any two race and/or Hispanic origin groupings is not advisable, other than comparing any one race or Hispanic origin category with White workers. Significance is in part due to the error around an estimate. While a point estimate may be reliable enough to be reported on its own, differences between races and Hispanic origin may not be significant because of the error around the estimate. Cells with "—" denote that the category's estimates were derived from fewer than 75,000 weighted observations and/or that the standard errors were high enough that the estimates were not considered reliable.

Question 2. What challenges have furloughed workers of color faced when seeking health care services, given that changes in their income have affected their ability to pay out-of-pocket costs for care?

This question cannot be answered completely either quantitatively or qualitatively, however CRS can provide answers and information regarding related questions. The rest of this response describes the

[7] 29 C.F.R. § 2590.702(d)(1).

limitations associated with answering the submitted question and provides answers to the related questions.

Quantitative Response

The Census Bureau has been conducting the Household Pulse Survey to measure household experiences during the COVID-19 pandemic.[8] The Census Bureau has been conducting the survey over six day periods (with the exception of the first survey period) and has been releasing data every week since May 20, 2020. The first data collection period occurred during 2020 from April 23-May 5 and the most recent data period was from June 4 -June 9.

With respect to this question, the Household Pulse Survey estimates the number of Americans aged 18 and older who report that they delayed getting medical care in the past four weeks because of the COVID-19 pandemic. It also estimates the number of Americans aged 18 and older who report that they did not get needed medical care (for a medical issue unrelated to COVID-19) in the past four weeks because of the COVID-19 pandemic. This data is presented by select characteristics including: age, sex, ethnicity, race, education level, marital status, presence of children in the household, whether the respondent or a household member experienced loss of employment income, whether the respondent is currently employed, and household income.

Given the newness of the data, CRS is still identifying the extent to which such data can be cross-tabulated to answer specific policy questions and still be statistically accurate. For example, to answer the asked policy question, CRS would need to be able to analyze the number of Americans aged 18 and older that delayed getting medical care in the past four weeks because of the COVID-19 pandemic by Hispanic origin and race, *and* whether the respondent or a household member experienced loss of employment income. At this time, CRS is able to answer questions regarding delayed medical care when controlling for one variable at a time. As such, the following questions have been answered:

What percentage of individuals (aged 18 and older), by race and Hispanic origin, have delayed getting medical care in the past four weeks because of the COVID-19 pandemic and how has this changed over time?

[8] U.S. Census Bureau, *Measuring Household Experiences during the Coronavirus (COVID-19) Pandemic*, https://www.census.gov/householdpulsedata.

Figure 1. Percentage of Individuals Who Reported that They Delayed Getting Medical Care in the Last Four Weeks Because of the COVID-19 Pandemic

Individuals Aged 18 and Older

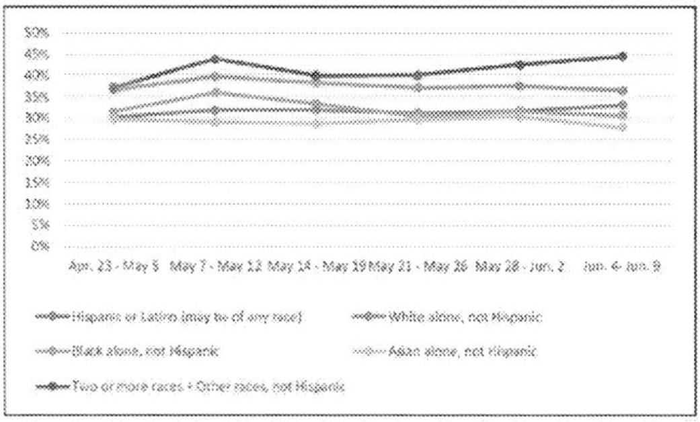

Source: CRS analysis of U.S. Census Bureau, Household Pulse Survey.

Notes: Time periods are associated with the survey date of the individuals, which took place in 2020. This chart displays the percentage of survey respondents that delayed medical care relative to all survey respondents (including those that did not answer this survey question). The racial and ethnic differences and changes over time were not evaluated for statistical significance.

What percentage of individuals (aged 18 and older), by race and Hispanic origin, did not get needed medical care in the past four weeks because of the COVID-19 pandemic and how has this changed over time?

Figure 2. Percentage of Individuals Who Reported that They Needed Medical Care for Something Unrelated to COVID-19 In the Last Four Weeks, But Did Not Get It Because of the COVID-19 Pandemic

Individuals Aged 18 and Older

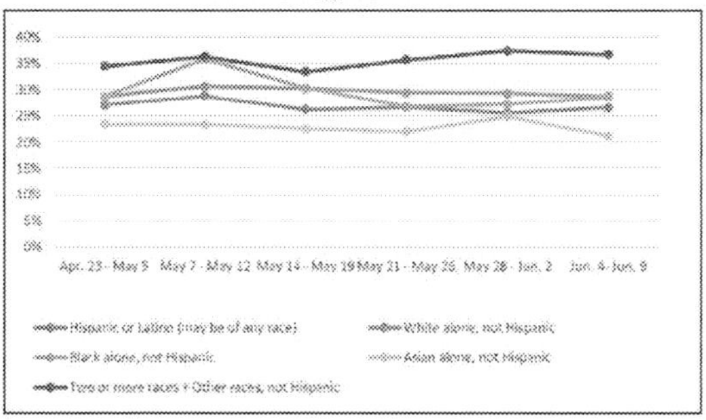

Source: CRS analysis of U.S. Census Bureau, Household Pulse Survey.

Notes: Time periods are associated with the survey date of the individuals, which took place in 2020. This chart displays the percentage of survey respondents that delayed medical care relative to all survey respondents (including those that did not answer this survey question). The racial and Hispanic origin differences and changes over time were not evaluated for statistical significance.

While the Census Bureau asked respondents to indicate whether they delayed care or did not receive needed care "because of COVID-19," it did not ask respondents for more specific reasons *why* they delayed or did not receive medical care.[9] Since there are multiple ways in which the COVID-19 pandemic may have caused an individual to delay or not receive care, CRS cannot speculate whether individuals delayed or did not receive care because the individual did not have access to a provider, had a nonemergency medical procedure delayed, lost their health insurance, did not have the resources to afford care, or had another reason (e.g., concerns about the risk of being exposed to the coronavirus during a visit).

Qualitative Response

In discussing this question with CRS, you indicated interest in a general explanation of health coverage options that may be available to individuals who lose employment. A given individual may have a range of options available to them, but the number and sources of such options will vary from person to person because different eligibility rules are associated with different public and private sources of coverage. The eligibility rules may take into account factors such as income, age, residency, disability status, immigration status, family composition, pregnancy status, duration of eligibility, other insurance coverage, and employer characteristics. Such eligibility criteria may lead to coverage gaps for certain individuals seeking health coverage. With this in mind, the following discussion identifies possible sources of public and private coverage; this discussion relies primarily on information provided in the CRS In Focus, *Health Insurance Options Following Loss of Employment*.

Job loss may not necessarily result in loss of employment-based health benefits. Some employers may continue to offer health benefits to such individuals, especially furloughed workers who are expected to return to their job. For example, an employer survey conducted by Mercer, a benefits consulting firm, found that of the employers who responded to the survey, one-third are considering furloughs within the next 60 days. And of those employers who are considering furloughs, one-half indicated that "they would continue health benefits while just 3% said they would not; the rest were still undecided."[10]

For workers who do lose health benefits due to job loss, they may be able to access other employment-based coverage, provided they meet applicable eligibility criteria. For example, a married individual whose spouse's employer offers health benefits to workers and dependents may be able to enroll in that coverage. Also, many employers are subject to federal COBRA continuation coverage requirements, which requires applicable employers to provide to certain former employees, their spouse, and their dependent children with temporary access to the former employer's health insurance. While certain individuals may have access to one or both of these coverage options, affordability may be a concern, due to the reduction in income following job loss. Affordability may be of particular concern for individuals seeking COBRA coverage. Federal law allows employers to charge the covered individual 100% of the premium (i.e., both the portion paid by the employee and the portion paid by the employer), plus an additional 2% administrative fee.

For individuals who are interested in seeking private health insurance outside of the employment setting, they may purchase individual insurance directly from an issuer in the individual health insurance market.[11] The individual market includes the health insurance exchanges (marketplaces) established under

---

[9] U.S. Census Bureau, *2020 COVID-19 Household Pulse Survey*, https://www2.census.gov/programs-surveys/demo/technical-documentation/hhp/2020_COVID-19_Household_Pulse_Survey-Week-of-6_11_2020_English.pdf.

[10] Mercer, "Poll Results: Furloughs, Lay-offs, and Health Benefit Decisions," April 9, 2020, at https://www.mercer.us/our-thinking/healthcare/poll-results-furloughs-lay-offs-and-health-benefit-decisions.html.

[11] For background information about the health insurance market, see the "Background" section of CRS Report R45146, *Federal Requirements on Private Health Insurance Plans*.

the ACA,[12] but individuals also can purchase coverage outside of the exchanges. Affordability may be a concern for those interested in obtaining individual insurance. While there is federal financial assistance, in the form of tax credits and cost sharing subsidies, that make insurance sold through exchanges more affordable, individuals must first meet income and other eligibility criteria in order to qualify for this assistance.[13] Moreover, individuals who do receive the financial assistance often are still required to pay some portion of their premium and cost-sharing. Loss of income due to unemployment may make this coverage option cost prohibitive.

Outside of private coverage, an individual[14] may be able to access public coverage through their state's Medicaid program. To be eligible for Medicaid, individuals must meet both categorical (i.e., a group listed in statute) and financial (e.g., income, assets) criteria in addition to requirements regarding residency, immigration status, and U.S. citizenship. Historically, Medicaid eligibility has been limited to low-income children, pregnant women, parents of dependent children, the elderly, and individuals with disabilities. However, since 2014, 36 states and the District of Columbia have taken up the option to cover non-elderly adults with income up to 133% of federal poverty level (FPL) through the ACA Medicaid expansion.[15] For some eligibility groups or *pathways*, state coverage is mandatory (e.g., low-income children up to 133% of the FPL, whereas for others it is optional (e.g., pregnant women with annual income between 133% and 185% of FPL). This results in variability in eligibility from state to state. For example, adult coverage differs between states with and without the ACA Medicaid expansion. A recent analysis by the Kaiser Family Foundation, shows the impact of state Medicaid eligibility decisions on "communities of color." According to the analysis, uninsured "Blacks" are more likely than uninsured "Whites" to fall in a coverage gap (15% vs. 9% as of April 2020) because a greater share of uninsured "Blacks" live in states that have not implemented the ACA Medicaid expansion, and they are not income eligible for subsidized coverage available through the exchanges.[16] Uninsured individuals in non-ACA Medicaid expansion states fall into a coverage gap when they earn too much to qualify for another Medicaid eligibility pathway, but too little to qualify for subsides to purchase health insurance coverage on the exchange. Subsidized coverage on the exchange typically applies between 100 percent and 400 percent of the federal poverty level. Beneficiary cost sharing (e.g., premiums and co-payments) is limited under the Medicaid program.[17]

Question 3. How has increased exposure to COVID-19 interfered with access to health enrollment assistance for communities of color?

The ACA requires a data-driven, coordinated eligibility determination and enrollment system across Medicaid, the State Children's Health Insurance Program (CHIP) and subsidized coverage available through the health insurance exchanges.[18] The ACA required states to screen for eligibility through a

[12] For more information about the ACA exchanges, see CRS Report R44065, *Overview of Health Insurance Exchanges*.

[13] For more information about the tax credits and cost-sharing subsidies, see CRS Report R44425, *Health Insurance Premium Tax Credits and Cost-Sharing Subsidies*.

[14] While some Medicaid eligibility pathways are specific to families and take into account household income, eligibility for Medicaid is generally determined on an individual basis.

[15] Medicaid and CHIP Payment and Access Commission (MACPAC), *Medicaid Expansion to the New Adult Group: State Medicaid Expansion Decisions. May 2020*, https://www.macpac.gov/subtopic/medicaid-expansion/.

[16] Samatha Artiga, Rachel Garfield, and Kandal Oegera, *Communities of Color at Higher Risk for Health and Economic Challenges due to COVID-19*, Kaiser Family Foundation, April 7, 2020, https://www.kff.org/coronavirus-covid-19/issue-brief/communities-of-color-at-higher-risk-for-health-and-economic-challenges-due-to-covid-19/. Analysis based on Kaiser Family Foundation analysis of 2018 American Community Survey, 1- year estimates and Kaiser Family Foundation, Status if State Action on the Medicaid Expansion Decision, as if April 2020.

[17] For more information on the Medicaid program, see CRS Report R43357, *Medicaid: An Overview*.

[18] Affordable Care Act (ACA, as amended; P.L. 111-148) Sections 1413, 2201 and 2202.

single, streamlined application that applicants can submit online, by phone, in-person, or mail and to enroll individuals in the appropriate subsidized health coverage that they might be eligible for. In addition, each program has its own unique eligibility requirements that also apply.[19]

Over time a number of enrollment facilitation strategies have been identified to find, enroll, and maintain eligibility among those eligible for the programs. Some of these policies are program specific,[20] others are intended to facilitate program enrollment across programs.[21] In general, these policies are designed to reach all eligible populations regardless of their demographic and/or health status, although the federal government and the states have worked to identify specific strategies to successfully find and enroll underserved, vulnerable and special needs populations, including minority populations and individuals who have experienced health disparities.[22]

Health Insurance Exchanges

Federal statute and regulations require that exchanges carry out certain consumer-assistance functions.[23] For example, exchanges must establish Navigator programs and certified application counselor (CAC) programs.[24] Under these programs, such assisters are trained to conduct public outreach and education activities; help consumers make informed decisions about their insurance options; and help consumers access exchange coverage and financial assistance or public coverage (e.g., Medicaid) if they qualify. In recent years, consumer assistance under many of these programs has undergone changes in funding and approach. As an illustrative example, in the fiscal year (FY) 2021 budget justification document submitted to congressional appropriators, CMS indicated in the line item for "Navigators Grants & Enrollment Assisters" that funding for such activities were reduced nearly 50% from FY 2016 to FY 2017.[25] In subsequent years, the funding for these activities have been further reduced. These actions have led some observers to question the potential impact of such changes on consumer experiences with the exchanges. For instance, with respect to the reduced funding and other specified changes in navigator funding, the Government Accountability Office (GAO) concluded that such actions

> [raise] the risk that navigator organizations will decrease the priority they place on fulfilling a range of other duties for which they are responsible, including providing assistance to traditionally underserved populations,

[19] For example, Medicaid and CHIP eligibility determinations can occur at any point during the year and are generally based on an individual's income at a certain point in time. Eligibility for coverage available through the health insurance exchange generally occurs during an open enrollment period, although certain changes in an individual's circumstances (e.g., loss of employment) can trigger a special enrollment period.

[20] For example, see Centers for Medicare and Medicaid Services, *Dear State Health Official: Dear State Medicaid Director: RE: Facilitating Medicaid and CHIP Enrollment and Renewal in 2014*, SHO #13-003; ACA #26, May 17, 2014, https://www.medicaid.gov/sites/default/files/Federal-Policy-Guidance/downloads/SHO-13-003.pdf.

[21] For example, when coordinating eligibility and enrollment across the low-income subsidy programs, states are permitted to enter into agreements to allow the health insurance exchange to make a final Medicaid eligibility determination, or they can require the health insurance exchange to determine potential Medicaid eligibility, and then transfer the application to the Medicaid agency for a final Medicaid eligibility determination.

[22] Centers for Medicare and Medicaid Services (CMS), *Serving Vulnerable and Underserved Populations*, 2018, https://marketplace.cms.gov/technical-assistance-resources/training-materials/vulnerable-and-underserved-populations.pdf.

[23] 42 U.S.C. §18031(i); 45 C.F.R. §155.205; 45 C.F.R. §155.210; and 45 C.F.R. §155.225.

[24] For the requirement to implement Navigator programs, see 45 C.F.R. §155.210. For the requirement to implement certified application counselor programs, see 45 C.F.R. §155.225.

[25] See CMS, "Health Insurance Exchanges Transparency Table," *Fiscal Year 2021: Justification of Estimates for Appropriations Committees*, at https://www.cms.gov/About-CMS/Agency-Information/PerformanceBudget/FY2021-CJ-Final.pdf. In this Transparency table, certain line items, including the one referenced above regarding "Navigator Grants and Enrollment Assisters," represent spending in federally-facilitated exchanges only. States that fully run their own exchanges, as well as states that administer their exchanges but utilize the federal information technology platform, Healthcare.gov, are responsible for funding their own Navigator programs and other consumer outreach activities. For additional information about these different types of exchanges, see CRS Report R44065, *Overview of Health Insurance Exchanges*.

which some navigator organizations we interviewed reported they had either decreased or planned to decrease due to reduced funding.[26]

In response to the GAO study, CMS stated that "their 2018 advertising approach was a success, noting that they cut wasteful spending on advertising, which resulted in a more cost-effective approach."[27] Moreover, in an FAQ concerning the most recent funding notice for Navigator grants posted on the CMS website, the agency notes that "eligible applicants may choose to partner with other entities and/or individuals…in order to target a larger total portion of the 'left behind' population who are disproportionately without access to health insurance coverage or care."[28]

Medicaid and CHIP

Under Medicaid and CHIP, there are a number of policies that states rely on to find and enroll eligible individuals. Many of these eligibility and enrollment facilitation strategies are available at state option, and as a result there is variability across states in their application. For example, under Medicaid, states are permitted to rely on presumptive eligibility[29] to immediately enroll certain individuals for a temporary period until a formal eligibility determination is made, and have flexibility in identifying qualified entities (e.g., hospitals, health care providers, community-based organizations, and schools) that are authorized to immediately enroll those who appear to be eligible.[30] States are permitted to rely on tools such as self-attestation to minimize the paperwork that individuals are required to submit as a part of their applications (e.g. income verification, residency, and date of birth). Under CHIP, states are permitted to eliminate waiting periods-- the length of time an applicant must be uninsured before they can enroll. States are also permitted to rely on Express Lane Eligibility to identify, enroll, and renew eligibility for children in Medicaid or CHIP by relying on eligibility findings from other means-tested programs (e.g., Head Start or SNAP). Conversely, the federal government and states rely on some of these same policy options to reduce the number of individuals eligible for and enrolling in these programs in an effort to control program costs, or as a part of program oversight efforts. For example, under Medicaid and CHIP, states are required to redetermine eligibility at least annually. However, with CMS approval, they are permitted to do so more frequently. State modifications to relax (or tighten) their Medicaid and CHIP enrollment facilitation strategies over time have been documented through a series of annual 50 state surveys.[31]

To assist states in responding to the COVID-19 public health emergency, CMS released a series of sub-regulatory guidance documents. Some of these guidance documents implement the Medicaid and CHIP provisions enacted under the Families First Coronavirus Response Act (FFCRA; P. L. 116-127)[32] and the Coronavirus Aid, Relief, and Economic Security Act (CARES; P.L.116-136),[33] and include information related to Medicaid and CHIP enrollment requirements as they apply to these laws (e.g., requirements

---

[26] GAO, GAO-18-565, Health Insurance Exchanges: HHS Should Enhance Its Management of Open Enrollment Performance, July 2018, p. 37, at https://www.gao.gov/assets/700/693362.pdf.

[27] Ibid, p. 23.

[28] The FAQ also addressed the diversity of persons and groups that may fall into the "left behind" designation. CMS, External Frequently Asked Questions for the 2019 Cooperative Agreement to Support Navigators in Federally-facilitated exchanges (Funding Opportunity), at https://www.cms.gov/CCIIO/Programs-and-Initiatives/Health-Insurance-Marketplaces/Downloads/2019-Navigator-NOFO-External-FAQ_.pdf.

[29] SSA §§ 1902(a)(47)(A); 1920A; 2107(e)(1).

[30] For more information, see https://www.medicaid.gov/medicaid/enrollment-strategies/presumptive-eligibility/index.html.

[31] For example, see Tricia Brooks, Lauren Roygardner, and Samantha Artiga, et al., *Medicaid and CHIP Eligibility, Enrollment, and Cost Sharing Policies as of January 2020: Findings from a 50-State Survey*, Kaiser Family Foundation, March 26, 2020, medicaid-and-chip-eligibility-enrollment-and-cost-sharing-policies-as-of-january-2020-findings-from-a-50-state-survey.

[32] For more information, see CRS Report R46316, *Health Care Provisions in the Families First Coronavirus Response Act, P.L. 116-127.*

[33] For more information, see CRS Report R46334, *Selected Health Provisions in Title III of the CARES Act (P.L. 116-136).*

related to "screen and enroll", outstation locations for the processing of applications, and the implementation of the maintenance of effort (MOE) eligibility requirements through the public health emergency period that were included as a condition for states to claim the temporary increase in the federal share of certain Medicaid benefit spending as authorized under FFCRA).[34] Other guidance documents specifically address Medicaid eligibility, enrollment, and other flexibilities that will be available to states during the public health emergency period (e.g., timeliness standards for processing Medicaid and CHIP applications and renewals, length of eligibility period, flexibility around requirements to obtain an applicant's signature, flexibilities to temporarily accept an assessment of Medicaid eligibility as a final Medicaid eligibility determination for states that rely on federally facilitated exchanges during the screen and enroll process).[35] Throughout these documents, CMS acknowledges an anticipated increase in Medicaid and CHIP program applications and enrollment due to changes in income related to job loss and demand for health care coverage tied to the pandemic. CMS also recognizes that the COVID-19 public health emergency has limited states' Medicaid and CHIP agency capacity to process eligibility applications and renewals.

In addition to the sub regulatory guidance, CMS provided states with time-limited, COVID-19-related state plan amendment (SPA) templates and waiver authorities to help states quickly respond to the public health emergency. Unlike other existing state plan and waiver authorities, these tools are intended to be temporary and are tied to the public health emergency period. Several of these authorities allow states to make changes to their Medicaid and CHIP eligibility and enrollment processes. The Medicaid and CHIP emergency SPA and waiver authorities include:

- *Medicaid and CHIP Disaster SPAs:* States are encouraged to use SPA templates to request CMS approval for temporary changes to their Medicaid and CHIP state plans. These streamlined SPA templates combine multiple, time-limited state plan options into a single SPA submission to eliminate the need for states to submit multiple Medicaid and/or CHIP SPAs for program changes related to eligibility, enrollment facilitation strategies, benefit coverage, cost sharing requirements, expansion of telehealth, provider payment rates, performance compliance timetables, requirements related to tribal consultation, etc. The Medicaid COVID-19 Disaster SPAs are retroactive back to March 1, 2020 (or as otherwise specified in the CMS approval letter) and will apply through the public health emergency period, including any extensions, or any earlier date as specified by the state.[36] CHIP COVID-19 Disaster SPAs are effective beginning at the start of the state or federally declared emergency through the end of the public health emergency, including any extensions.[37]
- *Section 1135 Waiver Authority*: Section 1135 of the Social Security Act allows the Secretary of Health and Human Services (HHS Secretary), under certain conditions, to temporarily waive specified program requirements and regulations to ensure that health

[34] Centers for Medicare and Medicaid Services, *Families First Coronavirus Response Act (FFCRA), Public Law No. 116-127 Coronavirus Aid, Relief, and Economic Security (CARES) Act, Public Law No. 116-136 Frequently Asked Questions (FAQs)*, April 13, 2020, https://www.medicaid.gov/state-resource-center/downloads/covid-19-section-6008-CARES-faqs.pdf.

[35] See Centers for Medicare and Medicaid Services, *COVID-19 Frequently Asked Questions (FAQs) for State Medicaid and Children's Health Insurance Program (CHIP) Agencies*, May 5, 2020, https://www.medicaid.gov/state-resource-center/downloads/covid-19-new-faqs.pdf. Also see, Centers for Medicare and Medicaid Services, *COVID-19 Frequently Asked Questions (FAQs) for State Medicaid and Children's Health Insurance Program (CHIP) Agencies*, May 5, 2020, https://www.medicaid.gov/state-resource-center/downloads/covid-19-faqs.pdf.

[36] CMS, *State Plan Flexibilities: Medicaid State Plan Disaster Relief State Plan Amendments; CHIP Disaster Relief SPAs*, March 2020, https://www.medicaid.gov/resources-for-states/disaster-response-toolkit/state-plan-flexibilities/index.html.

[37] CMS, COVID-19 Frequently Asked Questions (FAQs) for State Medicaid and Children's Health Insurance Program (CHIP) Agencies, May 5, 2020, https://www.medicaid.gov/state-resource-center/downloads/covid-19-new-faqs.pdf.

care items and services are available to enrollees in the Medicare, Medicaid, and CHIP programs during emergencies.[38] The Section 1135 waiver authority is retroactive back to March 1, 2020 (unless otherwise specified) and will apply through the public health emergency period, including any extensions, or any earlier date as specified by the state. In response to COVID-19, the Secretary of HHS has used this authority to waive Medicaid and CHIP program rules related to conditions of provider participation, licensure requirements, ability to pay out-of-state providers, ability to provide services in alternative settings, ability to suspend preadmission screening and annual resident review for certain residential care facilities, submission deadlines and public notice requirements for state plan amendments, etc.

- *Disaster Related Section 1115 Demonstration Authority*: Under the disaster related Section 1115 waiver opportunity, the Secretary of HHS has established a new Medicaid only (not CHIP) disaster-related Section 1115 demonstration opportunity for states to provide them with additional flexibility that will allow them to focus state operations to meet the health care needs of program enrollees during the COVID-19 public health emergency. Under these Medicaid disaster waivers, states are encouraged to extend home and community-based services (HCBS) flexibilities to beneficiaries receiving long-term supports and services (LTSS), to relax eligibility determination requirements, to target services to specific population and/or geographic areas, among other flexibilities.[39] The Medicaid disaster related demonstrations are retroactive to March 1, 2020 (unless otherwise specified), and will expire no later than 60 days after the end of the public health emergency, including any extensions.[40] Unlike most Section 1115 demonstration waivers,[41] federal costs under these disaster related demonstration waivers are not required to be budget neutral to the federal government as they are considered "likely to be otherwise incurred and allowable."
- *Section 1915(c) Home and Community Based Services (HCBS) Waiver Appendix K*: Appendix K is a standalone appendix to the Section 1915(c) Home and Community Based Services (HCBS) waiver template that may be utilized by states during emergency situations to request amendments to approved waivers and may be applied retroactively as needed by the state.[42] Requests can be made for single waivers, multiple waivers, or all waivers. The CMS template includes actions that states can take under the existing Section 1915(c) waiver authority in order to respond to an emergency. Other activities may require the use of various other authorities such as the Section 1115 demonstrations

---

[38] The Section 1135 waiver authority may be invoked when a declaration of emergency or disaster under the National Emergencies Act or Stafford Act and a Public Health Emergency Declaration Under Section 319 of the Public Health Service Act have been declared by the U.S. President, and a public health emergency has been declared by the Secretary of HHS, pursuant to section 319 of the Public Health Service Act [PHSA]. For more information, see CRS Legal Sidebar LSB10430, *Section 1135 Waivers and COVID-19: An Overview*.

[39] HHS, CMS , *DMDL # 20-002 RE: COVID-19 Public Health Emergency Section 1115(a) Opportunity for States*, March 22, 2020.

[40] CMS, *State Plan Flexibilities: Medicaid State Plan Disaster Relief State Plan Amendments: CHIP Disaster Relief SPAs*, March 2020, https://www.medicaid.gov/resources-for-states/disaster-response-toolkit/state-plan-flexibilities/index.html.

[41] In general, under Section 1115 of the Social Security Act, the Secretary has broad authority to waive Medicaid and CHIP program rules and to authorize federal Medicaid expenditures that are not otherwise permitted to grant demonstration projects that in the Secretary's judgement promote the objects of the program. Section 1115 demonstration projects are generally approved for a period of up to 5 years and must be budget neutral to the federal government.

[42] For more information on CMS' Emergency Preparedness and Response for Medicaid Home and Community Based (HCBS) 1915(c) waivers, see https://www.medicaid.gov/resources-for-states/disaster-response-toolkit/home-community-based-services-public-health-emergencies/emergency-preparedness-and-response-for-home-and-community-based-hcbs-1915c-waivers/index.html.

or the Section 1135 authorities. Under this appendix, the state or territory may temporarily expand setting(s) where services may be provided (e.g., hotels, shelters, schools, churches), modify provider qualifications, increase the pool of providers who can render services, among other activities. However, states are *not* permitted to include changes that are otherwise prohibited under the Medicaid statute, such as the inclusion of room and board costs.

Through the CMS guidance and the use of temporary state plan and waiver authorities, CMS is encouraging states to relax procedures that otherwise might restrict eligibility and enrollment facilitation in Medicaid and CHIP. CRS made preliminary estimates of the national totals of CMS approvals of state requests to temporarily modify their Medicaid and CHIP programs in response to the COVID-19 public health emergency as of May 12, 2020. They include: (1) 52 Medicaid Disaster SPAs in 29 states and 4 territories; (2) 12 CHIP Disaster SPAs in 12 states; (3) 71 Section 1135 waiver requests in 50 states, D.C., and 3 territories; (4) 1 Section 1115 Disaster Demonstration in 1 state; (5) 123 standalone Section 1915(c) Appendix K waivers in 28 states; and (6) 46 combined authority Section 1915(c) waivers in 31 states and the District of Columbia. These counts represent a rough estimate of current approvals as CMS has continued to approve state SPA and waiver requests since that time period. Given the time sensitive nature of this request, CRS does not have the resources to identify which of these CMS approvals explicitly make changes to Medicaid and CHIP eligibility and enrollment policies. However, outside organizations have begun to track state changes to Medicaid and CHIP enrollment policies in response to the COVID-19 pandemic through analysis of approved Medicaid and CHIP state plan amendments and information available on state websites. According to the analysis, 43 states have made changes to facilitate access to Medicaid and/or CHIP coverage in response to the COVID-19 beyond those that are required for states to access the enhanced federal funding that was included under the FFCRA, as of May 21, 2020. Changes include eligibility expansions, modifications to eligibility rules, elimination or waiving of premiums for program participation, and streamline application and enrollment processes.[43]

Question 4. How has COVID-19-related unemployment affected access to maternal health care and health insurance coverage for working mothers?

Medicaid and CHIP

Medicaid and CHIP are significant payers of maternal health services for low-income pregnant women, including coverage of labor and delivery services for undocumented individuals under emergency Medicaid. According to the CDC, Medicaid paid for 42.3% of all births in the United States, down 2% from 2017.[44] Among the key finding from the Medicaid and CHIP Payment and Access Commission's (MACPAC) June 2020 report to Congress, Medicaid pays for a greater share of births as compared to other payers for women (1) in rural areas, (2) under the age of 19, (3) with lower levels of educational attainment, (4) of racial and ethnic minorities, and (5) who are more likely to have pregnancy risk factors, such as obesity, hypertension, alcohol use during pregnancy, and cigarette smoking three months prior to or during pregnancy.[45] During periods of economic downturn, Medicaid enrollment increases at a faster

[43] For more information, see Rachel Dolan and Samantha Artiga, *State Actions to Facilitate Access to Medicaid and CHIP Coverage in Response to COVID-19*, Kaiser Family Foundation, May 22, 2020, https://www.kff.org/coronavirus-covid-19/issue-brief/state-actions-to-facilitate-access-to-medicaid-and-chip-coverage-in-response-to-covid-19/.

[44] Joyce A. Martin, M.P.H., Brady E. Hamilton, Ph.D., and Michelle J.K. Osterman, M.H.S., et al., *Births: Final Data for 2018*, Centers for Disease Control, National Vital Statistics, Volume 68, Number 13, November 27, 2019, https://www.cdc.gov/nchs/data/nvsr/nvsr68/nvsr68_13-508.pdf.

[45] Medicaid and CHIP Payment Access Commission (MACPAC), *Report to Congress on Medicaid and CHIP*, Chapter 5: Medicaid's Role in Maternal Health, June 2020, https://www.macpac.gov/wp-content/uploads/2020/06/June-2020-Report-to-Congress-on-Medicaid-and-CHIP.pdf. See also, Medicaid and CHIP Payment and Access Commission, *Access in Brief: Pregnant Women and Medicaid*, Issue Brief, November 2018, https://www.macpac.gov/wp-content/uploads/2018/11/Pregnant-

rate because job and income losses make more people eligible. In addition, those who were previously eligible but not yet enrolled may seek enrollment. These factors are likely to make Medicaid an even more important source of coverage for pregnant women during the COVID-19 related recession period.

Medicaid's Pregnancy Coverage

All states are required to provide Medicaid coverage for pregnant women with annual income at or below 133 percent of the federal poverty level, and are permitted to extend coverage to pregnant women at higher income levels at state plan option. According to MACPAC, the median Medicaid eligibility threshold was 195 percent of the FPL, as of April 2019.[46]

In general, Medicaid benefits for pregnant women differ by eligibility pathway both across and within states. Medicaid's poverty-related pregnant women pathway provides access to pregnancy coverage that may include full Medicaid benefit coverage, but in some cases is limited to prenatal care, labor and delivery, and 60 days of postpartum care. States also use the targeted pregnancy benefit coverage that is available through this Medicaid eligibility pathway to provide enhanced pregnancy-related benefits (e.g., postpartum home visits, dental care), but entitlement to these services terminates after the 60 days postpartum period.

Beyond the mandatory and optional poverty-related pregnant women pathway where Medicaid eligibility terminates after 60 days postpartum, there are a number of other mandatory and optional Medicaid eligibility pathways where a woman's pregnancy status is among the factors that make them Medicaid eligible. Some of these other Medicaid eligibility pathways allow for full Medicaid benefit coverage for a period of 12 months after which time the woman's Medicaid eligibility must be redetermined.[47]

CHIP Pregnant Women and Unborn Children

As of April 2019, 20 states provide coverage to pregnant women under CHIP. The three main ways that states may extend CHIP coverage to pregnant women (regardless of their age) are through: (1) the state plan option for pregnant women, (2) the Section 1115 waiver authority, and/or (3) the unborn child pathway. The unborn child pathway is the predominant pathway used by states for this purpose.[48]

As of April 2019, five states (Colorado, Missouri, New Jersey, Rhode Island and Virginia) extended coverage to pregnant women under Section 1115 waiver authority or the CHIP pregnant women state plan option. Under the Child Health Insurance Program Reauthorization Act of 2009 (CHIPRA; P.L. 111-3), states are permitted to cover pregnant women through a state plan amendment when certain conditions are met (e.g., the Medicaid income standard for pregnant women must be at least 185% FPL but in no case lower than the percentage level in effect on July 1, 2008; no preexisting conditions or waiting periods may be imposed; and CHIP cost-sharing protections apply). The period of coverage associated with the state plan option includes pregnancy through the postpartum period (roughly through 60 days postpartum), and benefits include all services available to CHIP children in the state as well as prenatal, delivery, and postpartum care. Infants born to such pregnant women are deemed eligible for Medicaid or CHIP, as appropriate, and are covered up to one year of age.

Women-and-Medicaid.pdf.

[46] Ibid.

[47] For more information on Medicaid pregnancy-related benefit coverage across states, see Kathy Gifford, Jenna Walls, and Usha Ranji, et al., *Medicaid Coverage of Pregnancy and Perinatal Benefits: Results from a State Survey*, Kaiser Family Foundation , April 27, 2017, https://www.kff.org/womens-health-policy/report/medicaid-coverage-of-pregnancy-and-perinatal-benefits-results-from-a-state-survey/.

[48] Medicaid and CHIP Payment and Access Commission, *MACSTATS Medicaid and CHIP Data Book*, EXHIBIT 35. Medicaid and CHIP Income Eligibility Levels as a Percentage of the FPL for Children and Pregnant Women by State, April 2019, https://www.macpac.gov/wp-content/uploads/2015/01/EXHIBIT-35.-Medicaid-and-CHIP-Income-Eligibility-Levels-as-a-Percentage-of-the-FPL-for-Children-and-Pregnant-Women-by-State-April-2019.pdf.

As of April 2019, 17 states provide CHIP coverage to pregnant women ages 19 and older by extending coverage to unborn children as permitted through federal regulation. Coverage available to such women may be limited to prenatal and delivery services, but is still the predominant form of coverage because it permits the extension of CHIP coverage to a pregnant woman regardless of her immigration status.

Medicaid and CHIP COVID-19 Related Response

In conversations with you in preparing this confidential memorandum, you noted that the Committee was interested in CMS policies and state activity in response to COVID-19 that are specific to pregnant and postpartum women. CMS addressed the implementation of the FFCRA provision to extend coverage of in vitro diagnostic products for the detection of SARS-CoV-2 or diagnosis of COVID-19 for pregnant women under Medicaid and CHIP and to extend Medicaid coverage for current enrollees through the public health emergency period for certain specified individuals who no longer meet the program specific eligibility criteria under the respective state plan.[49] However beyond these mentions, CRS is not aware of additional COVID related guidance specific to maternal health.

In addition, while states may use the emergency Medicaid and CHIP state plan amendment and waiver authorities (see discussion above in the previous response) that allow states to make changes to Medicaid and CHIP to quickly address the needs of Medicaid and CHIP program enrollees during the pandemic period, CRS was not able to identify any source that summarizes how states might be using these flexibilities specific to pregnant and postpartum women.

Private Health Insurance

As discussed in the answer to Question 2 above, individuals who lose employment may not necessarily lose employment-based health benefits; such individuals may be able to access coverage through their former employer or spouse's employer, if available. Outside of employment, individuals generally may purchase individual health insurance sold in the state in which they reside. In general, private health insurance typically includes coverage for maternal health care. Insurance offered through either the individual insurance market or the small group market is required under federal law to include maternity care.[50] While large group and self-insured plans are not subject to the same benefit mandate, "maternity coverage is nearly universal in employer plans."[51] Nevertheless, even when benefits are covered under private health insurance (such as maternal health care), the insured individual typically has some level of spending for use of covered services.[52] For individuals with little to no income due to unemployment, paying premiums for private insurance and the cost-sharing associated with maternity care may prove to be cost prohibitive.

Maternal Health Grant Programs

This part of the memorandum provides information about selected grant programs that address maternal and child health issues during the COVID-19 public health emergency. These programs—the Maternal and Child Health (MCH) Services Block Grant program and Maternal, Infant, and Early Childhood Home Visiting (MIECHV) program—are administered by the Health Resources and Services Administration

[49] Centers for Medicare and Medicaid Services, *Families First Coronavirus Response Act (FFCRA), Public Law No. 116-127 Coronavirus Aid, Relief, and Economic Security (CARES) Act, Public Law No. 116-136 Frequently Asked Questions (FAQs)*, April 13, 2020, https://www.medicaid.gov/state-resource-center/downloads/covid-19-section-6008-CARES-faqs.pdf.

[50] For additional information about these and other federal health benefit mandates, see CRS In Focus IF10287, *The Essential Health Benefits (EHB)*.

[51] Roland McDevitt, et al., "Group Insurance: A Better Deal For Most People Than Individual Plans," Health Affairs, Vol. 29, No. 1, p.162, at https://www.healthaffairs.org/doi/pdf/10.1377/hlthaff.2009.0060.

[52] For an example, see Michelle Moniz, et al., "Out-Of-Pocket Spending For Maternity Care Among Women With Employer-Based Insurance, 2008–15," Health Affairs, Vol. 39, No. 1, at https://www.healthaffairs.org/doi/10.1377/hlthaff.2019.00296.

(HRSA) at the Department of Health and Human Services. The MIECHV program is also administered by the Administration for Families at HHS. These programs are illustrative of HHS's response to COVID-19 in the context of maternal and child health, and do not provide an exhaustive overview of this response. For example, HRSA administers other grant programs such as the Rural Maternity and Obstetrics Management Strategies Program and the State Maternal Health Innovation Program that aim to address maternal health issues, including during the COVID-19 pandemic.[53]

On May 28, 2020, HRSA and ACF released a joint letter on COVID-19 to family support, maternal and child health, and early childhood programs.[54] The letter lists several ways program grantees may respond to the pandemic, including to (1) connect families to state and local resources or information, such as 211, crisis hotlines, or family resource centers for identified needs; (2) increase the frequency of visits or other check-ins to maintain connections with families, especially those identified at elevated risk, and communicate the availability of support to families; and (3) support families' capacity to connect with health and family support professionals through virtual, electronic, and telephonic means, including assisting families with access to technology and internet connectivity, among other supports.

Maternal and Child Health (MCH) Services Block Grant Program

The MCH Services Block Grant program aims to improve the health of the maternal and child population, particularly those with low incomes or limited availability of care.[55] MCH services generally are provided to pregnant women, mothers, children, and children with special health care needs (CSHCNs), some of whom are also eligible for and/or enrolled in Medicaid or CHIP. The MCH Services Block Grant program is composed of three funding programs. The first is the Block Grants to States program, which is the largest of the three funding programs. Formula-based grants are provided to states and territories (referred to collectively as *states*)[56] to enable them to coordinate programs, develop systems, and provide a broad range of health services to their respective maternal and child populations.[57] The second funding program is the Special Projects of Regional and National Significance (SPRANS) program. SPRANS is a competitive grant program that funds research and training projects that focus on low-income pregnant women, parents, and children including CSHCNs. The third funding program is the Community Integrated Service Systems (CISS) program. CISS is a competitive grant program that funds projects that support the development and expansion of integrated services at the community level.[58] Congress established the MCH Services Block Grant program under Title V of the Social Security Act (SSA, P.L.

---

[53] For more information on HRSA guidance related to the COVID-19 pandemic, see HHS, HRSA, *Coronavirus Disease (COVID-19) Maternal and Child Health Bureau Frequently Asked Questions*, updated June 19, 2020, available at: https://mchb.hrsa.gov/coronavirus-frequently-asked-questions. For more information about ACF guidance related to the COVID-19 pandemic, see HHS, ACF, ACF *COVID-19 Response & Resources*, https://www.acf.hhs.gov/coronavirus.

[54] Letter from Dr. Deborah Bergeron, Director, HHS, Administration for Children and Families (ACF), Office of Early Childhood Development and Office of Head Start; Ms. Shannon Christian, Director, HHS, ACF, Office of Child Care; Dr. Jerry Milner, HHS, ACF, Children's Bureau, et al., , May 28, 2020, https://www.acf.hhs.gov/sites/default/files/ecd/dear_colleague_letter_acf_mchb_covid_19_ada.pdf.

[55] Sections 501-509 of the Social Security Act (SSA; P.L. 74-271, as amended), codified in the *U.S. Code* at 42 U.S.C. 701-709. To learn more about the MCH Services Block Grant Program, see CRS In Focus IF10777, *Maternal and Child Health (MCH) Services Block Grant*.

[56] Referred to collectively as "states" in this memorandum, all 50 states and nine jurisdictions are eligible to apply for the MCH Services Block Grant. The nine jurisdictions consist of (1) American Samoa, (2) District of Columbia, (3) Federated States of Micronesia, (4) Guam, (5) Marshall Islands, (6) Northern Mariana Islands, (7) Palau, (8) Puerto Rico, and (9) U.S. Virgin Islands.

[57] SSA Section 501(a)(1).

[58] Health Resources and Services Administration (HRSA) of the Department of Health and Human Services (HHS), *Title V Maternal and Child Health Services Block Grant to States Program, Guidance and Forms for the Title V Application/Annual Report-Appendix of Supporting Documents*, p. 4, https://mchb.tvisdata.hrsa.gov/uploadedfiles/Documents/blockgrantguidanceappendix.pdf.

74-271, as amended). In FY2020, HRSA received $687.7 million for the MCH Services Block Grant program.[59]

Under the Block Grants to States program, states may redirect their funds to respond to the COVID-19 pandemic. According to HRSA, for example, a state may respond to the pandemic by:[60]

- Offering the support or leadership of Title V epidemiologists, in partnership with other state staff, to an outbreak investigation.
- Providing support in educating the MCH population about COVID-19 through partnerships with other state agencies, medical providers, and health care organizations.
- Working closely with state and local emergency preparedness staff to assure that the needs of the MCH population are represented.
- Funding infrastructure that supports the response to COVID-19. For example, Public Health Nurses who are routinely supported through the Title V program may be able to be mobilized, using Title V funds or separate emergency funding, to support a call center or deliver health services.
- Partnering with parent networks and health care providers to provide accurate and reliable information to all families.
- Engaging community leaders, including faith-based leaders, to educate community members about strategies for preventing illness.

Each state decides how it will use MCH block grant funds to respond to the pandemic.

Maternal, Infant and Early Childhood Home Visiting (MIECHV) Program

The MIECHV program is the primary federal program that focuses exclusively on home visiting.[61] The program—jointly administered by HRSA and ACF, also within HHS—seeks to strengthen and improve home visiting services and support to families residing in at-risk communities, while also referring families to services outside of the program. HHS provides MIECHV funding to states, territories, and tribal entities for home visiting services in at-risk communities, as identified by these jurisdictions. MIECHV prioritizes certain populations, including low-income families, young mothers, or individuals who have a history of substance abuse, among other risk factors. The ACA established the MIECHV program under SSA Section 511. Annual funding levels have been between $100 million and $400 million, including $400 million for FY2020. The most recent reauthorization of the program, the Bipartisan Budget Act of 2018 (P.L. 115-123), extended funding through FY2022.

HRSA has provided guidance to MIECHV grantees about topics related to the COVID-19 public health emergency. Beginning in mid-March, 2020, HRSA began disseminating this guidance to grantees, both through direct communications and on the HRSA website.[62] The website has been updated multiple times

---

[59] "Explanatory Statement Submitted by Mrs. Lowey, Chairwoman of the House Committee on Appropriations Regarding H.R. 1865, Furthering Consolidated Appropriations Act, 2020," House of Representatives, *Congressional Record*, vol. 165, part 204 (December 17, 2019), p. H11106.

[60] This list was adapted from HRSA, *Coronavirus Disease (COVID-19) Maternal and Child Health Bureau Frequently Asked Questions*, May 7, 2020, https://mchb.hrsa.gov/coronavirus-frequently-asked-questions.

[61] CRS Report R43930, *Maternal, Infant, and Early Childhood Home Visiting (MIECHV) Program: Background and Funding*. The New Parent Support Program, operated by the Department of Defense, also has a primary focus on home visiting; however, it is available only to military families.

[62] This is based on CRS correspondence with HHS, Office of the Assistant Secretary for Legislation (ASL), March 31, 2020.

through early June, 2020.[63] In general, HRSA guidance has provided information about the role of the program during the pandemic, the safety and well-being of home visitors, allowable expenses, and programmatic flexibilities related to COVID-19. The guidance has specified that the MIECHV program can help to:

- connect families to needed health, mental health, child care and other services;
- identify strategies for managing family stress and social isolation;
- keep families informed about current public health recommendations related to COVID-19; and
- promote family emergency planning strategies.

The guidance has emphasized that home visitors should determine whether to make a visit to families and to take certain precautions during any such visits. In addition, the guidance has outlined strategies for home visitors to manage stress. Regarding eligible expenses, HRSA has advised that grantees are generally not allowed to purchase emergency supplies; however, some emergency response activities—such as assisting families in emergency planning, providing parenting and other support, and distributing emergency supplies (e.g., baby food and diapers) in areas where transportation is a barrier—are within the scope of MIECHV funding.[64] HRSA has outlined flexibilities in the program, including advising that grantees may pursue alternative methods to visiting with families besides in-person visits, with the expectation that grantees make HRSA project officers aware of these changes. The guidance has also addressed performance of grantees during the COVID-19 period, noting that FY2020 "performance data, including participants served, benchmark performance measures, and caseload capacity data will be reviewed and interpreted with the recognition that many programs will continue to experience major service delivery disruptions."[65]

[63] HHS, HRSA, *Important Home Visiting Information During COVID-19*, updated on June 8, 2020, https://mchb.hrsa.gov/Home-Visiting-Information-During-COVID-19. (Hereinafter, HHS, HRSA, *Important Home Visiting Information During COVID-19*.)

[64] This is based on CRS correspondence with HHS, ASL, March 31, 2020.

[65] HHS, HRSA, *Important Home Visiting Information During COVID-19*.

Congressional
Research Service
Informing the legislative debate since 1914

MEMORANDUM June 19, 2020

To: House Committee on Education and Labor

From: Rebecca R. Skinner, Specialist in Education Policy, rskinner@crs.loc.gov, 7-6600
Benjamin Collins, Analyst in Labor Policy, bcollins@crs.loc.gov, 7-7382
Cassandria Dortch, Specialist in Education Policy, cdortch@crs.loc.gov, 7-0376
Kyrie E. Dragoo, Analyst in Education Policy, kdragoo@crs.loc.gov, 7-4421
Adrienne L. Fernandes-Alcantara, Specialist in Social Policy, afernandes@crs.loc.gov, 7-9005
Rita R. Zota, Analyst in Education Policy, rzota@crs.loc.gov, 7-9247

Subject: **Responses to Various Elementary and Secondary Education, Higher Education, and Homeless Youth Questions Related to the Ongoing Coronavirus Pandemic**

This memorandum has been prepared in response to your request for information about education-specific issues, specifically in the context of the Coronavirus Disease 2019 (COVID-19) pandemic. You initially provided a series of questions to the Congressional Research Service (CRS) as a starting point for this project; the final set of issues addressed in this memorandum is the result of discussions between you and CRS. Per your request, this memorandum specifically discusses issues related to elementary and secondary education, postsecondary education, and homeless youth.

Given that the pandemic is a recent event, real-time comprehensive national data about the effects of the pandemic on education are limited. Furthermore, given your time constraints, there was not sufficient time for us to do extensive research on these topics, collect any type of original data, or conduct original analyses. As such, CRS has synthesized relevant data and provided references to the original data sources.

Information in this memorandum may be of general interest to Congress. As such, this information may be provided by CRS to other congressional requesters, and may be published in CRS products for general distribution to Congress at a later date. Your confidentiality as a requester would be preserved in all cases.

Elementary and Secondary Education[1]

This section examines questions related to elementary and secondary education. Specifically, the questions address issues related to remote instruction and budgets for elementary and secondary education. The data discussed are based on surveys and studies, and in some instances estimates produced by third-party organizations are discussed, including estimates generated by education advocacy organizations. CRS did not review these third parties' methodologies and does not endorse their findings.

[1] This section was written by Becky Skinner, rskinner@crs.loc.gov.

They were included in this discussion in instances where limited alternative information is available, and because they speak directly to your requested issues.

Remote Education

There have been several surveys conducted to examine how schools and local educational agencies (LEAs) have transitioned to remote learning in response to the coronavirus pandemic. For example, the U.S. Census Bureau has been conducting weekly Household Pulse Surveys that ask adults living in households with at least one school-age child various questions about that child's educational experiences during the coronavirus pandemic. These surveys have been conducted weekly since April 23. *Education Week* conducted surveys in March and April, following the onset of the pandemic and compared their results from each survey. AASA, the Schools Superintendents Association, also conducted two surveys, one from March 20 through March 25 and one from May 5 to June 8.[2] The Center on Reinventing Public Education (CRPE) conducted a nationally representative survey of LEAs from April 6 to May 1. Results from each are discussed below.

U.S. Census Bureau Household Pulse Surveys

While the U.S. Census Bureau has been conducting weekly Household Pulse Surveys related to the education of school-age children since April 23, this discussion focuses on the survey conducted the week of May 21-26 as the more current data for June may be skewed by the school year ending in some locations.[3] Results are discussed only for the United States as a whole, but data are also available by state (50 states and the District of Columbia) and selected metropolitan areas (e.g., Boston metropolitan area, Seattle metropolitan area).[4]

Based on the data for the United States, respondents in households with children reported that 59.6 million children were enrolled in public or private education (**Table 1**). The average household reported spending 11.7 hours over the last seven days on all teaching activities with children. When examined by race/ethnicity, the hours spent on teaching activities ranged from 11.5 hours to 12.1 hours.[5] The average household also reported 4.4 hours of live virtual contact between students and teachers over the last seven days. When examined by race/ethnicity, the hours of live virtual contact ranged from 3.8 hours to 5.2 hours.

[2] The results from the two surveys are not compared, so only the results from the second survey are discussed in this memorandum. For the results of the first survey, see AASA, *AASA COVID-19 School Response Study*, April 6, 2020, https://aasa.org/uploadedFiles/AASA_Blog(1)/AASA_COVID_19_Report_FN_4_3_2020.pdf.

[3] U.S. Census Bureau, *Household Pulse Survey Data Tables*, 2020, https://www.census.gov/programs-surveys/household-pulse-survey/data.html. Data are included for all of the weekly surveys that have been conducted.

[4] Ibid.

[5] The Household Pulse Survey only asked about the race and ethnicity of the household member completing the survey. See Household Pulse Survey questionnaire at https://www2.census.gov/programs-surveys/demo/technical-documentation/hhp/household-pulse-survey-questionnaire-week1-5.pdf.

Table 1. Time Spent in Last Week on Home Based Education for Households with Children in Public or Private School: United States

(Week of May 21-26, 2020)

Hispanic Origin and Race[a]	Total Children in Public or Private School	Average Household Hours Spent in Last 7 Days on All Teaching Activities with Children	Average Household Hours Spent in Last 7 Days on All Live Virtual Contact between Students and Their Teachers
Hispanic or Latino (may be of any race)	12,562,900	11.9	5.2
White alone, not Hispanic	32,421,823	11.5	3.8
Black alone, not Hispanic	8,596,195	11.9	5.1
Asian alone, not Hispanic	3,376,835	12.1	4.5
Two or more races + other races, not Hispanic	2,618,257	12.4	4.8
Total	59,576,010	11.7	4.4

Source: Table prepared by CRS based on data available from U.S. Census Bureau, Household Pulse Survey: May 21 – May 26, Table 1, https://www.census.gov/data/tables/2020/demo/hhp/hhp4.html.

a. Reflects the race and ethnicity of the household member who responded to the survey

The survey also asked about how children were receiving instruction if their classes had moved to distance learning (**Table 2**). Overall, 44.4 million (74.6%) were reported as receiving online instruction and 11.5 million (19.3%) were reported as using paper materials that were sent home.[6] When examined by race/ethnicity, the majority of children in each group whose classes were moved to distance learning were using online resources. Across all racial/ethnic groups, a substantially smaller percentage of children were using paper materials that were sent home.

Table 2. Type of Distance Learning Provided If Classes Were Moved to a Distance Learning Format for Households with Children in Public or Private Schools: United States

(Week of May 21-26, 2020)

Hispanic Origin and Race[a]	Total Children in Public or Private School	Moved to Distance Learning Using Online Resources		Moved to Distance Learning Using Paper Materials Sent Home	
		Number of Children	Share of Total Children	Number of Children	Share of Total Children
Hispanic or Latino (may be of any race)	12,562,900	9,366,590	74.6%	1,872,919	14.9%
White alone, not Hispanic	32,421,823	24,904,893	76.8%	6,782,174	20.9%

[6] These are not mutually exclusive categories. Students could have been receiving online instruction and paper materials.

Hispanic Origin and Race[a]	Total Children in Public or Private School	Moved to Distance Learning Using Online Resources		Moved to Distance Learning Using Paper Materials Sent Home	
		Number of Children	Share of Total Children	Number of Children	Share of Total Children
Black alone, not Hispanic	8,596,195	5,422,046	63.1%	1,763,426	20.5%
Asian alone, not Hispanic	3,376,835	2,821,854	83.6%	486,679	14.4%
Two or more races + other races, not Hispanic	2,618,257	1,926,530	73.6%	568,811	21.7%
Total	59,576,010	44,441,913	74.6%	11,474,009	19.3%

Source: Table prepared by CRS based on data available from U.S. Census Bureau, Household Pulse Survey: May 21 – May 26, Table 2, https://www.census.gov/data/tables/2020/demo/hhp/hhp4.html.

Notes: Details may not add to totals as the question allowed multiple categories to be selected.

a. Reflects the race and ethnicity of the household member who responded to the survey

The survey also asked about the availability of a computer or digital device for educational use (**Table 3**). Overall, 69.1% of respondents indicated that a device was always, and 17.2% indicated that a device was usually, available (86.3% combined). While responses varied by the racial/ethnic group of the respondent, respondents in most racial/ethnic groups reported that a device was always or usually available.

With respect to devices used at home, the survey asked whether a computer or digital device that was available to children was provided by the children's school or school district to use outside of school; provided by someone in the house or family, or was the child's device; or provided by another source (**Table 4**). Overall 70.4% of respondents indicated that the device was provided by someone in the house or family or that it was the child's device, while 36.4% of respondents indicated the device had been provided by the child's school or school district and 1.8% reported that the device has been provided by an outside source.[7] When examined by race/ethnicity, similar trends were observed as respondents of all racial/ethnic backgrounds reported that having the device provided by someone in the house or family or that it was the child's device was the most common source of a device, followed by a device provided by a child's school or school district.

Data also were collected on the availability of the Internet for educational purposes (**Table 5**). Overall, 70.6% of respondents reported that the Internet was always available for educational purposes and 18.6% reported that the Internet was usually available (89.2% combined). Among respondents of different racial/ethnic groups, the percentage of respondents saying that the Internet was always or usually available for education purposes ranged from 79.0% to 93.3%.

Finally, the survey asked about whether Internet services made available for educational purposes were being paid for by the child's school or school district, someone in the household or family, or another source (**Table 6**). Overall, 92% of respondents indicated that someone in the household or family paid for Internet services. Across respondents from all racial/ethnic groups, the percentage of respondents indicating that someone in the household or family paid for Internet services ranged from 86.8% of to 94.0%.

[7] Respondents were able to select multiple responses.

Table 3. Availability of Computer for Educational Purposes in Households with Children Enrolled in Public or Private School: United States

(Week of May 21-26, 2020)

Hispanic Origin and Race[a]	Total Number of Children in Public or Private School	Computer Availability											
		Device Always Available		Device Usually Available		Device Sometimes Available		Device Rarely Available		Device Never Available		Did Not Report	
		Number of Children	Share of Total Children	Number of Children	Share of Total Children	Number of Children	Share of Total Children	Number of Children	Share of Total Children	Number of Children	Share of Total Children	Number of Children	Share of Total Children
Hispanic or Latino (may be of any race)	12,562,900	8,151,576	64.9%	2,307,842	18.4%	1,202,503	9.6%	383,618	3.1%	251,156	2.0%	266,204	2.1%
White alone, not Hispanic	32,421,823	23,289,360	71.8%	5,566,684	17.2%	2,246,641	6.9%	611,166	1.9%	367,269	1.1%	340,704	1.1%
Black alone, not Hispanic	8,596,195	5,732,224	66.7%	1,260,536	14.7%	831,250	9.7%	442,030	5.1%	271,463	3.2%	58,692	0.7%
Asian alone, not Hispanic	3,376,835	2,453,174	72.6%	575,641	17.0%	201,274	6.0%	80,420	2.4%	1,076	0.0%	65,250	1.9%
Two or more races + other races, not Hispanic	2,618,257	1,514,996	57.9%	520,703	19.9%	290,875	11.1%	81,346	3.1%	104,323	4.0%	106,014	4.0%
Total	59,576,010	41,141,330	69.1%	10,231,407	17.2%	4,772,543	8.0%	1,598,580	2.7%	995,286	1.7%	836,864	1.4%

Source: Table prepared by CRS based on data available from U.S. Census Bureau, Household Pulse Survey: May 21 – May 26, Table 3, https://www.census.gov/data/tables/2020/demo/hhp/hhp4.html.

Notes: Details may not add to totals due to rounding.

a. Reflects the race and ethnicity of the household member who responded to the survey

Table 4. Provider of a Computer or Digital Device Available to Children for Educational Purposes for Households with Children Enrolled in Public or Private School: United States

(Week of May 21-26, 2020)

Hispanic Origin and Race[a]	Total Number of Children in Public or Private School	Provider of Computer or Digital Device for Educational Purposes							
		Provided by the Children's School or School District to Use Outside of School		Provided by Someone in the Household or Family, or It Is the Child's		Provided by Another Source		Did Not Report	
		Number of Children	Share of Total Children	Number of Children	Share of Total Children	Number of Children	Share of Total Children	Number of Children	Share of Total Children
Hispanic or Latino (may be of any race)	12,562,900	5,357,022	42.6%	7,520,390	59.9%	182,473	1.5%	663,304	5.3%
White alone, not Hispanic	32,421,823	11,156,066	34.4%	24,454,028	75.4%	415,937	1.3%	967,403	3.0%
Black alone, not Hispanic	8,596,195	3,401,061	39.6%	5,471,677	63.7%	394,414	4.6%	507,767	5.9%
Asian alone, not Hispanic	3,376,835	874,578	25.9%	2,695,602	79.8%	42,422	1.3%	93,362	2.8%
Two or more races + other races, not Hispanic	2,618,257	913,809	34.9%	1,786,102	68.2%	66,018	2.5%	231,701	8.8%
Total	59,576,010	21,702,536	36.4%	41,927,800	70.4%	1,101,264	1.8%	2,463,538	4.1%

Source: Table prepared by CRS based on data available from U.S. Census Bureau, Household Pulse Survey: May 21 – May 26, Table 4, https://www.census.gov/data/tables/2020/demo/hhp/hhp4.html.

Notes: Details may not add to totals as the question allowed multiple categories to be selected.

a. Reflects the race and ethnicity of the household member who responded to the survey

Table 5. Internet Availability for Educational Purposes in Households with Children Enrolled in Public or Private School: United States

(Week of May 21-26, 2020)

Hispanic Origin and Race[a]	Total Number of Children in Public or Private School	Internet Availability											
		Internet Always Available		Internet Usually Available		Internet Sometimes Available		Internet Rarely Available		Internet Never Available		Did Not Report	
		Number of Children	Share of Total Children	Number of Children	Share of Total Children	Number of Children	Share of Total Children	Number of Children	Share of Total Children	Number of Children	Share of Total Children	Number of Children	Share of Total Children
Hispanic or Latino (may be of any race)	12,562,900	8,507,839	67.7%	2,521,896	20.1%	761,829	6.1%	309,769	2.5%	112,907	0.9%	348,661	2.8%
White alone, not Hispanic	32,421,823	24,084,423	74.3%	5,592,837	17.3%	1,429,593	4.4%	527,507	1.6%	352,930	1.1%	434,534	1.3%
Black alone, not Hispanic	8,596,195	5,446,476	63.4%	1,770,237	20.6%	684,644	8.0%	269,037	3.1%	189,778	2.2%	236,023	2.7%
Asian alone, not Hispanic	3,376,835	2,629,688	77.9%	521,970	15.5%	104,977	3.1%	46,618	1.4%	3,969	0.1%	69,614	2.1%
Two or more races + other races, not Hispanic	2,618,257	1,410,868	53.9%	656,985	25.1%	263,429	10.1%	75,097	2.9%	92,956	3.6%	118,922	4.5%
Total	59,576,010	42,079,293	70.6%	11,063,924	18.6%	3,244,471	5.4%	1,228,028	2.1%	752,541	1.3%	1,207,753	2.0%

Source: Table prepared by CRS based on data available from U.S. Census Bureau, Household Pulse Survey: May 21 -- May 26, Table 3, https://www.census.gov/data/tables/2020/demo/hhp/hhp4.html.

Notes: Details may not add to totals due to rounding.

a. Reflects the race and ethnicity of the household member who responded to the survey

Table 6. Provider of Internet Available to Children for Educational Purposes for Households with Children Enrolled in Public or Private School: United States

(Week of May 21-26, 2020)

Hispanic Origin and Race[a]	Total Number of Children in Public or Private School	Provider of Internet for Educational Purposes							
		Paid for by the Children's School or School District		Paid for by Someone in the Household or Family		Paid for by another source		Did not report	
		Number of Children	Share of Total Children	Number of Children	Share of Total Children	Number of Children	Share of Total Children	Number of Children	Share of Total Children
Hispanic or Latino (may be of any race)	12,562,900	656,043	5.2%	11,347,068	90.3%	248,992	2.0%	602,496	4.8%
White alone, not Hispanic	32,421,823	330,057	1.0%	30,487,987	94.0%	466,592	1.4%	1,352,016	4.2%
Black alone, not Hispanic	8,596,195	247,713	2.9%	7,537,467	87.7%	246,719	2.9%	703,588	8.2%
Asian alone, not Hispanic	3,376,835	38,030	1.1%	3,171,958	93.9%	49,586	1.5%	131,481	3.9%
Two or more races + other races, not Hispanic	2,618,257	41,958	1.6%	2,273,032	86.8%	37,212	1.4%	296,409	11.3%
Total	59,576,010	1,313,802	2.2%	54,817,513	92.0%	1,049,101	1.8%	3,085,991	5.2%

Source: Table prepared by CRS based on data available from U.S. Census Bureau, Household Pulse Survey: May 21 – May 26, Table 4, https://www.census.gov/data/tables/2020/demo/hhp/hhp4.html.

Notes: Details may not add to totals as the question allowed multiple categories to be selected.

a. Reflects the race and ethnicity of the household member who responded to the survey

Education Week Surveys

Education Week conducted two nationally representative surveys—one on March 24 and 25 and one on April 7 and 8—to examine disparities in remote learning among high poverty and low poverty LEAs.[8] Over 2,600 teachers and district leaders participated in the surveys. The surveys examined several topic areas, including gaps in basic technology access, whether teachers were continuing to teach, student truancy, the availability of live instruction, schools' ability to provide instruction to all students, types of communication tools used to reach students, and whether schoolwork was distributed online or in-person. For example, the first survey found that 67% of teachers teaching in high-poverty schools (75% or more students from low-income families) compared with 89% of teachers in low-poverty schools (25% or less of students from low-income families) were continuing to teach. By the second survey, these percentages had shifted to 85% and 95%, respectively. It is possible that these percentages continued to increase, but no additional data are available. *Education Week* also found that synchronous (live virtual) instruction was more readily available in low-poverty schools than in high-poverty schools, lack of access to technology hindered teaching to a greater extent in high-poverty schools than in low-poverty schools, and student truancy was higher in high-poverty schools than in low-poverty schools.

AASA Survey

More recently, AASA, The School Superintendents Association released the results of a national survey that addressed issues of remote learning among a variety of other issues related to education and the coronavirus pandemic.[9] AASA received about 500 responses from administrators across 48 states.[10] Below are responses to various survey questions that address, or at least partially address, the provision of remote learning.[11] These responses are taken directly from the document published by AASA and have not been edited for grammar, spelling, or clarity.

- When asked how districts are providing distance learning while schools are closed due to COVID-19, respondents replied "district owned laptop, tablets, and hotspots" (92%); "texts and phone calls home to students and families" (91%); "video casts/webinars" (89%); "work packets" (82%); "online test and quizzes" (70%); "interactive whiteboards & online platforms" (65%); "textbooks" (53%); "classroom blogs & wikis" (52%); "instant grading and feedback" (29%); and "podcast" (23%). (Q9)
- When asked to identify barriers that would prohibit their district from transitioning to a fully online-learning model, respondents answered "we lack adequate internet access at home (student homework gap)" (60%); "we do not have the instructional capacity for online learning (teacher technology proficiency, lack of online student learning portal/platform, etc.)" (40%); "we lack the resources to purchase a comprehensive

---

[8] Benjamin Herold, "The Disparities in Remote Learning Under Coronavirus (in Charts)," *Education Week*, April 10, 2020, https://www.edweek.org/ew/articles/2020/04/10/the-disparities-in-remote-learning-under-coronavirus.html.

[9] Letter from Chris Rogers, Policy Analyst and Noelle Ellerson Ng, Associate Executive Director, Advocacy & Governance, AASA, to AASA Members, Report of Initial Findings: COVID Survey 2 Impact on Public Schools, June 16, 2020, https://aasa.org/uploadedFiles/AASA_Blog(1)/COVID_School%20Response%20Survey%202_Intial%20findings_6_16_2020_FN.docx.

[10] AASA's discussion of its initial results does not discuss the specific survey respondents but does indicate that it had a response rate of 38%. In its first survey related to these issues, AASA noted that respondents were a non-random sample that included superintendents, associate superintendents, aspiring superintendents, and other school system leaders. For more information, see AASA, *AASA COVID-19 School Response Study*, April 6, 2020, https://aasa.org/uploadedFiles/AASA_Blog(1)/AASA_COVID_19_Report_FN_4_3_2020.pdf.

[11] CRS was unable to locate a public copy of the survey instrument within the deadlines associated with this request. While it appears that some of the questions included on the survey may have allowed respondents to choose more than one response from a list of options, CRS was unable to confirm this.

software program that could host all of our classes and data" (30%); "our educators and school personnel lack adequate connectivity and technology" (29%); "we offer one-to-one device programs in only certain grade spans/student clusters" (28%); "we do not have adequate bandwidth" (22%); "other" (18%); "we do not offer anyone to one device programs in our district" (14%). (Q14)

- When asked what percentage of their students are unable to participate in remote learning because they lack either internet access or a device at home, respondents replied "less than 10%" (47%); "11-20%" (22%); "21-30%" (12%), "31-40%" (6%); "41-50%" (3%); and "51% or greater" (6%).
- When asked how is their district paying for ed-tech services to deliver curriculum and instruction in the event of an extended COVID-19 outbreak, respondents replied "repurposing existing local funding" (61%); "repurposing existing state funding" (57%); "federal emergency education relief fund" (41%); "realize efficiencies within existing school budget" (41%); "federal E-rate program" (32%); "federal governors fund" (12%); "public-private partnerships" (12%); "private philanthropy or foundation" (10%); and "other" (6%). (Q20)

Administrators were also asked about general equity and funding issues in the AASA survey. Some of the responses addressed remote learning issues. When asked what they were doing to address equity issues during the coronavirus pandemic, 91% indicated that "devices are provided for students who need them" and 37% indicated that "home internet access is provided for all students."[12] When asked what their district was "finding hard to provide equitably" during the coronavirus pandemic, 52% of respondents said "access to online learning" and 27% said "devices for all students who need them." With respect to the costs that administrators are most concerned about, 47% responded "costs related to connectivity" and 41% responded "costs related to technology devices (laptops and personal devices)."

CPRE Survey

The Center on Reinventing Public Education (CRPE) also recently released the results of a national study examining the provision of remote learning in 477 LEAs.[13, 14] Overall, CRPE found that 33.5% of LEAs expected teachers to provide remote instruction to all students. With respect to tracking student engagement with remote learning, 27.4% of LEAs expected attendance to be taken, 36.9% expected teachers to check in with individual students, and 48.0% of LEAs expected that either attendance was taken or check-ins occurred. With respect to the monitoring of student progress and grading, 42.1% of LEAs expected grading for some or all students and 57.9% expected progress monitoring for some or all students.[15]

The CRPE study also examined differences by locality (city, rural, or suburban) and based on student eligibility for free and reduced-price lunch (FRPL). The researchers found that urban LEAs were more likely than rural LEAs to expect teachers to provide remote instruction to all students (51.3% compared with 27.2%, respectively), take attendance or check in with students (65.5% compared with 43.1%, respectively), monitor student progress for some or all students (79.6% compared with 52.6%, respectively), and provide grading for some or all students (57.2% compared with 39.8%, respectively). CPRE also examined the provision of synchronous (live virtual) instruction by LEAs with high FRPL

[12] AASA does not specify whether this means the school district provided home internet access for all students or only for the students who did not otherwise have home internet access.

[13] Betheny Gross and Alice Opalka, *Too Many Schools Leave Learning to Chance*, Center on Reinventing Public Education (CRPE), June 2020, https://www.crpe.org/sites/default/files/final_national_sample_brief_2020.pdf.

[14] The CPRE study does not discuss the specific survey respondents beyond indicating that districts responded to the survey.

[15] CRPE notes that expectations for grading and progress monitoring were usually for older students.

rates (rates of 71% and above) and low FRPL rates (rates of 34% and below). The researchers found that a greater percentage of LEAs with low FRPL rates required synchronous (live) instruction (28.8%) compared with LEAs with high FRPL rates (14.5%).

Estimates of State Budget Shortfalls, Education Funding, Job Losses, and the Costs of Reopening Schools, Prepared by Varied Groups

Various organizations have examined the economic costs of the coronavirus with respect to elementary and secondary education. This includes estimating state budget shortfalls over fiscal years 2020 through 2022 and how this might affect state funding for education. Related to the budget shortfalls, estimates of education-related job losses have also been produced. In addition, the possible additional costs of opening schools while complying with numerous safety requirements implemented in response to the coronavirus pandemic also have been examined.

The estimates and projections that follow are presented in response to your interest in work being generated by varied education groups. The methodologies employed are not reviewed in depth and may involve varied assumptions.

Estimated State Budget Shortfalls and Education Funding

Estimates have been published with respect to expected budget shortfalls over the next few years. For example, the Center on Budget and Policies Priorities (CBPP) has estimated that overall state budget shortfalls for state fiscal years 2020, 2021, and 2022 combined will be $615 billion.[16] CBPP formulated this estimate based on the Federal Reserve Board's summary of economic projections for June 2020 and the Congressional Budget Office's May projections. CBPP estimates that states may be able to use $100 billion provided through the Coronavirus Aid, Relief, and Economic Security Act (CARES Act; P.L. 116-136) to assist with these shortfalls. CBPP notes that states have reserves or "rainy day funds" that total $75 million. If states use all of their rainy day funds and the CARES Act funding to address the shortfall, CBPP estimates that the state budget shortfalls will be reduced to $440 billion.

According to the National Association of State Budget Officers, it is estimated that 24.9% of all state funds were used to support elementary and secondary education in FY2019.[17] If this share of funding were to hold through state fiscal years 2020 through 2022, elementary and secondary education's "share" of the budget shortfall, without accounting for CARES Act funding and rainy day funds, would be $153 billion. After accounting for the CARES Act funding and rainy day funds, it would be $110 billion. Neither the estimated overall state budget shortfall nor the estimated elementary and secondary education shortfall, however, take into account budget shortfalls at the local or tribal levels or for the outlying areas. Thus, the overall shortfall in funding for elementary and secondary education could be larger.

Budget cuts to elementary and secondary education in an individual state may begin in FY2020 or in subsequent fiscal years. For example, Governor DeWine has ordered all state agencies in Ohio to cut up to 20% of their budgets for the remainder of the fiscal year ending on June 30, 2020.[18] For elementary and

---

[16] Elizabeth McNichol and Michael Leachman, *States Continue to Face Large Shortfalls Due to COVID-19 Effects*, Center on Budget and Policy Priorities, June 15, 2020, https://www.cbpp.org/research/state-budget-and-tax/states-continue-to-face-large-shortfalls-due-to-covid-19-effects.

[17] National Association of State Budget Officers, *2019 State Expenditure Report*, November 21, 2019, https://www.nasbo.org/reports-data/state-expenditure-report.

[18] Valerie Strauss, "K-12 school leaders warn of 'disaster' from huge coronavirus-related budget cuts as layoffs and furloughs begin," *Washington Post*, May 8, 2020, https://www.washingtonpost.com/education/2020/05/08/k-12-school-leaders-warn-disaster-huge-coronavirus-related-budget-cuts-layoffs-furloughs-begin/.

secondary public schools, the governor's plans would require a $300.4 million reduction in funding with cuts targeted in the wealthiest districts.[19] In Georgia, Governor Kemp has told state agencies to cut 14% from their budgets for next school year.[20] In Texas, LEAs are retaining their full funding for the current school year but only because the Texas Education Agency is using funds provided under the CARES Act to make this possible.[21]

Estimated Job Losses

With respect to job losses, the American Federation of Teachers (AFT) stated that about 750,000 jobs in public education have already been lost due to the coronavirus pandemic based on federal jobs reports.[22] NEA estimates that about 1.9 million jobs in elementary, secondary, and higher education will be lost from FY2020 through FY2022 due to COVID-19.[23] (These estimates were not disaggregated by level of education or type of education-related jobs.)

Estimated Costs of Reopening Schools

Other organizations have examined the costs associated with reopening while meeting new requirements and needs related to COVID-19. AFT estimates that at least an additional $116.5 billion will be needed to open schools safely.[24] AFT developed this number based on estimated costs associated with, for example, increasing the number of instructional staff to meet social distance requirements that may necessitate reducing class sizes, purchasing personal protective equipment (PPE), providing transportation while meeting social distancing requirements, purchasing cleaning materials and health supplies, and providing needed technology to close the digital divide if instruction needs to continue online in some capacity.

AASA and the Association of School Business Officers International (ASBO International) also estimated the additional costs that an average LEA[25] may face in the fall to reopen while meeting safety guidelines related to COVID-19. These estimates take into account adhering to health monitoring and cleaning/disinfecting protocols, hiring staff to implement health and safety protocols, providing PPE, and providing transportation and child care. Based on these estimates, the additional costs for an average LEA would be $1,778,139. This breaks down to about $222,000 per school and $486 per student.

---

[19] Ibid.

[20] Ibid.

[21] Mari Salazar, "Texas school districts won't get supplemental CARES Act funds they were expecting; TEA puts money toward state funds," *KVUE*, June 9, 2020, https://www.kvue.com/article/news/local/texas-school-districts-cares-act-funds-tea-money-state-funds/269-3e09564f-afbb-4d7a-9acf-725011de20fb?fbclid=IwAR1snb3upmuUZE0llhZmY5fM6KOHUvsF_BwEKVjYlmu47m5UfgdwP3odaW0.

[22] American Federation of Teachers, "Statement by AFT President Randi Weingarten on Jobs Report," press release, June 5, 2020, https://www.aft.org/press-release/statement-aft-president-randi-weingarten-jobs-report.

[23] To determine potential job losses for elementary and secondary education, NEA used U.S. Census Bureau data from Current Spending of Public Elementary-School Education Finances: 2018 and the 2018 Survey of Public Employment and Payroll National Education Association. To calculate job losses for postsecondary education, NEA used data available from the *Digest of Education: 2018* published by the National Center for Education Statistics at the U.S. Department of Education. For selected states (CA, ID, IN, MN, NC, VT, and WA), potential job losses were capped at 28% of their total workforce. (*Health and Economic Recovery Omnibus Emergency Solutions (HEROES)*, June 10, 2020, https://educationvotes.nea.org/wp-content/uploads/2020/06/Revised-NEA-Estimates-in-Support-of-the-HEROES-Act-06-06-2020.pdf?_ga=2.119281344.891537264.1592333566-58023336.1585919363.)

[24] American Federation of Teachers, *Reopening Schools During the Time of a Triple Crisis: Financial Implications*, June 10, 2020, https://www.aft.org/sites/default/files/wysiwyg/reopen-schools-financial-implications.pdf.

[25] For the purposes of their estimates, AASA and ASBO International defined an average LEA as having 8 school buildings, 183 classrooms, 3,659 students, 329 staff members, and 40 school buses (transporting at 25% capacity).

Postsecondary Education

This section examines data on postsecondary outcomes, labor market outcomes, and student loan borrowing. It also discusses home internet access for postsecondary students.

Data on Postsecondary Outcomes, Labor Market Outcomes, and Student Loan Borrowing[26]

This section identifies sources that provide data on the intersection of race and the higher education issues in which you expressed interest. It focuses on data that were published by the National Center for Education Statistics (NCES). As is the case with other education data, these data precede the COVID-19 emergency and, in some cases, precede it by several years.

In accordance with your request, varied comparisons between minority students and White students are presented in this memorandum. The presentation follows the approaches used by the cited sources and typically reports data on Black and Hispanic students separately. Data on other minority student groups tend to be based on small samples and are generally not included. When referring to racial groups, this memorandum uses the terms used in the original source. This may, for example, result in cases where descriptions of some sources refer to "Hispanic" students and descriptions of others refer to "Hispanic or Latino" students.

In limited cases, third-party analyses that were conducted using NCES-commissioned data are discussed. These sources are included because they speak directly to your request. Due to your timeline, CRS did not have the ability to assess these sources' methodologies or re-create their findings. Their inclusion should not be considered a CRS endorsement.

Postsecondary Outcomes and Labor Market Outcomes

In February 2019, NCES published *Persistence, Retention, and Attainment of 2011–12 First-Time Beginning Postsecondary Students as of Spring 2017: First Look* (First Look). The First Look presents selected findings from the 2012/17 Beginning Postsecondary Students Longitudinal Study (BPS:12/17), a nationally representative survey of undergraduates who entered postsecondary education for the first time in the 2011–12 academic year and covering the experiences of these first-time beginning postsecondary students over six academic years. The report presents data that suggest, among first-time postsecondary students, differing rates of attainment in bachelor's degree programs by race and ethnicity: 43% of White students attain a bachelor's degree within six years of beginning their postsecondary education studies versus 23% of Black students and 24% of Hispanic students.[27]

In February 2019, NCES also published *Status and Trends in the Education of Racial and Ethnic Groups 2018* (Trends Report). The Trends Report uses data obtained from various surveys and administrative records, including surveys conducted by NCES and by the Census Bureau, to examine differences in educational participation and attainment of students and adults by race and ethnicity. Among many findings, the report suggests differing rates of persistence and bachelor's degree attainment by race and ethnicity in 2016: 35% of White adults aged 25 years or older had completed a bachelor's degree or higher compared to 21% of Black adults and 15% of Hispanic adults aged 25 years or older.[28]

---

[26] This section was written by Rita Zota, rzota@crs.loc.gov, and Benjamin Collins, bcollins@crs.loc.gov.

[27] U.S. Department of Education, National Center of Education Statistics, *Persistence, Retention, and Attainment of 2011-12 First-Time Beginning Postsecondary Students as of Spring 2017: First Look*, Table 1, February 2019, pp. 9-10, https://nces.ed.gov/pubs2019/2019401.pdf.

[28] Ibid, Figure 27.3, p. 162.

Additionally, 25% of Black adults aged 25 years or older completed some college but did not earn a degree relative to 21% of White adults and 18% of Hispanic adults.[29]

Additionally, the Trends Report presents information on labor market outcomes that is primarily sourced from the Current Population Survey. Specifically, the report indicates that, in 2017, higher shares of Black and Hispanic adults aged 18 to 24 are not enrolled in school or working relative to White adults in the same age group.[30] The report also indicates that, in 2016, Black and Hispanic adult full-time year-round workers aged 24-35 have lower median annual earnings relative to White adult workers in the same age group: in particular, Black and Hispanic workers have median annual earnings just shy of $34,000 compared to median annual earnings of $45,000 for White workers. This trend persists when median earnings data are disaggregated by educational attainment.[31]

Student Loan Borrowing and Repayment

In June 2019, NCES published *Baccalaureate and Beyond (B&B:16/17): A First Look at the Employment and Education Experience of College Graduates, 1 Year Later*.[32] This report used Baccalaureate and Beyond (B&B) data, which is a nationally representative data set of students who completed a bachelor's degree during the 2015-16 academic year. In this survey, Black students accounted for about 10% of the first-time bachelor's degree recipients and Hispanic students accounted for about 13%.[33] Among first-time bachelor's degree recipients, about 86% of Black students borrowed any kind of student loan, compared to 70% of Hispanic students and 67% of White students. Among borrowers, Black students borrowed an average of $36,900, compared to $26,900 for Hispanic borrowers and $30,500 for White borrowers.[34] The report did not include data on repayment, but did include data on unemployment. Twelve months after graduation, Black degree recipients reported an unemployment rate of 9.0%, compared to 8.2% for Hispanic students and 4.2% for white students.[35]

In March 2018, NCES published *Debt After College: Employment, Enrollment, and Student-Reported Stress and Outcomes*.[36] This report used data from a B&B survey which considered bachelor's degree recipients from the 2007-08 academic year with follow-up information from the 2012-13 period. Among other indicators, the report included data on borrowing for subsequent graduate education. Among the reference population of bachelor's degree recipients, 37% of Black students took out federal graduate loans, compared to 24% of Hispanic students and 22% of White students. Among borrowers, average cumulative borrowing for any postsecondary education was higher for Black students ($57,700) than for Hispanic or White students ($45,400 and $43,800, respectively).[37] The report also included a number of emotional and psychological indicators including self-reported "debt stress" and "perceived consequences of education cost" (e.g., "delayed buying a home"). On average, Black and Hispanic students were more

---

[29] U.S. Department of Education, National Center of Education Statistics, *Status and Trends in the Education of Racial and Ethnic Groups 2018*, Figure 27.2, February 2019, p. 161, https://nces.ed.gov/pubs2019/2019038.pdf.

[30] Ibid, Figure 29.1, p. 168.

[31] Ibid, Figures 30.1 and 30.2, pp. 170-171.

[32] U.S. Department of Education, National Center of Education Statistics, *Baccalaureate and Beyond (B&B:16/17): A First Look at the Employment and Education Experience of College Graduates, 1 Year Later*, June 2019, https://nces.ed.gov/pubs2019/2019241.pdf.

[33] Ibid, Table 1.

[34] Ibid, Table 3.

[35] Ibid, Table 5.

[36] U.S. Department of Education, National Center of Education Statistics, *Debt After College: Employment, Enrollment, and Student-Reported Stress and Outcomes*, March 2018, https://nces.ed.gov/pubs2018/2018401.pdf.

[37] Ibid, Table 1.

likely than White students to report their debt stress as "very high" or report delaying buying a home or having children.[38]

NCES has published analyses of longitudinal repayment, but these reports generally did not disaggregate students by race.[39] Third parties have used different versions of the previously-described BPS data to analyze borrowing and related issues by students' race. For example:

- In December 2019, the Center for American Progress used BPS data to analyze outcomes for students who began postsecondary education in the 2011-12 academic year through 2017 (six years).[40] Among all borrowers, the analysis found that 32% of Black borrowers defaulted on their loans compared to 20% of Hispanic or Latino borrowers and 13% of White borrowers. Among the subset of borrowers who did not complete a degree or certificate and were not enrolled in postsecondary education, the default rate was 55% for Black borrowers, 41% for Hispanic or Latino borrowers, and 33% for White borrowers. The analysis also reported that, among bachelor's degree recipients who borrowed, 34% of Black borrowers were enrolled in an income-driven repayment plan vs. 22% of Hispanic or Latino borrowers and 18% of White borrowers.
- In June 2018, the Brookings Institution published an analysis of student loan defaults using a prior version of BPS data for students who began postsecondary education in the 2003-04 academic year. The analysis considered defaults in the 12 years after initial college entry.[41] The analysis found that 49% of Black undergraduate borrowers defaulted within 12 years of entry, compared to 35% of Hispanic borrowers and 21% of White borrowers.[42] The analysis further reported that after controlling for various factors that are correlated with default such as parents' level of education and sector of the institution attended (e.g., public or for-profit), the gap between Black students and all students was reduced but that a statistically significant difference in default rates remained.[43]

As mentioned previously, CRS did not review these third parties' methodologies and does not endorse their findings. We include them in this discussion because they speak directly to your requested issues.

Home Internet Access for Postsecondary Students[44]

The available national data on the extent to which persons may have home internet access (which may serve as a proxy for home access to online postsecondary educational programming) precede the COVID-19 emergency. Data focused specifically on postsecondary students are not available. The primary sources of data on internet access are the U.S. Census Bureau (Census) and Federal Communications Commission (FCC). The FCC assesses broadband access by determining whether at least one home or business in a

[38] Table 2 and Table 6.

[39] See, for example, U.S. Department of Education, National Center of Education Statistics, *Repayments of Student Loans as of 2015 Among 1995-96 and 2003-04 First-Time Beginning Students*, October 2017, https://nces.ed.gov/pubs2018/2018410.pdf.

[40] Center for American Progress, "The Continued Student Loan Crisis for Black Borrowers," December 2019, https://www.americanprogress.org/issues/education-postsecondary/reports/2019/12/02/477929/continued-student-loan-crisis-black-borrowers/.

[41] The analysis supplemented BPS data with data from the National Student Loans Data Systems. Brookings Institution, *What Accounts for Gaps in Student Loan Default and What Happens After*, June 2018, https://www.brookings.edu/research/what-accounts-for-gaps-in-student-loan-default-and-what-happens-after/.

[42] Ibid, Figure 2.

[43] Ibid, Appendix Table A1.

[44] This section was written by Cassandria Dortch, cdortch@crs.loc.gov and Kyrie Dragoo, kdragoo@crs.loc.gov.

census block (not individual households) has broadband access.[45] FCC data are not provided because they do not reflect the number of persons with broadband access.

Calendar year 2018 Census data, however, indicate that, on average, 88% of the population are in a household that has a computer and a broadband internet subscription. Asians and Whites have the highest rate of access (94% and 89%, respectively) and access is lower among Blacks or African Americans (82%), American Indians and Alaska Natives (76%), Native Hawaiians and Other Pacific Islanders (84%), and Hispanics or Latinos (of any race) (86%). Census defines a computer to include desktop computers and smartphones. Smartphones may not be adequate for completing remote learning lessons, which means the data may overestimate access to remote learning.[46]

Youth Experiencing Homelessness[47]

This part of the memorandum provides information about rates of youth homelessness and access to services for youth experiencing homeless, including any variations by race, during the COVID-19 public health emergency.[48] National data about homeless youth are generally made publicly available a year or more after are they are collected. Therefore, no real-time data exist about homeless youth and the services they have received since the onset of the public health emergency. Nonetheless, one study has reported on the experiences of homeless youth during the COVID-19 period in a single community. The following sections discuss these sources as well as national data on homeless youth in the few years preceding the pandemic.

Experiences of Homeless Youth During the COVID-19 Public Health Emergency

Since national data on youth experiencing homelessness during the COVID-19 public health emergency are not currently available, CRS conducted a search of research and news publications between February 1, 2020 and mid-June 2020 to identify any information about the experiences of homeless youth over this period.[49] This review identified one study involving youth in a single community. While this source does not provide recent data on homeless youth, or address the specific experiences of African American youth, it includes anecdotal information about homeless youth and organizations that provide them with shelter and services.

The study—published by the University of California, Berkeley's School of Public Health—examined youth homelessness in Berkeley, California from July 2018 through June 2019 and in April 2020.[50] With

---

[45] For more information on FCC data, see CRS Report R45962, *Broadband Data and Mapping: Background and Issues for the 116th Congress*.

[46] U.S. Census Bureau, American Community Survey, 2018: ACS 1-Year Estimates Subject Table S2802, available at https://data.census.gov/cedsci/table?d=ACS%201-Year%20Estimates%20Subject%20Tables&tid=ACSST1Y2018.S2802&vintage=2018&hidePreview=true.

[47] This section was written by Adrienne Fernandes-Alcantara, afernandes@crs.loc.gov.

[48] There is no single federal definition of the term "homeless youth" or the related term, "runaway youth." See CRS Report, CRS Report RL33785, *Runaway and Homeless Youth: Demographics and Programs*, by Adrienne L. Fernandes-Alcantara.

[49] CRS Senior Research Librarian Sarah Caldwell searched ProQuest (which contains citations to and selected full text of academic journal articles, general news articles, policy papers, trade journals, conference proceedings, and more) using combinations of the following terms: homeless, runaway, run away, youth, teen, young adult, access, services, food, transportation, transit, counseling, therapy, prevention, health, medical, shelter, housing, drop-in center, crisis center, coronavirus, COVID-19, and pandemic. We also conducted a general internet search using the terms homeless youth, youth homelessness, services, or shelter, with coronavirus-related terms. We limited the searches to items published between February 1, 2020 and June 12, 2020. Please note that while we attempted to be thorough with our search, the results may not be comprehensive.

[50] Colette Auerswald et al., *On the COVID-19 Front Line and Hurting: Addressing the Needs of Providers for Youth*

respect to April 2020, when the pandemic was underway, researchers conducted interviews with representatives from 14 organizations in and around Berkeley that provide support for homeless youth to assess the needs of youth and providers during the public health emergency. However, the study did not examine any changes in rates of homelessness during April compared to previous periods. According to the study, some youth-serving organizations closed or moved their services online. In addition, shelters were no longer taking new residents to limit the spread of COVID-19. Some organizations had increased services for homeless youth during the pandemic and some staff were working longer hours to make up for other staff and volunteer shortages. Based on interviews with staff of these organizations, the study identified the following challenges for serving youth during the public health emergency: (1) a need for shelter and housing to appropriately practice social distancing; (2) a shortage of supplies and resources for staff and youth, such as access to masks, internet services, food, and phones for youth; (3) a need for physical and mental health services, including services for conditions not related to COVID-19; (4) inadequate resources to support staff in their work; and (5) a need for youth and staff to be better informed about how to safely shelter-in-place.

Homeless Youth in the Period Preceding the COVID-19 Public Health Emergency

National estimates of youth homelessness are available in the years preceding the COVID-19 public health emergency. These estimates depend on which definitions of homelessness are used and how counts take place, among other variables. The Department of Housing and Urban Development (HUD) is responsible for collecting and reporting data about the scale of homelessness. HUD also routinely reports two different estimates of homelessness in Annual Homeless Assessment Reports (AHAR). These estimates include point-in-time counts (PIT) and full-year estimates based on a sample of jurisdictions. Only PIT count data include homeless youth, referred to as unaccompanied youth; however, efforts are underway to collect data on homeless youth as part of the full-year estimates.[51] In addition, HUD has funded a national study of homeless youth known as *Voices of Youth Count*. Both the *Voices of Youth Count* and annual PIT counts include data on race and ethnicity of homeless youth.

The major federal programs that support homeless children and youth—the Runaway and Homeless Youth Act (RHYA) program, administered by the Department of Health and Human Services (HHS) and the Education for Homeless Children and Youths (EHCY) program, administered by ED—report data on homeless youth. While recent data do not include breakouts by race and ethnicity, HHS has reported in the past on race and ethnicity of youth served in the RHYA programs. HHS has also reported on the number of youth overall (and not broken out by race and ethnicity) who were unable to access services through the program.

HUD: PIT Count

HUD requires communities receiving funds through its Homeless Assistance Grants, which fund housing and services for homeless persons, to conduct annual PIT counts of people experiencing homelessness during the last week of January. Consistent with HUD's definition of "homeless individual," these PIT counts include people living in emergency shelter, transitional housing, and on the street or other places not meant for human habitation. They do not include people who are temporarily living with family or friends. The counts identify homeless youth, referred to as unaccompanied youth, under age 25 who are

---

Experiencing Homelessness in Berkeley and Alameda County, University of California, Berkeley School of Public Health, May 2020. Data were reported for the July 2018 through June 2019 period. According to the study, Berkeley's population is approximately 8% African American and 75% of homeless youth who received services in Berkeley during that time were black.

[51] U.S. Department of Housing and Urban Development (HUD), *The 2017 Annual Homeless Assessment Report (AHAR) to Congress, Report to Congress, Part 2*, p. X.

not part of a family. The PIT count for 2017 through 2019 for unaccompanied youth ranged from about 35,000 to 41,000 annually.[52] In each of these years, about 90% of youth were ages 18 to 24 with the remaining 10% under the age of 18.[53] **Figure 1** shows PIT counts of unaccompanied youth for 2017 through 2019 by race.[54] Though not shown in the figure, approximately one-quarter of homeless youth in each of 2017 through 2019 identified as Hispanic regardless of their race.

Figure 1. Race of Homeless Youth at Point-in-Time, 2017-2019

Based on a count of unaccompanied homeless individuals under age 25

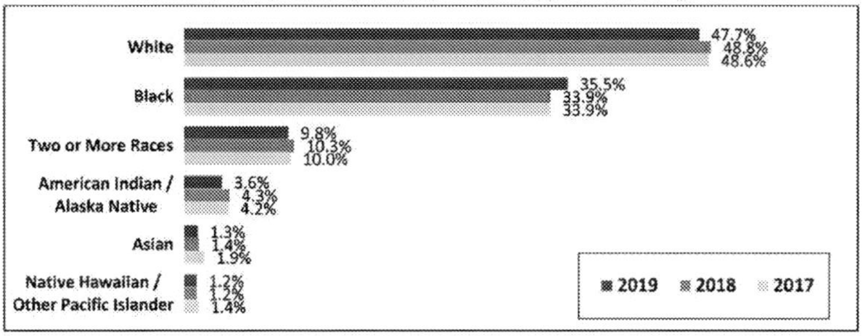

Source: Congressional Research Service, based on HUD, The 2019 Annual Homeless Assessment Report (AHAR) to Congress.

HUD: Voices of Youth Count

HUD has separately funded a research project known as *Voices of Youth Count* that is designed to better determine the number of homeless youth.[55] The study involved a nationally representative phone survey in 2017 of adults whose households had individuals ages 13 to 25 and respondents ages 18 to 25. Based on this study, researchers estimated that approximately 700,000 youth ages 13 to 17 and 3.5 million young adults ages 18 to 25 experienced homelessness within a 12-month period, meaning they were sleeping in places not meant for living, staying in shelters, or temporarily staying with others while lacking a safe and stable alternative living arrangement. The study also found that youth in rural and urban areas are affected by homelessness at similar levels. In addition, certain youth ages 18 to 25 were at heightened risk of experiencing homelessness, including those who are black or Hispanic; parenting and unmarried; or LGBTQ. With regard to race and ethnicity, and controlling for factors like income and

[52] This does not include parenting youth under the age of 25. The number of parenting youth was 9,434 in 2017; 8,724 in 2018; and 7,564 in 2019. Published data are not available on the race and ethnicity of parenting youth.

[53] The 2019 PIT count indicates that approximately half of the unaccompanied homeless youth were sheltered and the other half were unsheltered. As noted in the 2019 AHAR report, HUD and its federal partners selected the PIT counts from January 2017 as the baseline measure of homelessness among unaccompanied youth. Nearly 350 communities conducted unsheltered counts in 2018, but it was not required. The report indicates that 2019 will be the first year that HUD examines year-to-year trends in unaccompanied homeless youth.

[54] Among adults in the U.S. in 2018, 63% were non-Hispanic white, 12% were non-Hispanic black, 6% were non-Hispanic Asian, <.5% were non-Hispanic Native Hawaiian or Other Pacific Islander, 2% were two or more races and non-Hispanic. The remaining share of adults, 16%, were Hispanic or Latino. This methodology is distinct from the PIT count, which reports ethnicity as a separate category. The Annie E. Casey Foundation, *Kids Count Data Center*, "Adult Population by Race in the United States."

[55] Matthew H. Morton, Amy Dworsky, and Gina M. Samuels, *Missed Opportunities: Youth Homelessness in America. National Estimates*, University of Chicago, Chapin Hall, 2017.

education, the study found that older African American youth had an 83% increased risk of having experienced homelessness compared to youth of other races. Hispanic youth had a 33% increased risk of experiencing homelessness relative to non-Hispanic youth.

ED: Homeless Children and Youths Program

The Education for Homeless Children and Youth program provides assistance to homeless children and youth attending schools.[56] All local education agencies (LEAs) are required to report data annually to the Department of Education (ED) on the number of homeless students enrolled, regardless of whether or not they receive EHCY funds. Unaccompanied youth—homeless children or youth not in the physical custody of a parent or guardian—made up about 9% annually of the 1.3 to 1.5 million students in preschool through high school who were homeless in school years 2015-2016, 2016-2017, or 2017-2018.[57] Though published data are not available, ED appears to be moving forward with collecting race and ethnicity data for the program as of SY2019-2020.[58]

Runaway and Homeless Youth Act

The Runaway and Homeless Youth Act authorizes programs that provide short-term and transitional housing and supportive services for youth who are homeless.[59] HHS data indicate that in FY2018, Basic Center Program (BCP) grantees served 20,821 youth and Transitional Living Program (TLP) grantees served 3,082 youth, for a total of approximately 25,000 youth.[60] This is fewer than the number of youth who were homeless according to either the *Voices of Youth* study or the one-day PIT counts. FY2014 is the most recent year for which race and ethnicity data are available for RHYA programs. In that year, approximately one-third of youth in the BCP and nearly 40% of youth in the TLP were African American. Also in that same year, more than 8,000 youth were turned away by BCP and TLP grantees due to their lack of capacity in providing services (data were not further broken out by youth characteristics).[61]

[56] The program defines homeless children and youth in part by a reference to the definition of "homeless individual" in the McKinney-Vento Act, which refers to lacking a fixed, regular, and adequate nighttime residence, and by other criteria. These other criteria specify that children and youth eligible for the program are those who (1) share housing with other persons due to loss of housing or economic hardship; (2) live in hotels or motels, trailer parks, or campgrounds due to lack of alternative arrangements; (3) are awaiting foster care placement; (4) live in substandard housing; and (5) are the children of migrant workers. 42 U.S.C. §11434a(2).

[57] University of North Carolina Greensboro, National Center for Homeless Education, *Federal Data Summary School Years 2015-16 Through 2017-2018*. Data are excluded for Vermont for SY2017-2018 and for New Jersey for SY2015-2016 and SY2016-2017.

[58] University of North Carolina Greensboro, National Center for Homeless Education, *Guide to Collecting & Reporting Federal Data, Education for Homeless Children & Youth Program*, May 2019, p. 15. According to this publication, ED proposed a new data category on race and ethnicity for the program beginning with school year 2019-2020, and it had taken steps to solicit public comments on this new category. No further information appears to be available about the current status of this data collection effort.

[59] For purposes of the RHYA Basic Center program (BCP), "homeless youth" includes individuals under age 18 (or some older age if permitted by state or local law) for whom it is not possible to live in a safe environment with a relative and who lack safe alternative living arrangements. For purposes of the RHYA Transitional Living Program (TLP), "homeless youth" includes individuals ages 16 through 22 for whom it is not possible to live in a safe environment with a relative and who lack safe alternative living arrangements. 34 U.S.C. § 11279(3).

[60] U.S. Department of Health and Human Services (HHS), Administration for Children and Families (ACF), *FY 2021 Justification of Estimates for Appropriations Committees*, p. 137.

[61] Based on CRS analysis of FY2014 HHS data for the Runaway and Homeless Youth Act programs.

Congressional Research Service
Informing the legislative debate since 1914

MEMORANDUM June 19, 2020

To: House Education and Labor Committee

From: David H. Bradley, Specialist in Labor Economics, dbradley@crs.loc.gov, 7-7352
Sarah A. Donovan, Specialist in Labor Policy, sdonovan@crs.loc.gov, 7-2247
Julie M. Whittaker, Specialist in Income Security, jwhittaker@crs.loc.gov, 7-2587

Subject: **Equity Issues in the Labor Market and COVID-19**

This memorandum responds to your request for information on equity issues in the labor market prior to and during the Coronavirus Disease 2019 (COVID-19) pandemic. Specifically, you requested selected labor market statistics, disaggregated by race, and analysis in the context of the COVID-19 pandemic. Because race and Hispanic ethnicity are measured separately by the Bureau of Labor Statistics (BLS), a primary data source for this memorandum, the requested data and analysis are also provided for Hispanic and non-Hispanic workers, where possible.

You provided questions to the Congressional Research Service (CRS) as a starting point for this project; the final set of questions and issues addressed in this memorandum is the result of discussions between you and CRS. This memorandum is written in a Questions and Answers format to align with the memorandum request.[1]

In several cases you asked about differential labor market outcomes in the early stages of the COVID-19 pandemic. These patterns may change in the longer term as the pandemic and economic recession continue.[2] In addition, given the time constraints associated with this request, CRS's ability to perform original analysis was limited. The memorandum presents data trends and in some cases information on the correlation between data points. More sophisticated analysis, for example that control for multiple or unobservable factors, may produce a different or more nuanced set of responses.

Information in this memorandum may be of general interest to Congress. As such, this information may be provided by CRS to other congressional requesters, and may be published in CRS products for general distribution to Congress at a later date. Your confidentiality as a requester would be preserved in all cases.

[1] The questions were initially provided to CRS by email on June 8, 2020. The questions were subsequently clarified and reframed through additional communication on June 9 and June 10.

[2] A peak in economic activity in the U.S. economy occurred in February 2020, which marked the end of the previous expansion and the beginning of a recession. See Business Cycle Dating Committee of the National Bureau of Economic Research, *Determination of the February Peak in US Economic Activity*, Cambridge, MA, June 8, 2020, https://nber.org/cycles/june2020.html.

A Note on Terms and Concepts Used in this Memorandum

Race and Ethnicity. This memorandum follows the categorization used in the Current Population Survey (CPS) to describe a person's race. The main CPS categories are White, Black or African American, Asian, American Indian or Alaska Native, and Native Hawaiian or Other Pacific Islander. Most BLS publications using CPS data do not show separate estimates for American Indian or Alaska Native, and Native Hawaiian or Other Pacific Islander due to insufficient sample sizes, but individuals in these groups are included in the totals. As such, most presentations of race group shares do not sum to 100%. In addition, the terms Black and African American are used interchangeably in this memorandum. Hispanic or Latino ethnicity is a different demographic concept from race in the CPS data. Where data availability permits (e.g., **Table 6** and **Table 7**) we present statistics by race for *non-Hispanic* workers and separately for Hispanic workers to allow for comparisons across non-overlapping groups. Where such disaggregation is not possible, it is noted in the table "Notes". Individuals of Hispanic or Latino ethnicity may be of any race. Relative to its share of employment overall, a race or ethnic group is referred to as *overrepresented* in a given occupation if it accounts for *more* than its overall share of total employment and is *underrepresented* in a given occupation if it accounts for *less* than its overall share of total employment.

Periodicity of Data. To provide the most current descriptions of labor market outcomes, data from May 2020 are used when possible (the most recent available monthly BLS CPS data as of the publication of this memorandum). Comparing the most recent data to prior time periods, however, may vary depending on the type of data. For series in which seasonally adjusted data are available, data may be compared to any prior month.[3] For series in which seasonally adjusted data are not available, which includes the occupational data in this memorandum, comparisons are generally made to the same month in the prior year, to account for seasonal differences that vary from month-to-month. Thus for most occupation data in this memorandum, May 2020 data are compared to May 2019 data. In some cases, monthly data are not available due to insufficient sample sizes; for example, monthly data are not available on the racial composition of employment by occupation (national) or for demographic characteristics of state-level labor force data. In such cases, CRS provides annual average data (i.e., annual average of monthly data) for 2019.

What occupations are facing the largest layoffs? What is the racial composition of the workforce in occupations that have lost the most and least jobs?

Data in **Table 1** show the racial composition of occupations in 2019 (annual average) and the percentage change in employment by occupation from May 2019 to May 2020.

- In 2019, overall, White workers accounted for 77.7% of the total number of employed individuals, while Black workers accounted for 12.3% and Asian workers accounted for 6.5%. Relative to its share of employment overall, a race group is overrepresented in a given occupation if it accounts for *more* than its overall share of total employment and is underrepresented in a given occupation if it accounts for *less* than its overall share of total employment.
- Black workers are overrepresented in the following occupation groups: healthcare support, protective services, community and social services, transportation and material moving, personal care and services, building and grounds cleaning and maintenance,

[3] Seasonal adjustment is a statistical adjustment procedure that removes the effects of normal seasonal variations (e.g., increased hiring during certain holidays) from a data series and facilitates month-to-month comparisons.

office and administrative support, food preparation and serving, production, and healthcare practitioners.

- White workers are overrepresented in the management, business, financial, and professional occupations and underrepresented in most service occupations.
- While employment overall declined by 12.5% from May 2019 to May 2020, nine occupational groups experienced declines in employment of greater than 12.5%. Of these nine occupational groups with larger than average employment losses, Black workers were overrepresented in five.
- Of the three groups of occupations that did not see employment losses from May 2019 through May 2020 – business and financial operations, computer and mathematical, and life and social sciences – Black workers are underrepresented in all three.
- Of the three groups of occupations with the largest percentage decrease in employment – personal care and services, food preparation and serving, and building and grounds maintenance – Black workers are overrepresented in all three, with employment shares ranging from 13.9% to 16.1%.
- While the question asks specifically for disaggregation by race, **Table 1** also presents data by ethnicity with regard to Hispanic status. Similar to Black workers, Hispanic workers are overrepresented in the occupations experiencing the largest percentage decrease, notably food preparation, building and grounds maintenance, and personal care occupations.

Table 1. Occupation by Race, Ethnicity, and Change in Employment

May 2019 – May 2020

Occupation	Employment 2019	Share of Employment in 2019 (%)				*% Change May 2019-May 2020*
		White (of any ethnicity)	Black (of any ethnicity)	Asian (of any ethnicity)	Hispanic (of any race)	
Total, 16 years and over	157,538	77.7	12.3	6.5	17.6	*-12.5*
Management, Business, and Financial						
Management	18,985	83.6	7.8	6.1	10.7	*-1.4*
Business and financial operations	7,996	78.4	9.9	9.0	9.5	*3.8*
Professional and Related						
Computer and mathematical	5,352	65.7	8.7	23.1	7.8	*8.6*
Architecture and engineering	3,305	77.5	6.8	13.3	9.2	*-4.8*
Life, physical, and social science	1,485	76.9	6.3	14.4	9.5	*16.9*
Community and social service	2,717	72.9	20.1	3.6	13.0	*-0.8*
Legal	1,955	83.0	8.3	6.1	9.5	*-1.8*
Education, training, and library	9,455	81.7	10.2	5.3	11.0	*-13.5*
Arts, design, and entertainment	3,285	82.8	7.7	5.9	11.6	*-11.0*

Occupation	Employment 2019	Share of Employment in 2019 (%) White	Black (of any ethnicity)	Asian	Hispanic (of any race)	*% Change May 2019-May 2020*
Healthcare practitioners	9,684	75.3	12.5	9.6	9.0	*-1.4*
Service						
Healthcare support	3,758	64.2	26.7	5.1	19.1	*12.6*
Protective service	3,128	73.9	20.3	2.2	15.3	*-10.6*
Food preparation and serving	8,378	73.7	13.9	6.9	27.0	*-43.6*
Building and grounds maintenance	5,746	77.3	14.9	2.9	38.2	*-22.0*
Personal care and service	5,968	69.4	16.1	10.1	18.2	*-57.1*
Sales and Office						
Sales and related	15,582	79.8	11.2	5.4	16.7	*-19.4*
Office and administrative support	17,789	76.6	14.5	5.0	17.5	*-17.5*
Natural Resources and Maintenance						
Farming, fishing, and forestry	1,156	89.3	4.4	1.8	47.6	*-15.9*
Construction and extraction	8,325	87.1	7.3	1.6	36.4	*-15.4*
Installation, maintenance, and repair	4,862	84.0	9.1	3.3	20.3	*-10.8*
Production and Transportation						
Production	8,565	76.6	13.3	6.0	23.1	*-20.7*
Transportation and material moving	10,063	72.2	20.0	4.1	22.9	*-2.7*

Source: Prepared by CRS based on data from the Current Population Survey (CPS). Race composition data are from Bureau of Labor Statistics, U.S. Department of Labor, *Labor Force Statistics from the Current Population Survey*, Table 11. Employed persons by detailed occupation, sex, race, and Hispanic or Latino ethnicity, Washington, DC, January 22, 2020, https://www.bls.gov/cps/cpsaat11.htm. Occupational employment data are from Bureau of Labor Statistics, U.S. Department of Labor, *Labor Force Statistics from the Current Population Survey*, Table A-19. Employed persons by occupation, sex, and age, Washington, DC, June 5, 2020, https://www.bls.gov/web/empsit/cpseea19.htm.

Notes: Estimates for race groups do not sum to totals because data are not presented for all races. Estimates by race include workers of Hispanic and non-Hispanic ethnicity. Individuals of Hispanic or Latino ethnicity may be of any race. Data on share of employment by race and ethnicity are annual averages for 2019. Data on the change in employment by occupation are from May 2019 and May 2020 and are not seasonally adjusted. The changes in employment levels by occupation include both permanent and temporary employment changes.

Who is applying for unemployment benefits and who is receiving them, by racial group?

The U.S. Department of Labor (DOL), Employment and Training Administration (ETA), Office of Unemployment Insurance provides aggregated demographic information on regular Unemployment Compensation (UC) claimants each month.[4] The data are disaggregated by sex, ethnicity, race, age, industry, and occupation. The information is provided to the DOL by each state when it submits the ETA 203– Distribution of Characteristics of the Insured Unemployed Report. The ETA 203 Report contains information on continued regular UC claims filed during the week containing the 19th of the month, which would be attributed to unemployment from the prior week (containing the 12th of the month, just as the BLS *Employment Situation* reports employment statistics from the same week).[5] According to DOL, five states (California, Kentucky, Rhode Island, Utah, and Virginia) and the U.S. Virgin Islands reported generating information on a sample of UC claimants[6]; all other states reported generating the report on their full claimant population. **Table 2** below provides race and ethnicity breakdowns for regular UC beneficiaries who were reported being unemployed during the week of April 12, 2020 and were paid UC benefits paid the following week.[7] DOL does not publish the characteristics of claimants of any other UI benefit. In particular, it does not include information on the characteristics of individuals receiving benefits under the permanent law Extended Benefit (EB) payments. Additionally, it does not include information on individuals receiving one of the temporary Unemployment Insurance benefits created in Title II, Subtitle A, of the Coronavirus Aid, Relief, and Economic Security Act (CARES Act; P.L. 116-136).[8]

Table 2. ETA 203 – Distribution of Characteristics of the Insured Unemployed Report

April 2020

	Unemployment Compensation (UC) Claimants (In thousands)	Percent
Gender		
Male	8,175	47.1%
Female	8,972	51.7%

[4] Regular UC claimants only. The report does not include individuals receiving benefits under the permanent law Extended Benefit program.

[5] The ETA 203 Report is available at https://oui.doleta.gov/unemploy/chariu.asp.

[6] ETA provided guidance on sampling procedures in *UI Reports Handbook No. 401, 4th Edition*, ETA 203, "Characteristics of the Insured Unemployed," Washington, DC, https://oui.doleta.gov/dmstree/handbooks/401/4th/hb401_4.pdf. The most recent version (5th Edition) did not provide this guidance.

[7] Because 20% of beneficiaries have missing race data and 11% of beneficiaries have missing ethnicity data, it is difficult to ascertain if these number are disproportionate to the unemployed population. Using the underlying April data in **Table 7**, it appears that 74.4% of the unemployed were white (as compared to 58.4% of UC beneficiaries). Differences for both the Black (14.1% of all unemployed, 14.4% of UC beneficiaries) and Asian (6.2% of all unemployed, 58% of UC beneficiaries) race categories were much smaller in magnitude. While 22.8% of all unemployed were in the Hispanic category, they were 15.2% of all UC beneficiaries.

[8] For details of the temporary UI programs created in the CARES Act, see CRS In Focus IF11475, *Unemployment Insurance Provisions in the CARES Act*. For the week ending May 23, 2020, ETA reported over 19 million regular UC claims and over an additional 10 million receiving a benefit under a temporary CARES Act program. See Employment and Training Administration, *Unemployment Insurance Weekly Claims, Persons Claiming UI Benefits in All Programs (Unadjusted)*, June 11, 2020, p. 4, https://oui.doleta.gov/press/2020/061120.pdf.

	Unemployment Compensation (UC) Claimants (In thousands)	Percent
Information Not Available	200	1.2%
Ethnicity		
Hispanic or Latino	2,642	15.2%
Not Hispanic or Latino	12,782	73.7%
Information Not Available	1,923	11.1%
Race		
American Indian or Alaskan Native	169	1.0%
Asian	1,007	5.8%
Black or African American	2,478	14.3%
Native Hawaiian or Other Pacific Islander	106	0.6%
White	10,128	58.4%
Information Not Available	3,464	20.0%

Source: The ETA 203 Report is available at https://oui.doleta.gov/unemploy/chariu.asp.

Notes: The District of Columbia, Puerto Rico, and the Virgin Islands are considered to be states under federal UC law. The ETA 203 Report for April 2020 contains information on continued regular UC claims attributed to unemployment during the week of April 12-18, 2020.

What is the racial composition of workers in the following occupations, many of which are considered essential during the COVID-19 crisis: Health care; grocery, convenience, and drug stores; child care; public transit; trucking, warehouse, and postal service; building cleaning services; public safety; hazardous material; agriculture and food processing?

Data in **Table 3** show the racial composition of selected essential occupations.

- Overall, Black workers are overrepresented (i.e., comprise a larger share of employment than across all employment), in all selected occupational categories except farming, fishing, and forestry occupations and bakers.
- Among individual groups of essential occupations, Black workers make up more than one-third of postal service clerks and mail processors and more than one-quarter of workers in healthcare support, bus driver, and industrial truck and tractor occupations.
- Of the largest group of essential occupations – healthcare practitioners – Black workers comprise about the same share as in the overall labor force.
- Of the other occupational categories with at least 2 million employees, the share of Black workers ranges from 12.4% to 20.3%.

Table 3. Employment by Race and Ethnicity in Selected Essential Occupations

Annual Average 2019

Occupation	Employment (in thousands)	Shares of Employment (%)			
		White	Black	Asian	Hispanic
		(of any ethnicity)			(of any race)
Total, 16 years and over	157,538	77.7	12.3	6.5	17.6
Healthcare practitioners and technical	9,684	75.3	12.5	9.6	9.0
Healthcare support occupations	3,758	64.2	26.7	5.1	19.1
Cashiers	3,164	69.2	17.9	7.3	24.1
Retail salespersons	3,105	78.9	12.4	4.5	18.7
Protective service	3,128	73.9	20.3	2.2	15.3
Janitors and building cleaners	2,265	74.0	18.2	3.4	31.6
Childcare workers	1,193	76.0	17.4	3.3	24.6
Driver/sales workers and truck drivers	3,608	75.2	18.1	2.9	20.5
Bus drivers	546	67.2	27.0	3.1	15.0
Postal service mail carriers	331	72.7	19.6	5.5	14.4
Postal service clerks	96	47.4	35.8	13.0	6.7
Postal service mail sorters and processors	76	35.8	42.3	17.8	5.8
Laborers and material movers, hand	2,235	72.4	19.8	2.7	23.1
Packers and packagers, hand	628	69.2	19.0	7.7	41.5
Industrial truck and tractor operators	571	69.0	25.8	1.7	31.4
Refuse and recyclable material collectors	99	74.0	18.2	3.6	29.7
Farming, fishing, and forestry	1,156	89.3	4.4	1.8	47.6
Butchers and other meat processing workers	297	71.2	17.1	6.2	37.3
Bakers	228	74.0	11.7	9.6	30.7
Food processing workers, all other	147	72.1	18.1	7.0	38.8

Source: Prepared by CRS based on data from the Current Population Survey (CPS). Occupation and race composition data are from Bureau of Labor Statistics, U.S. Department of Labor, *Labor Force Statistics from the Current Population Survey*, Table 11.

Notes: Estimates for race groups do not sum to totals because data are not presented for all races. Estimates by race include workers of Hispanic and non-Hispanic ethnicity. Individuals of Hispanic or Latino ethnicity may be of any race. Data on share of occupational employment by race and ethnicity are annual averages for 2019.

What is the racial composition of those who can telework and those who must perform the jobs in person?

Data in **Table 4** show the share of workers, interviewed in 2017 and 2018, with access to telework.[9]

- Overall, 28.8% of workers are permitted to work from home at least some of the time. While a higher share of White (29.9%) and Asian (37.0%) workers have access to telework, only 19.7% of Black workers and 16.2% of Hispanic workers have such access.
- Worker access to telework also varies by earnings, with more than 60% of workers in the highest earnings quartile having access to telework and less than 10% of workers in the lowest earnings quartile having access to telework.
- The differences in worker access to telework is at least partly related to the racial composition of occupations and variation in access to telework by occupation. Workers in management, business, and professional occupations have the highest shares of access to telework, while these same occupations generally also have the lowest shares of Black workers.

Table 4. Access to Telework, by Race, Ethnicity, and Earnings

2017 – 2018 (Annual)

Characteristic	**Employment** (In thousands)	**Access to Telework** (In thousands)	**Share of Workers with Access to Telework** (%)
Race (workers are of any ethnicity)			
Total	144,295	41,571	28.8
White	115,129	34,390	29.9
Black	17,924	3,522	19.7
Asian	7,849	2,902	37.0
Ethnicity (workers are of any race)			
Hispanic or Latino	24,375	3,961	16.2
Occupation Group			
Management, business, and financial operations	22,754	13,679	60.1
Professional and related	40,284	17,108	42.5
Services	23,548	1,468	6.2
Sales and related	11,290	3,205	28.4
Office and administrative support	18,967	4,602	24.3
Farming, fishing, and forestry	n/a	n/a	n/a

[9] In the American Time Use Survey (ATUS), workers are asked if, as part of their job, they can work at home. Respondents are considered to have "workplace flexibility" (i.e., telework) if they answer "yes." See Bureau of Labor Statistics, U.S. Department of Labor, *Job Flexibilities and Work Schedules – 2017-2018, Data from the American Time Use Survey (ATUS)*, USDL-19-1691, Washington, DC, September 24, 2019, https://www.bls.gov/news.release/pdf/flex2.pdf.

Characteristic	Employment (In thousands)	Access to Telework (In thousands)	Share of Workers with Access to Telework (%)
Construction and extraction	5,853	469	8.0
Installation, maintenance, and repair	4,053	390	9.6
Production	8,560	374	4.4
Transportation and material moving	7,859	234	3.0
Usual Weekly Earnings			
Less than 25th percentile	25,200	2,314	9.2
25th to 50th percentile	26,521	5,337	20.1
50th to 75th percentile	27,193	10,148	37.3
Greater than 75th percentile	27,454	16,879	61.5

Source: Prepared by CRS based on data from Bureau of Labor Statistics, U.S. Department of Labor, *Job Flexibilities and Work Schedules – 2017-2018, Data from the American Time Use Survey (ATUS)*, USDL-19-1691, Washington, DC, September 24, 2019, https://www.bls.gov/news.release/pdf/flex2.pdf.

Notes: Estimates for race groups do not sum to totals because data are not presented for all races. Estimates by race include workers of Hispanic and non-Hispanic ethnicity. Individuals of Hispanic or Latino ethnicity may be of any race. Usual weekly earnings are for full-time wage and salary workers (single jobholders only). In the ATUS survey, workers are asked if, as part of their job, they can work at home. Respondents are considered to have "workplace flexibility" (i.e., telework) if they answer "yes."

Who is losing access to employer-provided healthcare by occupation and by racial group?

Data in **Table 5** show access to employer-provided healthcare by broad occupation groups.

- Overall, about 72% of workers had access to employer-provided health insurance in 2019.
- Workers in management, business, finance, and related occupations had the highest percentages of access to employer-provided health insurance. These occupations also have below average shares of Black workers.
- Service occupations have the least access to health insurance, 48%, while having a disproportionately high share of Black workers.
- The service occupations group experienced the largest loss of employment, both in percentage (-30.3%) and absolute terms (-8.3 million), from May 2019 to May 2020.

Table 5. Access to Employer-Provided Health Insurance by Race, Ethnicity, and Occupation

	Employment Share (%, 2019)					Employment (in thousands)		
Occupation Group	White	Black	Asian	Hispanic	Health Ins. Access (%)	May 2019	May 2020	% Change
	(of any ethnicity)			(of any race)				
Total, 16 years and over	77.7	12.3	6.5	17.6	72	157,152	137,461	-12.5
Management, Business, and Finance	82.1	8.4	7.0	10.4	94	26,534	26,592	0.2
Professional and Related	76.7	10.5	10.0	9.9	85	37,060	35,738	-3.6
Service	72.2	17.1	5.9	25.0	48	27,390	19,087	-30.3
Sales and Related	79.8	11.2	5.4	16.7	55	15,429	12,434	-19.4
Office and Administrative Support	76.6	14.5	5.0	17.5	79	17,568	14,497	-17.5
Natural resources, construction, and maintenance	86.2	7.7	2.2	31.9	74	14,355	12,362	-13.9
Production	76.6	13.3	6.0	23.1	81	8,660	6,868	-20.7
Transportation and Material Moving	72.2	20.0	4.1	22.9	73	10,156	9,883	-2.7

Source: Prepared by CRS based on data from the Current Population Survey (CPS) and the National Compensation Survey (NCS). Race composition data are from Bureau of Labor Statistics, U.S. Department of Labor, *Labor Force Statistics from the Current Population Survey*, Table 11. Employed persons by detailed occupation, sex, race, and Hispanic or Latino ethnicity, Washington, DC, January 22, 2020, https://www.bls.gov/cps/cpsaat11.htm. Occupational employment data are from Bureau of Labor Statistics, U.S. Department of Labor, *Labor Force Statistics from the Current Population Survey*, Table A-19. Employed persons by occupation, sex, and age, Washington, DC, June 5, 2020, https://www.bls.gov/web/empsit/cpseea19.htm. Healthcare data are from Bureau of Labor Statistics, U.S. Department of Labor, *National Compensation Survey: Employee Benefits in the United States, March 2019*, Bulletin 2791, Washington, DC, September 2019, https://www.bls.gov/ncs/ebs/benefits/.

Notes: Estimates for race groups do not sum to totals because data are not presented for all races. Estimates by race include workers of Hispanic and non-Hispanic ethnicity. Individuals of Hispanic or Latino ethnicity may be of any race. Data on share of employment by race and ethnicity are annual averages for 2019. Data on employment by occupation are from May 2019 and May 2020 and are not seasonally adjusted. As noted in the NCS benefit data, "healthcare" is a collective term medical, dental, vision, and outpatient drug coverage. If workers have access to at least one of these benefits, they are considered to have access to healthcare.

How have labor market outcomes varied by race since the onset of the COVID-19 pandemic?

The Department of Health and Human Services (HHS) declared a public health emergency for COVID-19 on January 31, 2020.[10] This section considers how labor market outcomes have varied by workers' race and Hispanic ethnicity over the early stages of the pandemic, and uses data for January 2020 as the baseline (i.e., pre-HHS declaration). **Table 6** provides recent BLS estimates of the labor force participation rate, employment-population ratio, and the unemployment rate. The labor force participation

[10] See https://www.hhs.gov/about/news/2020/01/31/secretary-azar-declares-public-health-emergency-us-2019-novel-coronavirus.html.

rate describes the share of the adult (16 years and older), non-institutionalized, civilian population that is in the labor force, i.e., that is employed or seeking employment. The employment-population ratio describes the share of that population that has a job.[11] The unemployment rate describes the share of the labor force that is unemployed.

All three indicators point to a sharp deterioration in labor market conditions since January 2020. Marked changes occurred across all groups shown in **Table 6** over the January to April 2020 period, with some recovery for certain groups between April and May 2020.[12] Notably, although the White (non-Hispanic) unemployment rate improved by 2.1 percentage points between April and May 2020, the Black unemployment rate and the Asian unemployment rate increased by 0.4 (16.2% to 16.6%) and 0.7 (14.2% to 14.9%) percentage points respectively. Hispanic and non-Hispanic workers' unemployment rates improved by 1.3 and 1.5 percentage points, respectively. However, Hispanic workers experienced a larger percentage point increase in their unemployment rate (from 4.3% to 18.9%) over the January to April 2020 period, when compared to non-Hispanic workers.

[11] The employment-population ratio is a summary indicator of labor market performance because it describes concurrently the proportion of the adult population *who want jobs* (i.e., the labor force participation rate) and the *success rate of this group in obtaining jobs* (i.e., the employment rate, or the complement of the unemployment rate). For more information, see CRS Report R44055, *An Overview of the Employment-Population Ratio*, by Sarah A. Donovan.

[12] Some studies have examined early-stage COVID-19 impacts on the labor market in greater detail. For example, Robert W. Fairlie, Kenneth Couch, and Huanan Xu study the impacts on unemployment and describe their main findings this way: "*First, we find that blacks had a somewhat favorable industry distribution that partially protected them from becoming unemployed in April 2020 relative to Whites. Second, we find that a less favorable occupational distribution and lower skills contributed to why Latinx experienced much higher unemployment rates than Whites. Finally, we find that occupational and educational differences contribute to why blacks have higher unemployment rates in the early stages of the pandemic.*" In other words, high shares of Black workers in industries like health and education services, which were not as hard hit by COVID-19 as others (like leisure and hospitality), provided them some protection from job loss. But this protection was countered by Black workers' concentration in service occupations, which had very high rates of job loss. Latinx workers were concentrated both in industries and occupations that had large increases in unemployment. Robert W. Fairlie, Kenneth Couch, and Huanan Xu, The Impacts of COVID-19 on Minority Unemployment: First Evidence from April 2020 CPS Microdata, NBER Working Paper No. 27246, May 2020, https://www.nber.org/papers/w27246.

Table 6. Selected Labor Market Indicators by Race and Hispanic Ethnicity

	Jan. 2020	Feb. 2020	Mar. 2020	Apr. 2020	May 2020	*Change: Jan. to April 2020*	*Change: April to May 2020*
All Workers (any race or ethnicity)							
Labor Force Participation Rate	63.4	63.4	62.7	60.2	60.8	-3.2	0.6
Employment-Population Ratio	61.2	61.1	60.0	51.3	52.8	-9.9	1.5
Unemployment Rate	3.6	3.5	4.4	14.7	13.3	11.1	-1.4
White, Not Hispanic							
Labor Force Participation Rate	61.8	62.0	61.6	59.4	60.2	-2.4	0.8
Employment-Population Ratio	59.9	60.2	59.4	51.8	53.7	-8.1	1.9
Unemployment Rate	3.1	3.0	3.5	12.8	10.7	9.7	-2.1
Black, Not Hispanic							
Labor Force Participation Rate	62.3	62.3	61.2	58.0	59.1	-4.3	1.1
Employment-Population Ratio	58.1	58.4	56.8	48.6	49.3	-9.5	0.7
Unemployment Rate	6.6	6.2	7.1	16.2	16.6	9.6	0.4
Asian, Not Hispanic							
Labor Force Participation Rate	63.2	64.2	63.6	60.1	60.4	-3.1	0.3
Employment-Population Ratio	61.2	62.6	61.0	51.5	51.3	-9.7	-0.2
Unemployment Rate	3.2	2.5	4.1	14.2	14.9	11.0	0.7
Hispanic (of any race)							
Labor Force Participation Rate	67.8	68.1	67.1	63.3	64.1	-4.5	0.8
Employment-Population Ratio	64.9	65.1	63.0	51.3	52.8	-13.6	1.5
Unemployment Rate	4.3	4.4	6.0	18.9	17.6	14.6	-1.3
Not Hispanic (of any race)							
Labor Force Participation Rate	62.1	62.3	61.7	59.3	60.1	-2.8	0.8
Employment-Population Ratio	59.8	60.1	59.1	51.3	52.8	-8.5	1.5
Unemployment Rate	3.7	3.6	4.2	13.6	12.1	9.9	-1.5

Source: CRS calculations using data from the Bureau of Labor Statistics, Current Population Survey Program.

Notes: All data are seasonally adjusted, with the exception of data for "Not Hispanic" workers. People of Hispanic origin may be of any race.

What is the percentage increase in unemployment by race since the beginning of the year?

Table 7 provides monthly data on the number of unemployed workers by race and Hispanic ethnicity. For each group, the number of unemployed workers more than doubled between January 2020 and May 2020. The number of total unemployed (i.e., all unemployed workers) more than tripled (i.e., increased by 256%) over that period. By racial group, the increase ranged from 137% for non-Hispanic Black workers to 354% for non-Hispanic Asian workers. Cumulative growth in the number of unemployed was higher for Hispanic workers (290%) than it was for non-Hispanic workers (213%).

Table 7. Unemployed Workers by Race and Hispanic Ethnicity

In thousands

	Jan. 2020	Feb. 2020	Mar. 2020	Apr. 2020	May 2020	% Change: Jan. to May 2020
All workers (any race or ethnicity)	5,892	5,787	7,140	23,078	20,985	256%
White, Non-Hispanic	3,123	3,037	3,472	12,308	1,0465	235%
Black, Non-Hispanic	1,290	1,201	1,348	2,936	3,057	137%
Asian, Non-Hispanic	316	253	416	1,356	1,434	354%
Hispanic	1,275	1,322	1,771	5,263	4,977	290%
Not Hispanic	4,998	4,779	5,529	17,378	15,662	213%

Source: CRS calculation using data from the Bureau of Labor Statistics, Current Population Survey Program.

Notes: All data are seasonally adjusted by BLS, with the exception of data for "Not Hispanic" workers. The number of unemployed workers in each racial group do not sum to the total number of unemployed workers in a given month, because monthly data on other groups (e.g., Native American, Native Alaska, Native Hawaiian) are not available. People of Hispanic origin may be of any race.

What share of the working age population is employed (employment to population ratio) by racial group?

Table 8 provides recent BLS estimates of the employment-population ratio for persons 25 to 54 years old (i.e., the "prime-age" or "working age" population). Overall, the prime-age employment-population ratio fell by nearly 11 percentage points over the January to April 2020 period, and improved by 1.7 points between April and May 2020.[13] A similar pattern of a sharp decline over the first four months followed by a partial improvement between April and May is seen for most groups of prime-age workers. The exception is Asian workers, for whom the prime-age employment-population ratio continued to decline through May 2020.

Table 8. Prime-Age Employment-Population Ratio by Race and Hispanic Ethnicity

	Jan. 2020	Feb. 2020	Mar. 2020	Apr. 2020	May 2020	*Change: Jan. to April 2020*	*Change: April to May 2020*
All	80.6	80.5	79.6	69.7	71.4	*-10.9*	*1.7*
White	81.5	81.5	80.6	71.1	73.2	*-10.4*	*2.1*
Black	75.9	75.9	75.4	64.4	65.7	*-11.5*	*1.3*
Asian	77.0	78.2	77.6	68.9	68.2	*-8.1*	*-0.7*
Hispanic	77.6	78.0	75.9	63.9	65.6	*-13.7*	*1.7*
Not Hispanic	81.3	81.2	80.6	71.1	72.8	*-10.2*	*1.7*

Source: CRS calculation using data from the Bureau of Labor Statistics, Current Population Survey Program.

Notes: "Prime Age" refers to persons 25-54 years old. All data are seasonally adjusted, with the exception of data for Hispanic and Not Hispanic workers. Estimates by race include workers of Hispanic and non-Hispanic ethnicity. People of Hispanic origin may be of any race.

[13] For perspective, the lowest value of the prime-age employment-population ratio during the Great Recession (December 2007-June 2009) and its recovery was 74.8 in December 2009.

What is the percentage loss of employment by the self-employed?

Figure 1 shows that between January 2020 and May 2020, the number of unincorporated self-employed workers fell by approximately 8.2% from 9.46 million (January 2020) to 8.68 million (May 2020).[14] Some self-employed workers may have transitioned from self-employment to wage and salary (i.e., employee status) over this period; data on these transitions are not available.

Figure 1. Employed Self-Employed Workers

In thousands

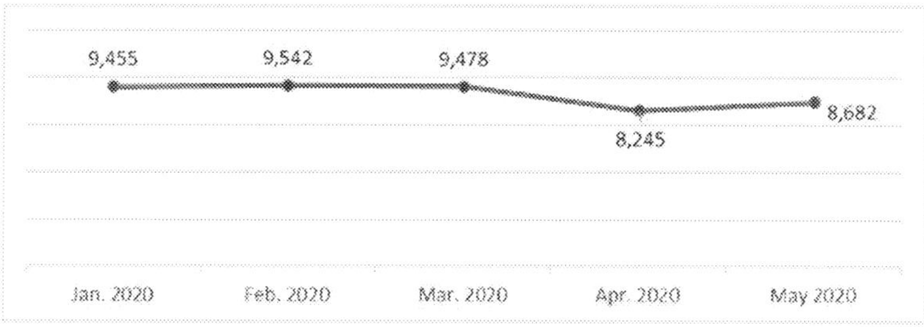

Source: Figure created by CRS using data from the BLS CPS program (employment-population ratios).

Notes: Self-employed refers to unincorporated self-employed workers. Data are seasonally-adjusted.

[14] Information on BLS self-employment concepts, including why most BLS self-employment statistics do not include incorporated self-employed workers, is at https://www.bls.gov/cps/definitions.htm#selfemployed.

At the state level, is there a relationship between the degree of job loss since January 2020 and the share of people of color in the labor force?

Table 9 presents state-level data on the non-White share of the labor force in 2019 and recent changes in unemployment.[15] In 2019, the share of non-White workers ranged from 4.8% in Maine to 77.5% in Hawaii. The number of unemployed workers doubled in nearly all states between January and April 2020, with the increase in unemployment over this period ranging from 95% in Connecticut to 686% in Hawaii.

Table 9. State Labor Force Racial Composition in 2019 and Recent Unemployment Data

	Non-White Share of the Labor Force, 2019	Monthly Unemployment			Percentage Point Change in the Unemployment Rate, Jan.-April 2020
		January 2020	April 2020	% Change	
Alabama	28.6%	61,069	283,787	365%	10.2
Alaska	34.5%	20,931	43,683	109%	6.9
Arizona	16.5%	162,073	445,461	175%	8.1
Arkansas	18.1%	48,068	133,962	179%	6.7
California	27.6%	753,269	2,885,334	283%	11.6
Colorado	11.0%	79,407	347,832	338%	8.8
Connecticut	19.1%	72,224	140,743	95%	4.2
Delaware	29.2%	21,577	44,874	108%	5.9
District of Columbia	44.4%	19,398	66,665	244%	10.3
Florida	22.8%	291,383	1,217,964	318%	10.1
Georgia	39.8%	159,611	581,820	265%	8.8
Hawaii	77.5%	17,792	139,892	686%	19.6
Idaho	5.1%	24,748	102,975	316%	8.7
Illinois	21.8%	227,789	1,004,365	341%	12.9
Indiana	14.3%	106,776	545,909	411%	13.8
Iowa	8.9%	49,726	175,306	253%	7.4
Kansas	12.2%	46,871	168,317	259%	8.1
Kentucky	11.7%	90,232	318,274	253%	11.1
Louisiana	34.3%	111,315	281,572	153%	9.2
Maine	4.8%	21,208	70,753	234%	7.5
Maryland	40.1%	109,061	304,444	179%	6.6
Massachusetts	19.6%	106,249	515,658	385%	12.3
Michigan	19.5%	187,209	1,048,250	460%	18.9
Minnesota	12.9%	98,778	249,453	153%	4.9
Mississippi	38.8%	69,795	183,012	162%	9.9

[15] Non-White workers may be Black or African-American, Asian, Native American or Alaska Native, Native Hawaiian or other Pacific Islander, or another non-White race. Estimates by race include workers of Hispanic and non-Hispanic ethnicity.

	Non-White Share of the Labor Force, 2019	Monthly Unemployment			Percentage Point Change in the Unemployment Rate, Jan.-April 2020
		January 2020	April 2020	% Change	
Missouri	14.9%	110,281	292,690	165%	6.2
Montana	6.9%	18,678	58,919	215%	7.8
Nebraska	9.2%	30,613	87,550	186%	5.4
Nevada	27.3%	56,299	400,520	611%	24.6
New Hampshire	5.9%	19,940	117,568	490%	13.7
New Jersey	26.5%	172,261	685,545	298%	11.5
New Mexico	19.5%	45,670	104,408	129%	6.5
New York	27.8%	364,511	1,320,297	262%	10.7
North Carolina	29.6%	184,891	573,118	210%	8.6
North Dakota	11.1%	9,335	34,802	273%	6.2
Ohio	17.6%	238,438	957,366	302%	12.7
Oklahoma	24.7%	60,607	242,677	300%	10.4
Oregon	14.1%	69,814	300,420	330%	10.9
Pennsylvania	16.9%	307,029	975,740	218%	10.4
Rhode Island	15.0%	18,946	90,310	377%	13.6
South Carolina	29.1%	56,599	288,022	409%	9.7
South Dakota	11.9%	15,811	48,081	204%	6.8
Tennessee	21.2%	111,930	471,212	321%	11.4
Texas	22.2%	494,392	1,656,638	235%	9.3
Utah	7.8%	40,039	155,810	289%	7.2
Vermont	4.9%	8,305	54,490	556%	13.2
Virginia	28.3%	118,315	453,923	284%	7.9
Washington	21.1%	155,468	610,721	293%	11.5
West Virginia	6.4%	40,537	117,134	189%	10.2
Wisconsin	10.3%	109,603	437,359	299%	10.6
Wyoming	6.8%	10,739	27,358	155%	5.5

Source: CRS calculations using BLS Local Area Unemployment Statistics (LAUS) program data.

Notes: Share "non-White" is a residual estimate, i.e., it is 100% minus the share of the state labor force that reports "White" as their race. Estimates by race include workers of Hispanic and non-Hispanic ethnicity. State unemployment data for April 2020 are preliminary.

Despite Hawaii having both the highest labor force share of non-White workers in 2019 and the highest percentage increase in the number of unemployed workers between January and April 2020, scatter plot analysis of these variables do not reveal a clear relationship. **Figure 2** plots the share of non-White workers against the percentage increase in unemployment (top figure) and the percentage point increase in the unemployment rate (bottom panel); Hawaii is omitted from both figures because it is an outlier. The plots show a small negative correlation between the non-White share and the percentage increase in the number of unemployed workers, and a small positive correlation between the non-White share and the percentage point increase in the unemployment rate. In terms of magnitudes, the top figure trend line formula predicts that a 10 percentage point increase in the non-White share is associated with about a 16 percentage point reduction in unemployment growth, and the bottom figure trend line predicts that a 10 percentage point increase in the non-White share is associated with about a 0.3 point increase in the change in unemployment rate. The R^2 (goodness of fit) statistic is low in both cases, indicating that other factors are important determinants to the change in unemployment. Scatter plot analysis is a basic analytic tool and does not rule out a relationship between labor force composition and labor market outcomes. A more sophisticated analysis of these relationships may produce different findings.

Figure 2. Scatter Plots of the Share of Non-White Workers in the 2019 State Labor Force and the Change in State Unemployment Level and Rate between January and April 2020

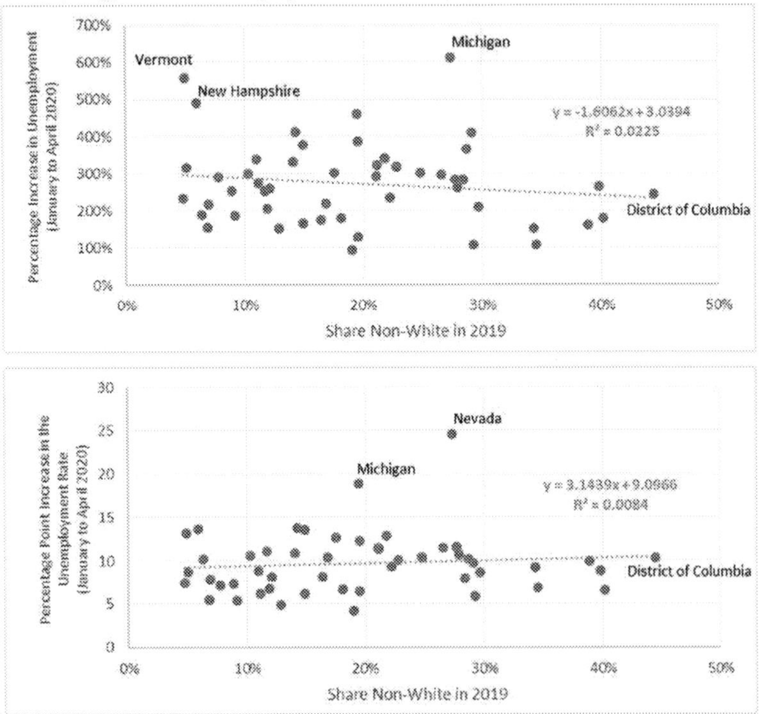

Source: Figure created by CRS using data from the BLS LAUS program.

Notes: Data for Hawaii are omitted because it is an outlier. The dotted line is a linear regression trend line fitted to the state data (without Hawaii). The trend line formula and R^2 (goodness of fit) statistic are shown in light blue.

Following the 2007-2009 recession, how long did it take for labor-market metrics to recover their pre-recession levels across racial groups?

Figure 3 shows the seasonally-adjusted monthly unemployment rates for Black, White, and Asian workers over the January 2007 to December 2019 period.[16] At the start of the 2007-2009 recession in December 2007, Asian workers' unemployment rate was 3.7%, White workers' was 4.4%, and Black workers' was 9.0%. Rates rose considerably for all groups, but the increase was particularly large for Black workers whose unemployment rate reached 16.8% in March 2010. White workers' unemployment returned to prerecession rates in August 2015. Black and Asians workers' rates have more fluctuation than White workers', making the exact monthly of recovery hard to identify. Black workers' unemployment rate returned to 9.0% in October 2015 and fluctuated around that rate before trending downward. Similarly, Asian workers' unemployment rate reached 3.9% in June 2015 with some fluctuation thereafter.

Figure 3. Monthly Unemployment Rate for Selected Racial Groups

Seasonally Adjusted Data, January 2007 to December 2019

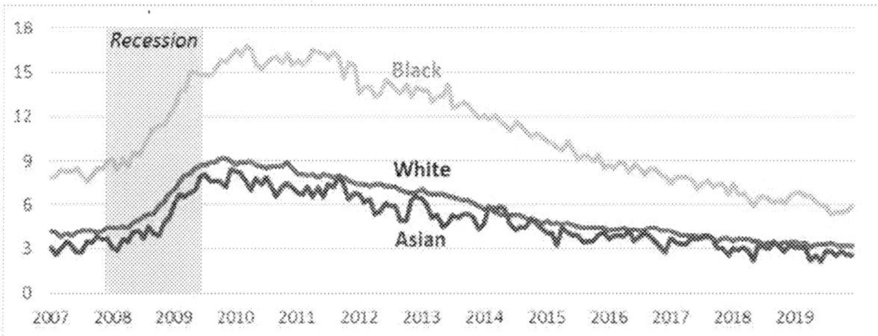

Source: Figure created by CRS using data from the BLS-CPS program (unemployment rate) and the National Bureau of Economic Research (NBER) (recession).

Notes: Unemployment rates are for the adult (age 16 years and older) non-institutionalized civilian population. Estimates by race include workers of Hispanic and non-Hispanic ethnicity.

The employment-population ratio for White, Black, and Asian workers declined over the Great Recession and early years of the expansion (**Figure 4**).[17] Black workers experienced particularly sharp losses as a share of their adult population following the onset of the recession, falling from 57.8 in December 2007 to 51.0 in July 2011. Black workers' employment-population ratio returned to prerecession rate around September 2017. White workers' ratios declined from 63.5 (December 2007) to 59.0 (November 2010), and Asian workers' ratios fell from 64.2 (December 2007) to 59.0 (February 2012). Ratios for White and Asian workers did not return to their prerecession rates, despite lower unemployment rates. This trend of simultaneous drops in the employed share of the population and the unemployed share of the labor force is driven by declining labor force participation rates.[18]

---

[16] Analysis of labor market patterns since the 2007-2009 recession for Hispanic and non-Hispanic workers is in CRS Report R45330, *Labor Market Patterns Since 2007*, by Sarah A. Donovan and Marc Labonte.

[17] Ibid.

[18] For more information, see CRS Report R44055, *An Overview of the Employment-Population Ratio*, by Sarah A. Donovan.

Figure 4. Employment-Population Ratio for Selected Racial Groups
Seasonally Adjusted Data, January 2007 to December 2019

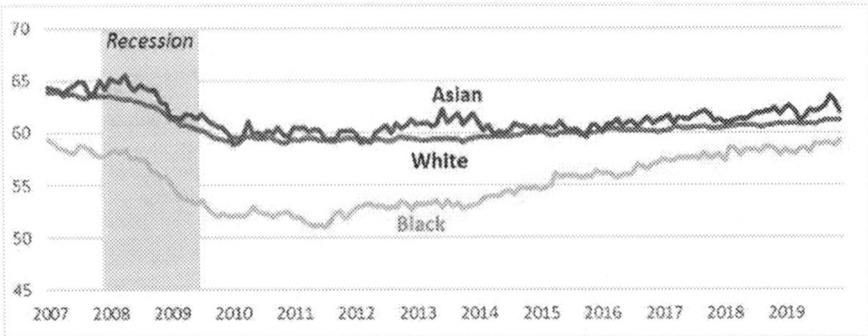

Source: Figure created by CRS using data from the BLS-CPS program (employment-population ratios) and NBER (recession).

Notes: Employment-population ratios are for the adult (age 16 years and older) non-institutionalized civilian population. Estimates by race include workers of Hispanic and non-Hispanic ethnicity.

In the states that have reopened (or plan to reopen), what percentage of the currently unemployed population are people of color and what percentage are women?

This question is challenging to answer for several reasons. According to analysis by the National Governors Association, all states had allowed some businesses to reopen to some degree by early June 2020. Some business openings are accompanied by restrictions, which can vary across business type.[19] For this reason it is difficult to separate states into a few well-defined groups based on opening status. It is similarly difficult to create a timeline of state openings, as states did not reopen all types of businesses at once, some counties were permitted to open certain businesses before others within the same state, and, as noted, reopenings in most states were not unconditional. Further, BLS state-level demographic data are available only as annual averages and the most recent data are for 2019.

Some insights on the demographic composition of unemployment across states can be gleaned from regular state UC claims data, which are presented in **Table 10**.[20] These data indicate, for example, that although women tend to make up less than half of the labor force in each state, they represent more than half of regular UC claimants in April 2020 in most states.[21] However, it should be stressed that while approximately 17 million unemployed persons claimed regular UC for unemployment during the week of April 12-18th, 2020, over 23 million persons were estimated to be unemployed during the period. Additionally, the permanent law EB program and the temporary UI programs created in the CARES Act cover many unemployed workers who would not typically be insured or otherwise eligible for regular UC

[19] See https://www.nga.org/coronavirus-business-reopenings/.

[20] A discussion of the unemployment compensation claim data is in the "Who is applying for unemployment benefits and who is receiving them, by racial group?" section of this memorandum.

[21] Table 10 provides data only on regular unemployment compensation claimants. It does not include the permanent law Extended Benefit program nor does it include any of the temporary benefits authorized under the CARES Act.

benefits, as well as some insured unemployed workers have exhausted regular UC benefits. While EB was not active in most states in April and the temporary UI programs created under the CARES Act had just begun to be offered in a handful of states those beneficiaries, approximately 1.2 million of those beneficiaries are not included in Table 10 because they did not receive a regular UC benefit.[22]

[22] For details of the temporary UI programs created in the CARES Act, see CRS In Focus IF11475, *Unemployment Insurance Provisions in the CARES Act*. For the week ending April 18, 2020, see Employment and Training Administration, *Unemployment Insurance Weekly Claims, Persons Claiming UI Benefits in All Programs (Unadjusted)*, May 7, 2020, p. 4, https://oui.doleta.gov/press/2020/050720.pdf.

Table 10. Selected Characteristics of Unemployment Compensation Claimants, April 2020

	Total Claims in April 2020	% Non-White	% Female	% Hispanic
Alabama	173,855	45%	59%	4%
Alaska	42,551	40%	50%	6%
Arizona	198,435	--	56%	--
Arkansas	109,159	34%	58%	6%
California	1,886,140	--	51%	45%
Colorado	219,166	--	55%	26%
Connecticut (March 2020)	44,015	--	42%	38%
Delaware	44,977	44%	53%	17%
District of Columbia	57,688	--	53%	17%
Florida	556,966	27%	59%	34%
Georgia	758,856	--	--	--
Hawaii	68,479	--	56%	--
Idaho	61,568	--	57%	--
Illinois	682,580	--	51%	25%
Indiana	254,166	19%	50%	22%
Iowa	174,152	--	57%	10%
Kansas	119,962	24%	52%	--
Kentucky	190,030	15%	49%	--
Louisiana	294,701	52%	56%	8%
Maine	74,123	9%	55%	--
Maryland	224,232	--	56%	14%
Massachusetts	498,570	--	51%	19%
Michigan	992,005	--	40%	--
Minnesota	410,848	24%	53%	14%
Mississippi	164,081	53%	57%	4%
Missouri	261,645	--	55%	--
Montana	54,202	10%	56%	10%
Nebraska	76,795	--	60%	13%
Nevada	274,850	--	51%	--
New Hampshire	107,461	10%	59%	10%
New Jersey	621,753	--	55%	32%
New Mexico	80,633	--	54%	57%
New York	1,614,107	--	48%	--
North Carolina	490,296	38%	59%	13%
North Dakota	35,167	20%	48%	8%
Ohio	765,006	22%	52%	10%

	Total Claims in April 2020	% Non-White	% Female	% Hispanic
Oklahoma	134,550	--	53%	10%
Oregon	284,486	--	54%	15%
Pennsylvania	915,154	--	47%	10%
Rhode Island	96,663	--	57%	--
South Carolina	245,951	46%	55%	12%
South Dakota	22,467	18%	60%	7%
Tennessee	336,096	--	52%	5%
Texas	954,490	--	54%	--
Utah	106,094	--	54%	22%
Vermont	69,914	--	--	--
Virginia	411,987	45%	58%	9%
Washington	542,596	--	48%	--
Wisconsin	320,952	--	56%	--
West Virginia	146,566	--	52%	--
Wyoming	16,207	--	49%	17%

Source: CRS calculations using Department of Labor, Characteristics of the Unemployment Insurance Claimants data https://oui.doleta.gov/unemploy/chariu.asp.

Notes: Claimant data are reported to the Department of Labor by state agencies and are based on a sample or on the universe of those who file a continued claim in the week containing the 19th of the month, which reflects unemployment during the week containing the 12th. The ETA 203 Report for April 2020 contains information on continued regular UC claims attributed to unemployment during the week of April 12-18, 2020. A double dash (--) indicates a share is not reported because 10% or more claims were missing data on the characteristics of interest (e.g., the share of non-White claimants is not provided in the table if 10% or more claims for a state did not contain data on the claimant's race). Share "non-White" is a residual estimate, i.e., it is 100% minus the share of the state labor force that reports "White" as their race. Estimates by race include workers of Hispanic and non-Hispanic ethnicity. People of Hispanic origin may be of any race.

[Questions submitted for the record and their responses follow:]

COMMITTEE ON
EDUCATION AND LABOR
U.S. HOUSE OF REPRESENTATIVES
2176 RAYBURN HOUSE OFFICE BUILDING
WASHINGTON, DC 20515-6100

July 8, 2020

Mr. John B. King, Jr.
President and CEO
The Education Trust
1250 H Street NW, Suite 700
Washington, D.C. 20005

Dear Mr. King:

I would like to thank you for testifying remotely at the June 22, 2020 Full Committee hearing entitled *"Inequities Exposed: How COVID-19 Widened Racial Inequities in Education, Health, and the Workforce."*

Please find enclosed additional questions submitted by Committee Members following the hearing. Please provide a written response no later than Wednesday, July 22, 2019, for inclusion in the official hearing record. Your responses should be sent to Ijeoma Egekeze of the Committee staff. She can be contacted at 202-225-3725 should you have any questions.

I appreciate your time and continued contribution to the work of the Committee.

Sincerely,

ROBERT C. "BOBBY" SCOTT
Chairman

Committee on Education and Labor
"Inequities Exposed: How COVID-19 Widened Racial Inequities in Education, Health, and the Workforce"
Monday, June 22, 2020 12:00 p.m.

Representative Gregorio Kilili Camacho Sablan (D-MP)

- Secretary King, can you speak to your concerns regarding life outcomes for Black students and students with disabilities, such as educational, career, socio-emotional and health outcomes, due to the combination of the COVID-19 pandemic and the possibility of gaping holes in state education budgets for several years?

- Secretary King, what is the impact of a lack of quality early learning on student outcomes later in life?

Representative Joseph Morelle (D-NY)

- Secretary King, given racial inequities in internet services and educational technology, what actions need to be taken to prevent further deepening of the academic achievement gap, particularly as we head into the summer months?

Representative Haley Stevens (D-MI)

- Secretary King, last month I co-introduced the Child Care is Essential Act with many of my colleagues here on this Committee to ensure all providers survive the pandemic and continue providing services to our nation's children. The bill would help child care providers who serve historically underserved populations and ensure those providers receive funding as swiftly as possible. How is COVID-19 exacerbating racial inequity in access to quality early childhood education, including child care? What else should we be considering as we look toward economic recovery?

U.S. House Committee on Education and Labor
Hearing: "Inequities Exposed: How COVID-19 Widened Racial Inequities in Education, Health, and the Workforce"
Questions for the Record
June 22, 2020

Responses of John B. King Jr., President and CEO, The Education Trust

The responses of John B. King Jr. are denoted in text that is not bolded.

Representative Gregorio Kilili Camacho Sablan (D-MP)

Secretary King, can you speak to your concerns regarding life outcomes for Black students and students with disabilities, such as educational, career, socio-emotional and health outcomes, due to the combination of the COVID-19 pandemic and the possibility of gaping holes in state education budgets for several years?

The long-term effects of this crisis could be incredibly detrimental for low-income students and students of color, including Black students, who are at greater risk of learning loss, thanks to the digital divide and racial and socioeconomic inequities that also mean their parents are more likely to be frontline workers with less time and fewer resources to devote to the academic success of their children. Students with disabilities are also at greater risk for lasting negative impacts from the pandemic and related educational spending cuts, which could undermine critical services that they need to receive the free and appropriate education their schools must provide to them under law.

The inequities within our system that impact Black students are very likely to be exacerbated by the pandemic and looming budget cuts. Before the pandemic, 79% of White households had broadband access, while only 66% of Black families had broadband service at home. That has impacted, and will continue to impact, Black students' ability to participate in online learning, as schools opt to continue distance learning or implement hybrid learning plans this fall amid the ongoing pandemic. Students of color are also at higher risk of losing their teachers to state and local education budget cuts, as we learned during the last downturn. While funding cuts to education were widespread following the Great Recession, an analysis of layoffs in Los Angeles found that Black elementary students were 72% more likely to have their teacher laid off. Ed Trust's California poll revealed that Black parents were less likely than parents of all other racial groups to have been contacted by their child's teacher. Research shows that teachers are the single greatest in-school factor influencing student success, so preventing further disruption for Black students will be predicated on Congress providing federal aid to states and districts, so they can keep teachers in the classroom.

At the collegiate level, a recent poll by The Education Trust and the Global Strategy Group found that roughly three-quarters of the undergraduate students surveyed said they are worried about being able to stay on track and graduate, and those shares were higher among Black students. Another survey showed that 24% of Black students have canceled or delayed their education plans due to the pandemic. Two-thirds of Black students rely on Pell Grants every year; if state budget cuts produce tuition hikes, the Pell Grant will cover even less of those students' college costs going forward.

Many students with disabilities face serious challenges as well. Before the pandemic, they were already twice as likely to live in poverty, more likely to experience homelessness, more likely to experience anxiety and depression, and less likely to graduate than their peers without disabilities. All of these disparities may become worse during this crisis. Distance learning has been particularly challenging for many students with disabilities. Only 20% of parents of children with disabilities reported that their children were receiving special education services guaranteed to them under IDEA, while 39% said their children were receiving no support at all, putting them at greater risk of falling behind during the pandemic. Parents were also twice as likely to report having increased concerns about the mental health of their children with disabilities; and those parents reported significantly higher stress, anxiety, and depression levels during the pandemic compared to parents of children without disabilities. Even a temporary loss of special education services or individualized instruction could impact some students with disabilities into adulthood, as employment training and work experiences in high school are critical factors in successful postsecondary transitions, and have become much more difficult to provide during the pandemic. We need robust supports to ensure these risks don't increase and to uphold IDEA and Section 504 [of the Rehabilitation Act of 1973] to protect students' rights to a free and appropriate education.

In response to these challenges, and in addition to state and local stabilization dollars, Congress should allocate dedicated funds to help schools facilitate expanded learning time, via summer school (online or in-person, based on the most recent public health guidance available), extended day or year-long initiatives, intensive tutoring, or other evidence-based approaches that support students in completing unfinished learning and accelerating new learning. Congress should also should allocate at least $4 billion to the Federal Communications Commission's E-Rate program to provide hotspots and devices for students who need them, and create a separate $1 billion program to provide home internet access to low-income college students. This funding should be put toward closing the equity gaps we know have been exacerbated by COVID-19 and prioritize students from low-income backgrounds and students of color, including Black students, students with disabilities, English learners, and students experiencing homelessness or in foster care, who have been most directly impacted. In particular, the National Center for Learning Disabilities has provided comprehensive policy guidance to educators, schools, districts, and states on how best to serve students with disabilities during the pandemic.

Secretary King, what is the impact of a lack of quality early learning on student outcomes later in life?

In order to understand how a lack of quality in early learning can impact student outcomes later in life, it's important to recognize the racial inequities in our early childhood education systems, which may manifest before students of color even enter kindergarten. This is especially important given that more than half of babies in the U.S. are children of color and 42% of babies in the U.S. are from low-income families. Young children of color face many barriers to accessing high-quality early care and education, while disproportionately living in poverty. Infant care can consume up to 116% of a low-income family's total income, yet few families receive financial child care assistance: For instance, only 7% of eligible infants and toddlers are served by Early Head Start programs. Child care subsidies through the Child Care and Development Block Grant (CCDBG) serve a very small portion of potentially eligible children of color: only 15% of Black children and 6% of Latino children. In fact, accessing any type of child care is challenging for many families of color: 57% of Latino families and 60% of American Indian and Alaska Native families live in child care deserts.

Those inequities are preventing millions of young children ages zero to 5 from obtaining tools for upward mobility and becoming a part of our highly educated, skilled workforce later in life. Research on comprehensive, high-quality, birth-to-5 early childhood programs for disadvantaged children found that they yielded a 13% return on investment per child annually, through better education, economic, health, and social outcomes. However, when states do fund high-quality preschool programs, access is often lower for Black and Latino children, who are underrepresented in several such programs. Compared to early learning programs attended by White children, programs attended by Black children are, on average, lower quality, and therefore aren't associated with the many positive outcomes linked to high-quality early learning opportunities. Young children of color who do have access to early childhood education are pushed out of the classroom at alarming rates: Black children, and especially Black boys, are disproportionately suspended and expelled from early learning settings, even though such practices are associated with negative educational and life outcomes. It is not enough to provide access to early childhood education; stakeholders must be vigilant in assessing inequities and proactive in enacting policies that provide equitable access.

Congress should make significant investments in the early childhood education system by passing the Child Care for Working Families Act (H.R. 1364), which would subsidize child care for families within 150% of the poverty line, ensuring they spend less than 7% of their income on child care. The bill would also fund pre-K expansion. While Congress may be unlikely to adopt the bill before the end of this term, it should be a priority for a new Congress in 2021.

Representative Joseph Morelle (D-NY)

Secretary King, given racial inequities in internet services and educational technology, what actions need to be taken to prevent further deepening of the academic achievement gap, particularly as we head into the summer months?

It is virtually certain that distance education or hybrid models (that combine in-person and online learning) will continue through the summer and into the beginning of next year and could be used intermittently until the virus is brought under control. The results of recent parent surveys are alarming. For example, a poll of California parents found that 38% of low-income families and 29% of families of color are concerned about access to distance learning because they lack reliable internet at home. Before the pandemic, 79% of White households had broadband access, while only 66% of Black families and 61% of Hispanic families had broadband service at home. More than one-third of all households with school-age children and incomes of less than $30,000 annually lack high-speed internet access. The lack of equitable broadband access is not only an online learning issue, but also an emergency preparedness issue in the event of further widespread closures.

The pandemic also has had detrimental effects on college students who were forced to vacate campuses and return home to learn remotely, and especially on those who were working while enrolled and have lost income that is essential to continuing their education. A recent poll by The Education Trust and the Global Strategy Group found that roughly three-quarters of the undergraduate students surveyed said they are worried about being able to stay on track and graduate, and those shares were higher among Black and Latino students. Another survey showed that 32% of Latino students, 24% of Black students, and 21% of Asian American students have canceled or delayed their education plans in light of the pandemic. Many college students are also being impacted by the digital divide, as they return to homes that may not have reliable broadband access.

Any upcoming Congressional COVID response legislation must contain funding to expand emergency broadband access for K-12 students and provide for higher education emergency broadband access as well. Congress should address the lack of emergency K-12 online learning access by ensuring that any upcoming COVID response legislation includes the Emergency Educational Connections Act. That bill allocates $4 billion through an Emergency Connectivity Fund via the Federal Communications Commission's federal E-Rate program to expand access to broadband services, Wi-Fi hotspots, and devices to ensure that all students have the ability to access online learning at home in the event of continued disruptions. Additionally, Congress should include the Supporting Connectivity for Higher Education Students in Need Act in upcoming legislation, which would direct $1 billion to institutions that primarily serve students of color and students from low-income backgrounds, thereby ensuring that students at those institutions can get the home internet access they need to continue their postsecondary education. Finally, in the interest of inclusivity, Congress should also encourage districts to implement multilingual digital learning platforms and provide professional development opportunities for educators, so they can effectively teach, assess, and connect with their students remotely. Congress should also encourage private companies to provide free home broadband access to students who would not otherwise have it during the pandemic.

Representative Haley Stevens (D-MI)

Secretary King, last month I co-introduced the Child Care is Essential Act with many of my colleagues here on this Committee to ensure all providers survive the pandemic and continue providing services to our nation's children. The bill would help child care providers who serve historically underserved populations and ensure those providers receive funding as swiftly as possible. How is COVID-19 exacerbating racial inequity in access to quality early childhood education, including child care? What else should we be considering as we look toward economic recovery?

There are clear racial and socioeconomic inequities within our early child educational system that begin before children enter kindergarten. Chief among them is grossly unequal access. Young children of color are particularly hurt by this, as their families disproportionately live in poverty. Child care deserts are far too common in America today, and 57% of Latino families and 60% of American Indian and Alaska Native families reside in them. In fact, the areas that are least likely to have child care shortages are high-income suburban neighborhoods, which tend to be predominantly White. Even when families of color have access to child care services, the cost – which may take up to 116% of a low-income family's household income – can be prohibitive without financial assistance. Unfortunately, financial subsidies provided by programs like Early Head Start and the Child Care and Development Block Grant (CCDBG) don't reach enough low-income children or children of color. Early Head Start provides access to only 7% of eligible infants and toddlers, and only 15% of Black children and 6% of Latino children receive CCBDG. Furthermore, Black and Latino children are underrepresented in several publicly funded, high-quality preschool programs, and the quality of the programs that most Black children have access to tends to be lower than that of programs attended by their White peers, showing that the issue goes beyond the obvious financial barriers. As in other parts of our educational system, systemic racism is present within early childhood education: Black children, and especially Black boys, are disproportionately suspended and expelled from early learning settings.

The COVID-19 crisis has compounded these inequities and has pushed many early care and learning providers toward collapse. Two-fifths of child care providers – half of them minority-owned businesses –

report that they will permanently close if they do not receive more public funding. That could have deleterious consequences for families of color with young children and an early childhood workforce that's disproportionately made up of women of color. Nearly half of child care providers have closed down due to the pandemic, and we could permanently lose over four million child care slots. We support efforts such as the Child Care Is Essential Act, which would help parents and providers alike, and we thank the Congresswoman for her leadership in this area.

In addition to taking these steps to support our nation's child care providers, the Education Trust recommends the following legislative actions be taken to stabilize education budgets and increase educational equity for students most impacted by the pandemic:

- Congress should allocate at least $500 billion for state and local budget stabilization, including at least $175 billion for K-12 education, and at least $50 billion for higher education. It should also allocate those dollars in an equitable manner by including maintenance of effort and maintenance of equity provisions and maintaining positive formula reforms contained in the HEROES Act.
- Congress should include $4 billion for the E-Rate program to bolster online K-12 learning access for millions of students during the pandemic, as detailed in the Emergency Educational Connections Act (S.3690). Congress also should include $1 billion for a higher education emergency broadband connectivity fund for students from low-income backgrounds, as detailed in the Supporting Connectivity for Higher Education Students in Need Act (S.3701).
- Congress should double the Pell Grant in upcoming legislation.
- Congress should extend the Pandemic Electronic Benefits Transfer (P-EBT) program through the summer and into the next academic year, as well as expand the program to cover children under 5 years old.
- Congress must protect students' civil rights in upcoming legislation by not permitting blanket waivers to key civil rights laws, like the Every Student Succeeds Act (ESSA) and Individuals with Disabilities Act (IDEA), and by enforcing the historic interpretation of the Title I equitable services provision in administering the CARES Act and future funds.

Chapter 2

Management Report: Preliminary Information on Potential Racial and Ethnic Disparities in the Receipt of Unemployment Insurance Benefits During the COVID-19 Pandemic*

United States Government Accountability Office

June 17, 2021

The Honorable Martin J. Walsh
Secretary,
United States Department of Labor

Dear Secretary Walsh:

The unemployment insurance (UI) system provides a vital safety net for individuals who become unemployed through no fault of their own, and this support is essential during widespread economic downturns. States design and administer their own UI programs within federal parameters, and the Department of Labor (DOL) oversees states' compliance with federal requirements, such as by ensuring states pay benefits when they are due. During the pandemic, the CARES Act supplemented the regular UI program by creating three federally funded temporary UI programs that expanded benefit eligibility and enhanced benefits.[1] These three programs—Pandemic Unemployment Assistance (PUA), Federal Pandemic Unemployment Compensation (FPUC), and Pandemic Emergency Unemployment

* This is an edited, reformatted and augmented version of the United States Government Accountability Office Report, Publication No. GAO-21-599R, dated June 17, 2021.

[1] These programs were amended by the Consolidated Appropriations Act, 2021 and the American Rescue Plan Act of 2021.

Compensation (PEUC)—are set to expire on September 6, 2021.[2] We are currently conducting several ongoing reviews of these programs and will issue reports in the coming months.[3]

The purpose of this chapter is to inform DOL about potential racial and ethnic disparities in the receipt of UI benefits, which we have identified in our preliminary data analysis for our ongoing work. According to DOL, ensuring equitable access to UI benefits is a top priority for the agency, and in March 2021, Congress appropriated $2 billion to DOL to promote equitable access to UI benefits, among other purposes.[4] We recognize that the complexity of these issues may take time to examine in depth. However, given that PUA and the other temporary UI programs are scheduled to expire in September 2021, we are sharing this preliminary information for DOL to consider in determining whether it needs to engage with states at this point to ensure equitable access to the UI system.

Specifically, as part of our ongoing work on the various UI programs during the pandemic, we analyzed data from the U.S. Census Bureau's (Census) COVID-19 Household Pulse Survey (Household Pulse Survey), phase 3.[5] The phase 3 survey asked respondents whether they had applied for

---

[2] PUA, which is generally available through September 6, 2021, generally authorizes up to 79 weeks of UI benefits to individuals not otherwise eligible for UI benefits, such as self-employed and certain gig economy workers, who are unable to work as a result of specified Coronavirus Disease 2019 (COVID-19) reasons. FPUC generally authorized an additional $600 weekly benefit through July 2020, and authorizes a $300 benefit for weeks beginning after December 26, 2020, and ending on or before September 6, 2021, for individuals eligible for weekly benefits under the regular UI and CARES Act UI programs. PEUC, which is generally available through September 6, 2021, generally authorizes an additional 53 weeks of UI benefits to those who exhaust their regular UI benefits. At least 25 states, as of June 1, 2021, have announced that they will terminate participation in pandemic UI programs prior to their September 2021 expiration dates.

[3] We are conducting these reviews under the CARES Act, which includes a provision for GAO to report on its ongoing monitoring and oversight efforts related to the COVID-19 pandemic. Pub. L. No. 116-136, § 19010, 134 Stat. 281, 579-81 (2020).

[4] The American Rescue Plan Act of 2021 appropriated $2 billion to DOL to detect and prevent fraud, promote equitable access, and ensure the timely payment of benefits in UI programs, including the CARES Act UI programs. Pub. L. No. 117-2, § 9032, 135 Stat. 4, 121.

[5] The Household Pulse Survey, an experimental data product, is an interagency federal statistical rapid response survey to measure household experiences during the COVID-19 pandemic. The survey is conducted by Census in partnership with seven other agencies from the Federal Statistical System. Phase 3 surveys were conducted on a biweekly basis from October 28, 2020, through March 29, 2021 (a total of 10 surveys). National level weighted response rates for the phase 3 biweekly surveys ranged from 5.3 to 7.5 percent. For example, for the final phase 3 survey (week 27), 1,040,111 housing units were randomly sampled and 77,104 respondents answered the survey questionnaire (the national level weighted response rate was 7.2 percent). In March 2021, Census published the results of a nonresponse bias analysis that identified evidence of response patterns that could result in biased estimates. The report also

UI benefits since March 13, 2020, and if so, whether they had received UI benefits. Because the questions refer broadly to UI benefits, they likely cover regular UI, PUA, and the other temporary UI programs. To determine whether there were differences in the receipt of benefits by race and ethnicity, we calculated the percentage of UI applicants who reported receiving UI benefits by racial and ethnic group, and tested differences for statistical significance.[6] We determined these survey data are sufficiently reliable for the purpose of identifying preliminary information for DOL's consideration.[7] In addition, as part of our ongoing review of the PUA program, we obtained data from five selected states on: (1) the number of unique individuals by race and ethnicity who received PUA benefits at any time during 2020, and (2) the number of individuals by race and ethnicity who submitted initial claims for PUA in 2020.[8] We used these states' data to calculate the percentage of PUA claimants who received benefits by racial and ethnic group. We are in the process of assessing the reliability of these states' data, but we determined that the data used in this chapter are sufficiently reliable for the purpose of identifying preliminary information for DOL's consideration.[9] Our ongoing work is being conducted in accordance with generally accepted government auditing standards.

According to our analysis of data from the Household Pulse Survey, nationwide, a higher percentage of White applicants reported receiving benefits from UI programs during the pandemic than certain other racial and ethnic groups. For example, among the most recent phase 3 survey

concluded that Census found evidence that its adjusted sampling weights help mitigate, though may not completely eliminate, nonresponse bias in the final survey estimates. U.S. Census Bureau, *Nonresponse Bias Report for the 2020 Household Pulse Survey* (March 24, 2021).

6 For this analysis, we created a combined race/ethnicity variable using the "rrace" and "rhispanic" variables in the Household Pulse Survey. Our combined variable had the following values: Asian, non-Hispanic/Latino; Black, non- Hispanic/Latino; Hispanic or Latino (any race or multiple races); White, non-Hispanic/Latino; Other or multiple races, non-Hispanic/Latino.

7 We assessed the reliability of these data by reviewing survey documentation, Census reports on the survey data's accuracy and potential nonresponse bias in the data, and written responses to questions we sent to Census.

8 Our ongoing review of the PUA program is examining how states' implementation of the PUA program has varied, how the pandemic has affected contingent workers in selected states, and how the PUA program has assisted those workers. We selected five states to include variety across several characteristics, including the volume of PUA claims, the timing of PUA implementation, and the percentage of the overall workforce that is self-employed.

9 We have assessed the reliability of these data by interviewing knowledgeable state officials and conducting manual testing to check for logical errors, and we have sent some related follow-up questions to state officials. Although these efforts are ongoing, the time-sensitive nature of this issue warranted sharing our preliminary results with DOL.

respondents, 80.2 percent of White, non-Hispanic/Latino UI applicants reported receiving UI benefits, as compared to 73.0 percent of Black, non-Hispanic/Latino applicants (see table 1).[10] We did not control for other characteristics that could be correlated with race/ethnicity and receipt of UI benefits, such as education or occupation, and we cannot determine the cause of differences between groups. Various factors could explain these differences, such as differences in UI eligibility that may be correlated with race and ethnicity.

For example, according to DOL, claimants' attachment to the workforce can affect their eligibility for regular UI benefits; thus, if certain racial and ethnic groups tend to have less continuous employment than other groups, they might receive regular UI benefits at lower rates.[11] However, another potential explanation for the disparities we identified is that states could be approving or processing UI claims differently for applicants in different racial and ethnic groups.[12] Although we cannot determine causality, these possible explanations provide context for DOL to consider in determining whether to engage with states to ensure equitable access to the UI system.

---

[10] The percentages represent responses to the final phase 3 survey (week 27), which collected data from March 17, 2021 through March 29, 2021. The difference in the rate of reported UI benefit receipt is statistically significant at the 95 percent confidence level. We also examined responses from each of the 10 phase 3 surveys (weeks 18-27). We found that applicants in the following racial and ethnic groups reported receiving UI benefits at a lower rate than White, non-Hispanic/Latino applicants, and these differences were statistically significant in multiple surveys: 1) Black, non-Hispanic/Latino UI applicants (this difference was statistically significant in 8 of the 10 phase 3 surveys); 2) Hispanic or Latino UI applicants (this difference was statistically significant in 2 of the 10 surveys); 3) Other or multiple races, non-Hispanic/Latino UI applicants (this difference was statistically significant in 4 of the 10 surveys). In all remaining surveys, each of these groups reported receiving benefits at a lower rate than White, non- Hispanic/Latino applicants, but the differences were not statistically significant.

[11] According to DOL, to be eligible for regular UI benefits, jobless workers must demonstrate, among other things, workforce attachment, which is usually measured by amount of wages and/or weeks of work. U.S. Department of Labor, *Unemployment Compensation: Federal-State Partnership*, May 2019. PUA eligibility requirements differ from regular UI. Because the questions in the Household Pulse Survey refer broadly to UI benefits, they likely include applicants for regular UI and PUA benefits.

[12] Because of how the survey questions were asked, differences in rates of UI benefit receipt could be due to differences in claim approval rates or delays in payments. For example, all groups' claims may have been approved at similar rates, but certain groups may have had to wait longer to receive payments or may have had their claims approved more recently and thus were still waiting to receive benefits.

Table 1. Percent of UI applicants who reported receiving UI benefits at any time from March 2020 through March 2021, by race and ethnicity

Racial/ethnic group	Percent of UI applicants who reported receiving UI benefits	Difference compared to White, non-Hispanic/Latino significant at p<. 05
White, non-Hispanic/Latino	80.2 (+/- 1.9)	N/A
Asian, non-Hispanic/Latino	79.1 (+/- 5.0)	No
Hispanic or Latino (any race or multiple races)	77.4 (+/- 3.9)	No
Black, non-Hispanic/Latino	73.0 (+/- 4.8)	Yes
Other or multiple races, non-Hispanic/Latino	71.0 (+/- 6.5)	Yes

Source: GAO analysis of data from the U.S. Census Bureau's COVID-19 Household Pulse Survey, phase 3, week 27. | GAO-21-599R.

Notes: Confidence intervals at the 95 percent level are shown in parentheses. The week 27 survey collected data from March 17, 2021, through March 29, 2021. The relevant survey questions asked respondents whether they applied for and received UI benefits since March 13, 2020.

In addition to our findings from the Household Pulse Survey, our preliminary analysis of data obtained from the five selected states in our ongoing review of the PUA program identified some racial and ethnic disparities in the receipt of PUA benefits.[13] In two of the five states, the percentage of White PUA claimants who received benefits in 2020 was considerably higher than the percentage of Black PUA claimants who received benefits that year (both groups consist of non-Hispanic/Latino claimants).[14] In one of these states, the percentage of White, non- Hispanic/Latino PUA claimants who received benefits in 2020 was also considerably higher than the percentage of Hispanic or Latino PUA claimants (of any race) who received benefits that year. This analysis of state-provided data is preliminary, and we are continuing to explore these issues with the selected states, including potential reasons for the disparities and the reliability of these data.[15] We plan to report on the PUA program in more detail in early 2022.

---

[13] Unlike the Household Pulse Survey, the state data is aggregated population data and has no margin of error associated with it.

[14] Among the three remaining states, for one state our preliminary analysis did not observe such large disparities in the receipt of PUA benefits, and for the other two states we had significant data reliability questions that we are following up on.

[15] As noted above, various factors could explain these disparities, such as differences in PUA eligibility that may be correlated with race and ethnicity, or differences in how states are approving or processing PUA claims for applicants in different racial and ethnic groups. These disparities in the receipt of PUA benefits could also reflect fraudulent claims. For example, in

Sincerely yours,

Thomas M. Costa
Acting Director
Education, Workforce, and Income Security

a given state, the individuals who submitted fraudulent PUA claims could have disproportionately used identities stolen from Black or Hispanic/Latino individuals relative to that state's PUA applicants. To the extent that states identified these claims as fraudulent and denied them, it could appear as though Black or Hispanic/Latino applicants received PUA benefits at a lower rate.

Index

D

E

I

J

L

M

S

T

U

V

W